Props for Yoga

A Guide to Iyengar Yoga Practice with Props
Volume II: Sitting Āsanas and Forward Extensions

Eyal Shifroni, Ph.D.

Co-Author: *Michael Sela*

Based on the teachings of
Yogacharya B.K.S. Iyengar, Geeta S. Iyengar and Prashant S. Iyengar
at the Ramamani Iyengar Memorial Yoga Institute (RIMYI), Pune, India.

Photography Aviv Naveh and book team
Text Editing Pauline Schloesser
Models Ravit Moar, Eleanor Jacobovitz, Anat Rachmel, Michael Sela & Eyal Shifroni
Graphic Design Aviv Gros-Allon, ViV design
Props Illustrations Kym Ben-Yaakov

No part of this publication may be reproduced, stored in a retrieval system, or transmitted in any form or by any means, electronic, mechanical, photocopying, recording, scanning, or otherwise, without the prior written permission of the author.
Copyright © 2015 by Eyal Shifroni

The author of this book is not a physician and the instructions, procedures, and suggestion in this guide are not intended as a substitute for the medical advice of a trained health professional. All matters regarding your health require medical supervision. Consult your physician before adopting the procedures suggested in this guide, as well as about any condition that may require diagnosis or medical attention. The author and the publisher disclaim any liability arising directly or indirectly from the use of this guide.
All rights reserved © 2015

Acknowledgments and Gratitude

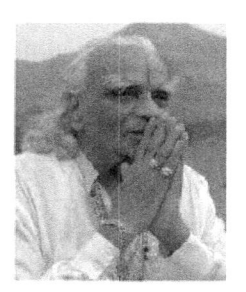

1918 - 2014

The source of all the knowledge presented in this guide is my Guru, Yogācharya B.K.S Iyengar, the founder of the Iyengar Yoga method. The use of props in yoga practice was introduced by Mr. Iyengar (Guruji). The various apparatus which he invented and adapted over the years were created to enrich practice and to enable every person to benefit from the gift of Yoga. It is already more than a year since Guruji has left us, nevertheless, every day, when I return to my practice mat, I remember him with great appreciation, gratitude and Love, and I thank him from the bottom of my heart for the precious gift of Yoga he had given to us. I feel that when I practice he still lives inside of me, and his voice echoing in my head, calling me to improve my practice, to be more attentive, to dive deeper to the heart of any āsana without any compromise. I feel that as long we continue to practice seriously, as he taught us, he will continue to live in our hearts. I wish to express my deep admiration and gratitude to Guruji, not only as my personal teacher, but also for making yoga accessible to millions worldwide.

I wish to thank Prashant and Geeta Iyengar for their guidance and inspiration in their teaching in RIMYI[1].

I have been very fortunate to have come across many inspiring teachers who have shared their deep knowledge with me and who have shed light on Yoga in general and on the use of props in particular. They are too many to list their names here. However, I am indebted to each and every one of them and wish to express my deep gratitude to them all. I have done my best to convey to you readers, the rich knowledge transmitted to me by all these talented and knowledgeable teachers – if, however, my presentation includes mistakes, then I am the one to be blamed, not the teachers I have learnt from!

This Guide owes its conception and delivery to my friend and colleague, Michael Sela, who helped conceive it and formulate its structure. Michael went through the text over and over again and contributed substantially to its clarity and flow. I wish to express deep appreciation for his collaboration on this project.

I wish to thank Pauline Schloesser, Ph.D., from Alcove Yoga at Houston, Texas (http://alcoveyoga.com/) for contributing many important ideas and clarifications; she did a wonderful job in improving the style of my writing to make it more fluent and clear.

[1] Ramāmaṇi Iyengar Memorial Yoga Institute – the home and teaching site of the Iyengars in Pune, India.

Thanks to all the teachers at the Iyengar Yoga Zichron-Ya'acov center who contributed many beneficial ideas and feedbacks; special thanks go to Ravit Moar, Anat Rachmel and Eleanor Jacobovitz for spending so many hours modeling for the photos in this guide. As yoga teachers your contribution goes much beyond mere modeling – you gave many insights and ideas that improved the contents of this guide.

I extend many thanks to my students, who helped testing and developing new ideas of using props during classes and workshops. Their willingness to try out these ideas and their enthusiastic feedback encouraged me to write this guide.

And, last but not least, thanks to my wife, Hagit, for her continuous love and support which made this guide (and many other things) possible.

Eyal, September, 2015

Table of Contents

Acknowledgments and Gratitude / III
Introduction / IX
About the Use of Props / X
About this Guide / XII
The Structure of the Guide / XIII
How to Use this Guide / XIV

Chapter 2: Centering Down - Sitting Poses (Upaviṣṭha Sthiti) / 1

Chapter 3: Surrendering to Mother Earth - Forward Extensions (Paśchima Pratana Sthiti) / 71

Appendix 2.1 Practice sequences / 141

1. A Short Sequence for Beginners	142
2. A Sequence with a long belt	144
3. Long stays in sitting & forward extensions	148
4. Forward bends for beginners	150
5. Forward bends & Twists – an advanced sequence	152

Index 1: Listing by Prop type, Asana and Variation / 157

Index 2: Listing by Asana names / 165

Detailed Contents of Chapter 2: Centering Down - Sitting Poses

(Upaviṣṭha Sthiti)

About Sitting Poses The Three Diaphragms	2
Daṇḍāsana	4
About Daṇḍāsana	4
1: Avoiding rounded back: Sitting on a raised plane	5
2: Making the spine Concave: Holding a belt	6
3: Bracing the legs: Belt from heels to sacrum	7
4: Opening the backs of the legs: Heels on block	8
5: Activating the feet: Feet against wall	9
6: Turning the thighs in: Block between thighs	10
7: Stabilizing the legs : Tying belts around legs	11
Baddha Koṇāsana	12
About Baddha Koṇāsana and Upaviṣṭha Koṇāsana	12
Maintaining the Length of the Trunk	
1: Lifting the pelvis to descend the knees: Sitting on a height	13
Moving the Heels closer to the Pelvis	
2: Moving the heels to the pelvis: Bracing the shins and the thighs	14
3: Moving the pelvis to the heels: Supporting the palms with blocks	15
Increasing the opening of the thighs	
4: Opening the thighs: Using belts behind the knees	16
5: Supporting the knees: Bracing the pelvis and the knees	17
6: Further opening of the groins: Block between soles	18
Restorative Baddha Koṇāsana	
7: Supporting the back: Using a chair	19
8: Opening the chest: Using a wall rope	20
Advancing in the Pose	
9: Preparing for Kandāsana: Raising the feet	21
Upaviṣṭha Koṇāsana	22
1: Stabilizing the back: Holding belts	22
2: Stabilizing the legs: Bracing the pelvis and legs	23

3: Further opening of the inner legs: Feet against a wall	24
4: Opening the backs of the legs: Heels on blocks	25

Swastikāsana (Sukhāsana) — 26
About Swastikāsana — 26

Supporting the Buttocks
- 1: 'Standard' Swastikāsana: Regular blanket support — 27

Using the Palms to Extend the Trunk
- 2a: Supporting the palms on a folded blanket — 28
- 2b: Supporting the palms on blocks — 29
- 3: Supporting the shins with a blanket — 30
- 4: Spreading the buttock bones: Sitting on a rolled mat — 31
- 5: Arrangement for long sittings: Using a high support — 32
- 6: Sensitizing the buttocks area: Sitting on a block — 33
- 7: Bracing the legs — 34
- 8: Compacting the base: Bracing the pelvis with a belt — 36
- 9: Moving the sacrum in: Block between sacrum and wall — 37
- 10: Stabilizing the base: Pulling the shins — 38

Opening the Upper Body
- 11: Supporting the chest: A block between wall and back — 39
- 12: Aligning the spine: Sitting against an external corner — 40
- 13: Supporting the back: Using a hooked rope — 41
- 14: Rolling the shoulders back: Crossed "shoulder jacket" — 42
- 15: Stabilizing & resting the arms: Belt on elbows — 43
- 16: Checking the upright alignment: A block on top of the head — 44
- 17: Sensitizing the chest: A belt around the chest — 45
- 18: Supporting the chin in Pranayama: Using a rolled belt — 46

Vajrāsana — 47
About Vajrāsana and Vīrāsana — 47
- 1: Joining the ankles and knees: Using belts — 48
- 2: Improving feet flexibility: Stretching the toes inward — 49
- 3: Anchoring the roots of the legs: A belt from groins to ankles — 50
- 4: Doing the pose when the ankles are stiff: Adding support for the shins — 51
- 5: Extending the ankles: Lifting the metatarsals — 52

Vīrāsana — 53
- 1: Spreading the calves from the thighs: Entering into Vīrāsana — 53
- 2: Compacting the base: Strapping the legs — 55
- 3: Compacting the base: Strapping the pelvis and knees — 56
- 4: Supporting the hands in Vīrāsana: Bolster on thighs — 57

Padmāsana — 58
About Padmāsana — 58

A Preparation Sequence for Padmāsana
- 1: Adho Mukha Swastikāsana — 60
- 2: Baddha Koṇāsana & Adho Mukha Baddha Koṇāsana — 61
- 3: Ardha Baddha Padmottānāsana — 62
- 4: Akunchanāsana — 63
- 5: Sitting Akunchanāsana — 64
- 6: Akunchanāsana with chair supporting the leg — 65
- 7. Standing Akunchanāsana — 66
- 8: Supta Ardha Padmāsana (or Ardha Matsyāsana) — 67
- 9: Matsyāsana (or Supta Padmāsana) — 68
- 10: From Ardha Padmāsana to full Padmāsana — 69

Detailed Contents of Chapter 3: Surrendering to Mother Earth - Forward Extensions (Paśchima Pratana Sthiti)

About the Forward Bends — 72

Adho Mukha Vīrāsana — 73
About Adho Mukha Vīrāsana
- 1: Anchoring the pelvis: Partner pulls back with a rope — 74
- 2: Stretching forward: Anchoring the legs and palms on blocks — 75
- 3: Stretching forward: Partner extends the trunk forward — 76
- 4: Overcoming stiffness in the ankles: Raising the shins — 77
- 5: Stretching the sacral band: Keeping the knees together — 78
- 6: Restorative Adho Mukha Vīrāsana: Supporting the body — 79

Supta Pādāṅguṣṭhāsana I — 80
About Supta Pādāṅguṣṭhāsana
- 1: Bones vs. Muscles: Basic usage of belt — 81

2: Learning to keep the leg straight: Entering from Daṇḍāsana	83
3: Activating the lifted leg: Bracing the body and the leg	84
4: Creating space in the lifted leg side: Hooking a belt from heel to groin	85
5: Creating space in the lifted leg side: Partner pulls the leg	86
6: Supporting the leg at 90°: Using a wall corner	87

Supta Pādāṅguṣṭhāsana II (lateral) — 88
About Supta Pādāṅguṣṭhāsana II — 88

1: Stabilizing the pelvis: Holding a belt with two hands	89
2: Activating the leg: Bracing the body and the leg	90
3: Creating space in the pelvis: Hooking a belt from heel to groin	91
4: Creating space in the stretched leg side: Partner pulls the leg	92
5: Moving the femur head into the hip joint: Side foot against wall	93
6: Moving the femur head into the hip joint: Partner pulls the buttock	94
7: Restorative Supta Pādāṅguṣṭhāsana II: Supporting the outer thigh	95

Paschimottānāsana — 96
About Paschimottānāsana — 96

Activating the Legs

1: Activating the legs: Block between the thighs	97
2: Activating the feet: Block against the soles	99
3: Compacting the legs: Using belts	100
4: Opening the sides: Belt around feet	101
5: Opening the backs of the legs: Heels on block	102
6: Anchoring the hands: Feet on inverted chair	104
7: Lifting the sides: Supporting the hips	105

Entering the pose with bent legs

8: Sliding back into the pose: Hands grasping hooks	107
9: Rolling the pelvis forward: Belt around pelvis and heels	108
10: Rolling the pelvis forward: Two Belts around pelvis and heels	109
11: Anchoring the base: Partner pulls back and down	110
12: Bending deeper into the pose: Belt around thighs and back	111

Restorative Paschimottānāsana

13: Opening the sides of the body: Supporting the elbows with blocks	112
14: Relaxing the head: Forehead on chair	113
15: Relaxing the head: Forehead on bolster	114
16: Using gravity: Sitting on a chair	115

Using Wall Ropes

1: Ūrdhva Mukha Paschimottānāsana I: Using wall ropes	116
2: Ūrdhva Mukha Paschimottānāsana II: Using wall ropes	117
3: Ūrdhva Mukha Paschimottānāsana II: Helper presses down	118

Jānu Śīrṣāsana — 119
About Jānu Śīrṣāsana — 119

1: Turning sideways: Using a belt	120
2: Rolling the bent leg out: Using bolster against the heel	121
3: Rolling the bent leg out: Partner pulls the thigh back	122
4: Keeping the bent knee backward: Knee against wall	123
5: Keeping the bent knee backward: Bracing the right leg	124
6: A different way to enter the pose: Sliding the knee back	125
7: Folding into the pose: Start by bending the Daṇḍāsana leg	126
8: Activating the straight leg: Foot against a block	127
9: Aligning the trunk: Rolled blanket on top thigh	128

Upaviṣṭha Koṇāsana — 129

1: Stabilizing the base: Supporting the lower abdomen	130
2: Restorative bending forward: Supporting the trunk	131

Mālāsana — 132
About Mālāsana

1: Preparation: Using chair	133
2: Preparation: Supporting the heels	134
3: Preparation: Sitting on a bolster	135
4: Preparation: Sacrum against the wall	136
5: Flexing the ankles: Holding a wall anchor	137
6: Preparation: Partner pushing the knees	138
7: Mālāsana I with a belt	139

Introduction

Yoga was revealed by the ancient sages as a way of spiritual realization and transformation; it was transmitted to us by a succession of sages (*rishis*) and *Gurus*. Texts like *The Yoga Sutras of Patañjali*, the *Bhagavad Gita* and the *Shiva Samhita* define and describe the essence of yoga, the yogic state, and yogic conduct. Many interpretations of these ancient texts have evolved over the years, including several books by my own teacher, Yogācharya B.K.S. Iyengar.

Yoga is not just a theory; it is a practical philosophy, a path to be travelled with intention, action, sensitivity and dedication. Only by putting the *sutras* into practice in our own lives can their full meaning and significance be revealed to us. Mere theoretical study of the texts will not lead to transformation and liberation. Mr. Iyengar's brilliant contribution has been in formulating ways in which the practice of āsana and Pranayama can be used to transform our bodies and minds through self-reflection, seeking to achieve the yogic state of knowing the eternal soul within.

Āsanas are not mere exercises; they enable us to study our bodies and minds and to get acquainted with our limitations, tendencies and potentialities. Iyengar has developed the practice of āsana to a level of art and science. In his book The Tree of Yoga, he writes:

"Mahatma Gandhi did not practice all the aspects of yoga. He only followed two of its principles – non-violence and truth, yet through these two aspects of yoga, he mastered his own nature and gained independence for India. If part of yama could make Mahatma Gandhi so great, so pure, so honest and so divine, should it not be possible to take another limb of yoga – āsana – and through it reach the highest level of spiritual development? Many of you may say that performing āsana is a physical discipline, but if you speak in this way without knowing the depth of āsana, you have already fallen from the grace of yoga." [2]

[2] *The Tree of Yoga* in the chapter: The depth of asana

In this book, he shows how all the eight limbs of *Ashtānga Yoga* can be experienced through a deep practice and study of the third and fourth limbs (āsana and Pranayama). Of course, practicing āsana as physical exercises has its own merit; it may keep your body flexible, healthy and light, but if you do not accompany your practice by observing and studying your mind, you will miss the opportunity to develop your intelligence and to uplift your consciousness (By 'intelligence' I do not refer merely to one's IQ level but rather to one's ability to perceive one's self and one's surroundings without biases; to act skillfully in the pursuit of good according to one's own values and sense of truth).

Looking at āsana practice in light of B.K.S. Iyengar's teachings, we can understand the role of yoga props in his method. It is because such props – a wide range of equipment and accessories that he invented to aid the practice – allow people of all age groups and health conditions to enjoy the gifts of yoga. Indeed, the introduction of props, together with B.K.S Iyengar's detailed instructions and thorough interpretation of ancient yoga texts have enabled millions to realize his vision of "Yoga is for All".

About the Use of Props

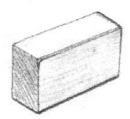

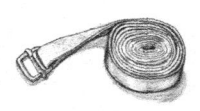

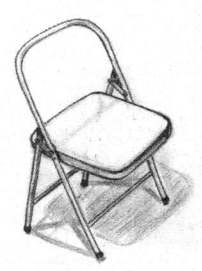

This is how Iyengar explains why he introduced props into his practice and teaching:

"I was preoccupied trying various ways to improve and perfect my own practice. I used to pick up stones and bricks lying on the roads and used them as 'supports' and 'weight bearers' to make progress in my mastery of asana…

Props help to perform the asanas with ease… The student understands and learns asana faster on props as the brain remains passive. Through passive brain one learns to be alert in body and mind. **Props are guides to self-learning**[3]. *They help accurately without mistakes."* (In 70 Glorious years of Yogacharya B.K.S.. Iyengar, page 391)

Christian Pisano adds to that:

"Props thus allow us to unfold the space of an asana and acquaint us with certain asanas that may otherwise be too difficult to practice. Props create understanding of the correct gesture (mudra) and attitude (bhava) of asana. Props let us stay longer in an asana, thus permitting deeper penetration of unexplored bodily regions." [4]

[3] *Highlighted by present author*
[4] *The Hero's Contemplation*

While props are an important characteristic of Iyengar Yoga, they should not be confused with its essence. Props are means for achieving ends - such as alignment, stability, precision, and prolonged stays in asanas.

The usage of props covered here is intended to direct awareness to different aspects of the asanas and to different parts of the body, in order to deepen and enhance the understanding of the asanas. At the same time, practitioners should be careful not to develop dependency on props; rather, props should be employed intelligently in pursuit of a mature and mindful practice of asanas.

Iyengar continues his description:

"Now, talking of the pros and cons of using props, one of the criticisms leveled against props is that one becomes habituated and lacks the will to attempt doing independently. Is this the fault of props? Certainly not! Props are to feel the asana. But I never say that they should be used on a permanent basis. Props give the sense of direction. When sense of direction sets in, I want my pupils to do the asanas independently sooner or later… The props are meant to give a sense of direction, alignment and understanding of the asana."[1]

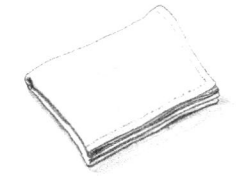

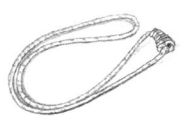

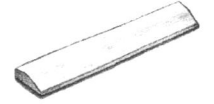

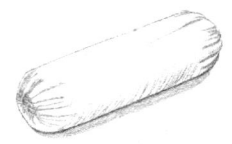

Ultimately the body and mind are also external props to help 'the seer to dwell in his own true splendor' (*Yoga Sutras of Patanjali*, I.3), or as Pisano expresses it:
"… Props can be regarded as an outer weave that points to the very essence of the asana, in a purely subjective way. There will therefore always be some swaying between using an external prop and using the body itself as a prop. Ultimately, the body-mind is itself only an external prop."[2]

To sum it up, props make it possible for every person to enhance his/her *Sadhana* (study and discipline of yoga), regardless of physical limitations. By using props adequately one can:

- Perform asanas which are difficult to perform independently
- Achieve and maintain correct alignment during the practice
- Stay longer and relax in challenging asanas, thus attaining their full benefit
- Study and investigate asanas on a deeper level
- Continue practice and improve one's condition despite illness, injury, or chronic condition

[1] *Ibid.*
[2] *Ibid.*

About this Guide

This is the 2nd volume in a series about the use of props in Iyengar Yoga practice. The series is the fruit of my 35 years of *Yoga Sādhanā*. In the course of these rewarding years of daily practice and study, every day brings with it a new feeling, a new observation, a new insight. This book has evolved from this continuous journey of practice and study, be it in my own studio; at RIMYI, under B.K.S Iyengar, Geeta and Prashant; in countless workshops that I took or gave in Israel and around the world; and last but not least – from the daily work with teachers and students at my own Iyengar Yoga Center in Israel.

Often, when preparing a class or a workshop, I search for new ways of highlighting the principles of āsana practice using props. I believe that many of my colleagues share a similar need. *Props for Yoga* is my modest attempt to address this need.

Since the original publication of *Light on Yoga*, the book which laid the foundation of the 'Iyengar Method', many books have been written in an attempt to elaborate and explain the wealth of knowledge embedded in that fundamental and by now classic text. The most prominent one is the beautiful book by B.K.S. Iyengar himself: *Yoga – the Path to Holistic Health*. Geeta's book: *A Gem for Women* and her booklets: *Yoga in Action, Preliminary* and *Intermediate-I* courses are important additions to that body of knowledge. Other books like *Yoga the Iyengar Way* by Silva, Mira & Shyam Mehta further clarify and specify the method. Most of these books, however, are intended for the general public, and cover mostly the basic usage of props. There are also several books showing the use of props specifically for Yoga Therapy. The present guide is intended primarily for teachers and experienced practitioners of the Iyengar method. It presents and explores a much greater variety of ways to use props. While some of the variations may be well known, many others are new and innovative ways that have not yet been documented.

My first book, *A Chair for Yoga*, focused on the use of a single prop in the practice of a wide variety of āsana. In contrast, each volume of the *Props for Yoga* series focuses on one family of āsana (or two) but utilizes a variety of prop types. I purposefully limit the discussion to the simple, most commonly available props such as blocks, belts, blankets, walls, bolsters, ropes, etc.

The present book is the second in the series. Volume I focused on standing āsana, while this volume contains two chapters: Chapter 2 - covers Sitting poses and Chapter 3 - Forward extensions. Future volumes will focus on other families of āsana and will include additional practice sequences of various lengths and levels. These sequences demonstrate how to use specific props for a complete practice session. This Volume contains five such sequences (see Appendix 2.1).

The Structure of the Guide

Each chapter in this guide begins with a short introduction followed by a number of representative āsanas. For each āsana a number of variations with different props are offered. Each variation is presented in the following order:

a. Props in use
b. Short introduction
c. Step-by-Step Instructions
d. Effects of practicing this variation
e. Tips – special points to observe in this variation
f. Applicability – in what other asanas the prop can be used in this way

The **Step-by-Step Instructions** (part c), illustrated by many photos, provide the technical information needed in order to position the body and use the props. The **Effects** section explains why the specific variation is given. It tells what we can learn from using the prop in the specified manner or how it might help us avoid common mistakes in alignment. The **Tips** section gives some clues regarding physical as well as mental actions you should do while staying in the asana in order to get the desired effect.

Note: *Āsana practice works on many levels. Our presentation refers mostly to the seen and explicit level, the anamayakośa (the structural, anatomic body). However āsana also affect the more internal kośas including the organic-physiological sheath (pranamayakośa) and the psychological sheath (monomayakośa). This text, being a practical guide, focuses on the technical aspects of the practice. This does not mean that the deeper effects of the practice are less important. We leave it for you – the reader - to pursue and experiment on your own to experience these internal effects.*

How to Use this Guide

Keep the following in mind when using this guide:

- This guide is not a substitute for learning with a certified Iyengar Yoga teacher. The subtleties of the instructions in the Iyengar method cannot adequately be captured in a book. So, while it can help you study and explore the asanas, please remember that no guide can observe you and correct the mistakes you may perform while doing a variation.

- Work by comparison and analysis: Do the pose several times with and without the props. Observe your sensations when doing the pose with the prop and then try to recreate those sensations without the prop. Do not use the props habitually, but rather use them for learning in a creative and innovative way; study and compare the effects to enhance your understanding. Do not develop dependency on props; rather, employ them mindfully. Always remain fresh and alert!

- The possibilities are virtually endless; use your imagination and creativity to find new ways of using props.

You should also note the following:

1. For the sake of clarity, each variation we present focuses on the use of a single prop, or on one specific way to work on an asana. However, some of the variations can be practiced in combination or in sequence. To avoid confusion, we do not show such combinations, but rather encourage you to try it on your own.

2. To facilitate quick access to the material in the guide use the detailed **Index** and the **Table of Contents**. The **Index** contains references to the variations according to the prop used and the asana taken – this is helpful if you wish to see all the variations that use a certain prop.

3. When working in pairs, it is recommended to work with a partner of the same gender and, as much as possible, of the same size and flexibility. Always be watchful and prudent when helping other people.

4. Certain variations refer to plates in *Light on Yoga*. Those are marked by the symbol LOY followed by the plate number. For example "LOY Pl. 100" refers to plate number 100 in *Light on Yoga*.

5. The guide shows only a sample of what can be done with props. In particular, the number of variations using a chair is limited. For extensive use of chairs in Iyengar Yoga practice, please refer to *A Chair for Yoga – A complete guide to Iyengar Yoga practice with a chair*, by the same author.

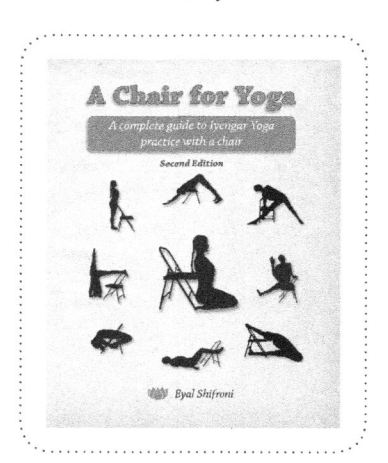

CAUTION Users of this guide must have a solid foundation in yoga practice, preferably obtained through regular classes with a certified Iyengar Yoga teacher. Some of the variations shown in this guide are advanced and should not be attempted without guidance and supervision. The author takes no responsibility for any injury or damage that may occur due to improper use of the material presented.

Enjoy your practice!

If you have any comments or feedback...I'd love to hear it.
Please write to me at:
eyal@theiyengaryoga.com

Chapter 2
Centering Down – Sitting Poses

About Sitting Poses

(11) "He should sit in a clean place, his firm seat neither too high nor too low, covered with sacred grass, a deerskin and a cloth, one over the other."

(13) "Holding the body, head and neck erect and still, looking fixedly at the tip of his nose, without looking around."

The Bhagavad Gita, Ch. 6 (from Radhakrishnan)

These famous *slokas* from the *Bhagavad Gita* describe how a Yogi should sit. Indeed, sitting is fundamental for yoga practice; we sit for meditation, we sit for practicing Pranayama and we sit for chanting OM at the beginning of every Yoga class to prepare mentally for the practice and study. Sitting āsanas allow for long stays with stability, balance and evenness. They help develop correct alignment, extension and openness as well as concentration and mindfulness.

The root of the word āsana in Sanskrit, *as*, means 'sitting' - so, in a sense, we should do all the other āsanas – standing poses, forward bends, backward bends, twists and so on - with the qualities of stability, comfort and balance that are characteristic of sitting.

Sitting is like coming home; returning to ourselves; when we sit properly, not only the body sits, but also the mind joins in and sits with the body. With our center of gravity closer to Mother Earth we become stable and quiet. In this relaxed, neutral state we can observe our tendencies: face our impatience, boredom, restlessness, agitation, etc. We can also follow our breath and just enjoy being in the 'here and now', savoring the present (gift) of being present at the present moment.

In *The Hero's Contemplation*, Pisano writes:

"The organs of action (arms and legs) are conditioned to ensure survival. In sitting āsana, the legs are reposed in different ways and learn to become quiet and free from the desire for movement linked to defense, aggression or escape"." [3]

This quote is equally true for the other organs of action (speech, elimination and reproduction organs) which are also become quiet in sitting.

[3] *See page 258*

The Three Diaphragms

Proper alignment in sitting means that if we drop an imaginary plumb from the crown of the head its line will go straight down through the center of the chest to the center of the perineum. In any sitting pose we have to be aware to the positioning of the three diaphragms: the pelvic diaphragm (or pelvic floor), the thoracic (or respiratory) diaphragm and the cervical (or vocal) diaphragm (which is referred anatomically as the thoracic inlet). These diaphragms form the base of the three main spaces, or cavities of the body: the abdomen, the chest and the throat. The thoracic diaphragm (which is often just called 'the diaphragm') separates the thoracic cavity containing the heart and lungs, from the abdominal cavity and performs an important function in respiration. The vocal diaphragm separates the thoracic cavity from the cervical region and performs an important function in voice generation through the vocal cords. In all sitting poses these three diaphragms should be vertically aligned over each other and be soft, wide and released. We should sit in a way that expands those three cavities. The various supports used in the Iyengar method are meant to help us achieve this.

To ensure left to right alignment we should sit evenly on the two buttock bones (the ischial tuberosity) and extend evenly both sides, from the pelvis extremities up to the armpits. To ensure front to back alignment we should sit on the heads of the buttock bones and lift both the sacrum and the pubic plates and keep them vertical and parallel to each other.

A proper base allows the abdomen and lungs to lengthen, widen and soften. The respiratory diaphragm can then move freely and breathing becomes rhythmical and smooth. Correct sitting will bring about a sense of symmetry, stability, harmony and poise.

Correct sitting requires flexibility in the joints of the legs (ankles, knees and hips) and a strong and stable spine. When there is tightness in these places, it is difficult to lift the spine. People with short hamstrings and stiff back groins will find it impossible to sit correctly on the floor. These people must sit on a higher support in order to sit erect. You will need to raise your seat if you sit on the back of the buttock bones and you cannot lift the spine from the sacrum.

For many people, achieving comfort in sitting āsana is more challenging than performing standing āsana. When we stand we can use our feet and legs to align the pelvic area and to lift the trunk from the pelvic floor. But when we sit the legs cannot be used in the same way. The actions we need to do in order to extend and stabilize the spine are subtler and more intricate. We need to activate deeper layers of our torso muscles. This is developed as we mature in our practice. However, even beginners can sit for a few minutes; over time – as flexibility, stability and strength are developed, the duration of the sitting can be naturally extended.

Dandāsana

About Dandāsana

Dandāsana is the basis for the sitting and forward extensions, much like what Tādāsana is for the standing poses. This symmetrical, simple pose is a good place to learn how to extend and activate the legs, to lift the trunk and to open the chest while sitting.

We should always sit centered on the pointed tips of the buttock bones – if we sit on the front edges of these bones, the lumbar spine tends to move excessively forward (exaggerated lordosis); if we sit on the back edges of these bones (as many beginners do), the lumbar spine is drawn too much backward and cannot be lifted up.

> **CAUTIONS**
>
> If your spine has a tendency to sag or if you are experiencing a severe attack of asthma, support your spine against a wall (see photo 4, Variation 7 in page 11)

Dandāsana

Variation 1
Avoiding rounded back: Sitting on a raised plane

Effects
Raising the buttocks eases the tension of the hamstrings and makes it easier to keep the lower back erect. The spine extends and creates space in the abdominal and the thoracic cavities.

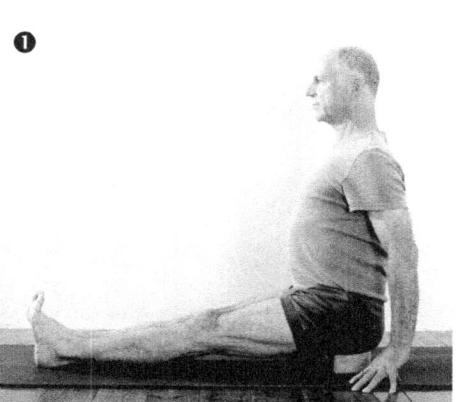

Props
folded blanket, block, bolster or chair.
Optional: 2 additional blocks, wall hook and rope

Different types of 'under-the-buttocks' support induce different effects. For example, bolsters are soft, so the buttocks sink slightly into the seat and thus receive some lateral support. Blocks are harder, so the buttock bones do not sink and it is easier to extend the spine vertically up. In addition you can sense exactly what part of the bone touches the seat. Choose the prop according to the height you need and the effect you want to bring about. Feel free to combine props; experiment and find out which prop enables a better lift of the spine from its base. Remember that both the sacrum and pubic bones should be lifted and held perpendicular to the floor.

Here are two examples for support, using a block ❶ and a chair ❷

⚠ CAUTIONS
To prevent slippage when sitting on a chair: 1. Use sticky mats under the chair and on the seat, and 2. Support your feet against a wall.

T i p If the palms do not reach comfortably the floor, place them on blocks as in ❸.

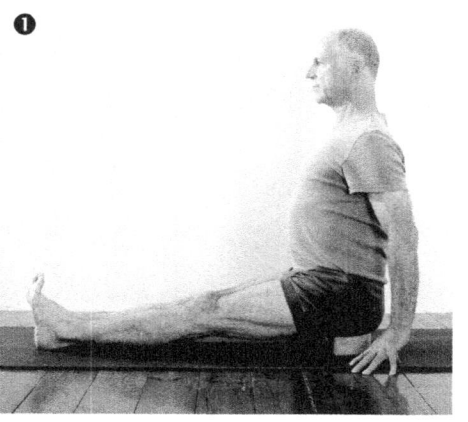

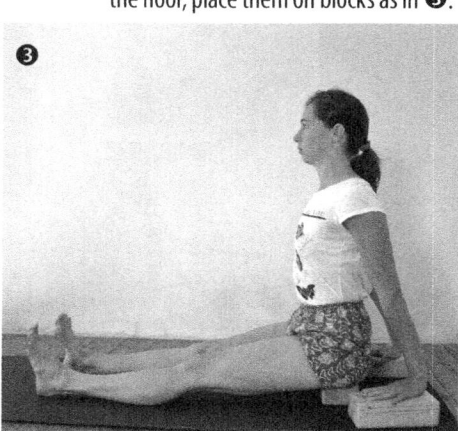

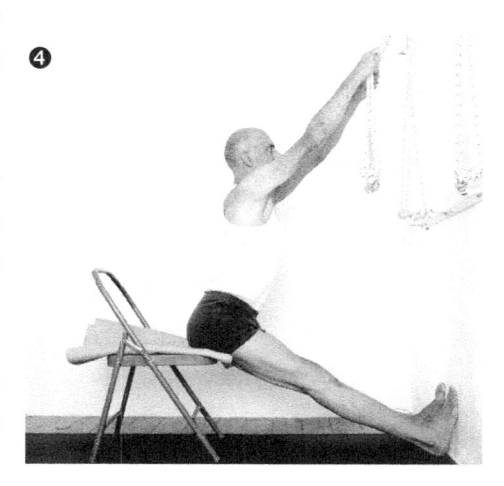

Tips
- Learn to balance your body weight on the two buttock bones: identify which buttock feels lighter and release it further onto the seat until both sides take an even load.

- Learn to identify the sensation in your lower abdomen when the body weight is distributed evenly between the two sides.

- In order to extend the spine up and open the chest, you can use a rope attached to the wall ❹.

Effects
The hard surface creates a sharp sensation in the buttock bones. A chair gives a more substantial sitting height and is useful when the back of the legs are tight or when there is back pain due to compression in the lower back.

Effects
Pulling the rope helps to extend the spine; it is recommended for stiff people and for those suffering from back pain.

Dandāsana

Variation 2
Making the spine Concave: Holding a belt

Effects
The legs extend against the resistance of the belt and become more active. Holding and pulling the belt helps to move the shoulder blades and to make the thoracic dorsal spine concave. These actions open the chest.

Props
belt

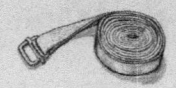

⟶ Loop a belt around the heels and hold it.

> Pull the belt to open the chest and move the area between the shoulder blades into the body. This is called: making the upper back (thoracic dorsal spine) concave.

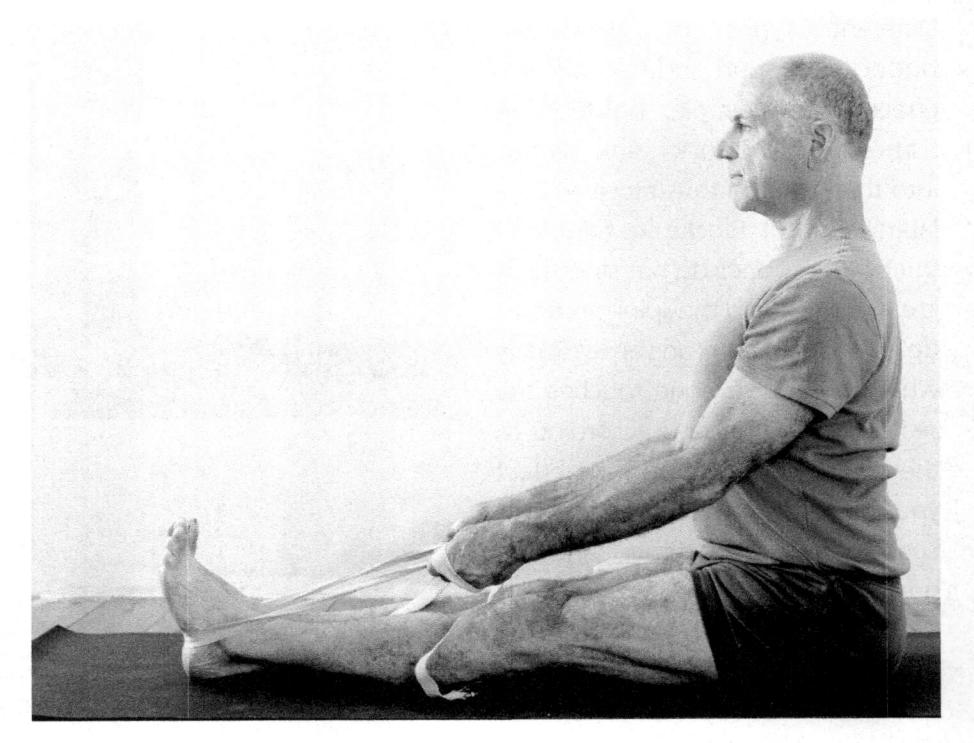

Dandāsana

Variation 3
Bracing the legs: Belt from heels to sacrum

Effects
The belt supports the sacrum and serves as an external framework to the pose. The legs work against the resistance of the belt and become more active. This structure enables the spine to extend with less effort and relaxes the lower abdomen. It makes the pose quiet and relaxed.

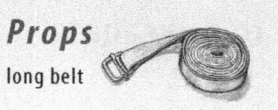

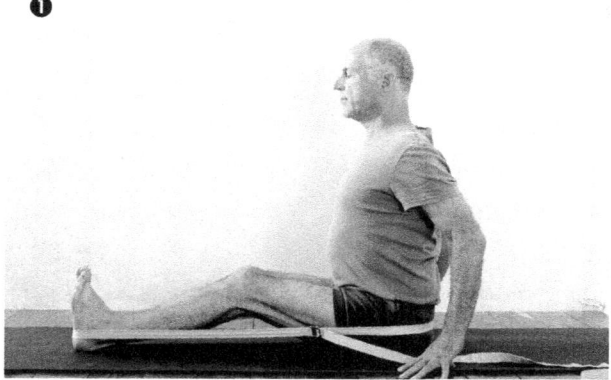

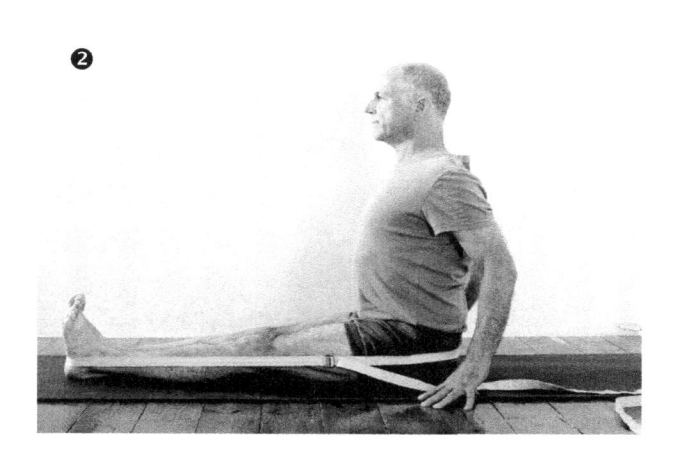

Props
long belt

In Dandāsana the sacrum should move into the pelvis and towards the heels, the legs should be active and the feet should open.

⟶ Loop a belt around the heels and the sacrum (long-legged people may need a long belt).

> Slightly bend the knees and tighten the belt ❶.

> Straighten the legs against the resistance of the belt ❷.

> Push the feet against the belt. Broaden the feet and open the skin of the soles from inside out.

Tips

✓ Imagine that the soles of the feet form a wall and move the sacrum towards this wall.

✓ If moving the sacrum in is difficult, spread your legs to pelvis width; this broadening helps to move the sacrum in.

Dandāsana

Variation 4
Opening the backs of the legs: Heels on block

Effects
Pressing the heels down to the block activates the front muscles of the thighs and stretches the backs of the legs. The hard surface of the block sharpens the sensation of the heel bones.

Props
1-2 blocks

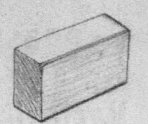

→ Sit in Dandāsana with the heels on a block.

› Extend the Achilles tendons, open the feet and press the back bones of the heels down against the block ❶.

› Pull the kneecaps toward the body and open the backs of the legs.

The same variation can be done while sitting on a block ❷.

Tips

✓ Imagine you have heavy weights on the thighs; learn to activate the quadriceps without shortening them; tighten these muscles down into the bones in order to move the bones down.

✓ Learn to keep the symmetry of the pose by equating the pressure of the left buttock and heel to that of the right buttock and heel.

If the calf muscles drop too much down to the floor, then the knees are hyper-extended ❸. This is unhealthy for the knees.

If you cannot prevent the calf muscles from moving down, support them with a rolled blanket to prevent unhealthy locking of the knees ❹. Once the calves are supported, contract the quadriceps and move the front thighs down towards the floor.

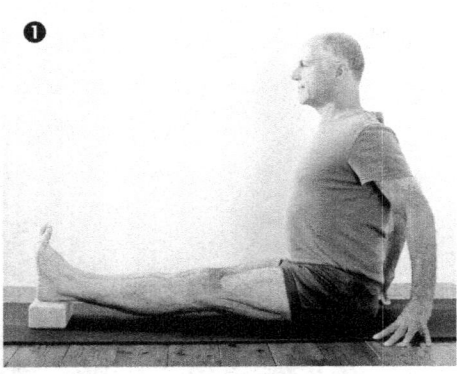

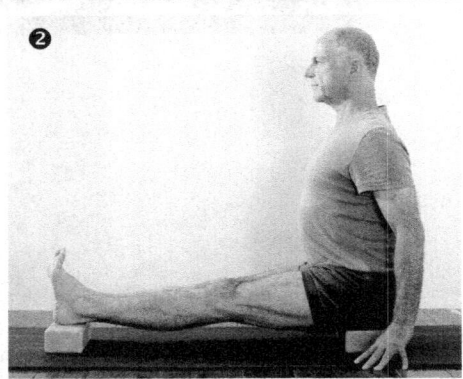

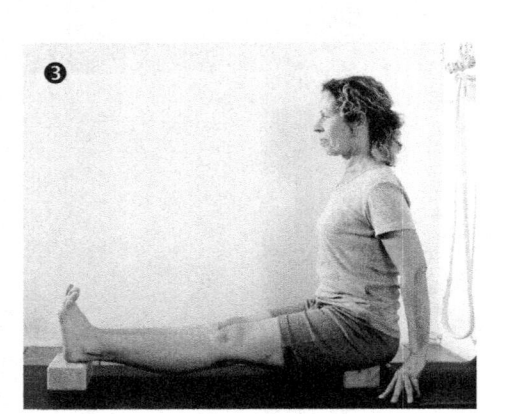

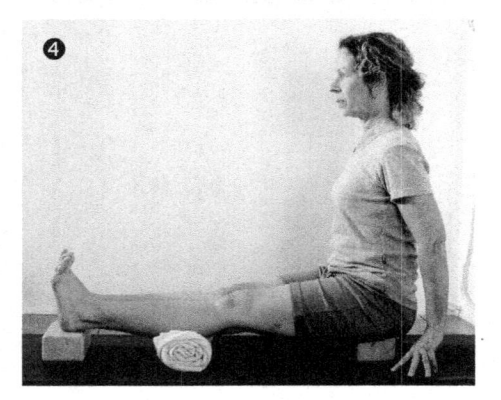

Effects
The hard surface of the block sharpens the sensation of the buttock bones.

Dandāsana

Variation 5
Activating the feet: Feet against wall

Effects
Pressing the feet against resistance activates the inner feet and teaches how to extend the inner legs.

Props
wall

This variation helps to activate the inner and the outer legs simultaneously.

⇒ Sit in Dandāsana with the feet against the wall and the knees slightly bent ❶.

▷ Straighten the legs against the resistance of the wall. Open the feet and press the heels and the toe mounds against the wall ❷.

Option: Spreading the legs

▷ Spreading the legs to pelvis width as in ❸ and ❹ helps to create width in the pelvis and lower abdomen.

▷ If a hook is available, use it to extend the trunk as in ❺

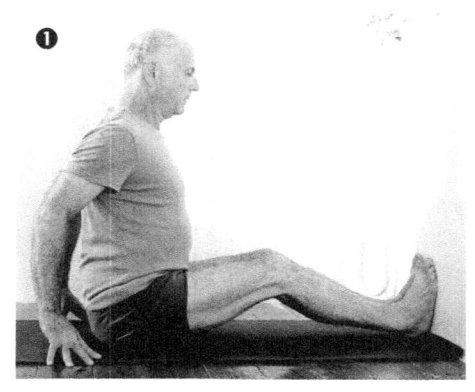

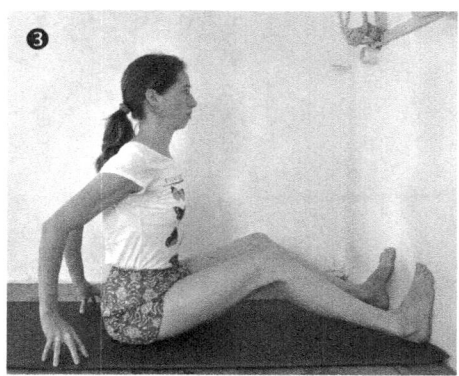

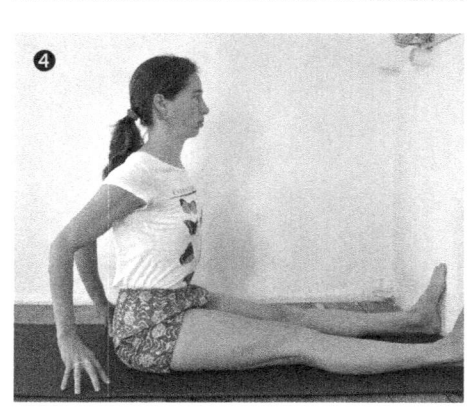

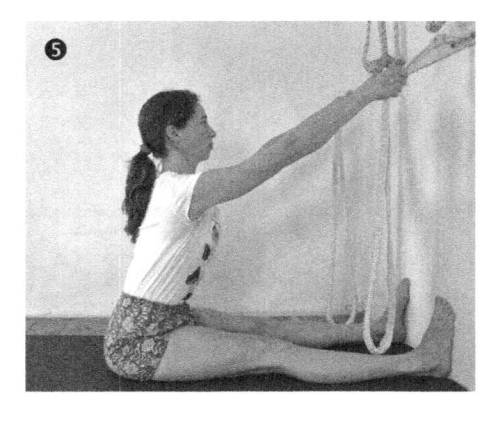

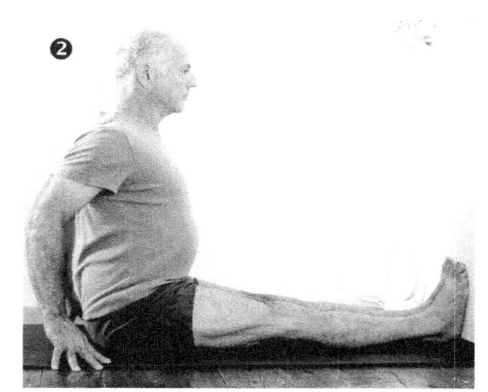

Tips

✓ When straightening the legs do not 'slam' the knees but rather expand the space between the thighs and the shins. Stretch the calf muscle toward the heels and the thigh muscles toward the hips.

✓ Suck the kneecaps deeply into the knee.

✓ Broaden the space between the big toe and the second toe; spread all the toes.

✓ Press equally the outer edges of the feet, the big toe mounds and the heels.

Dandāsana

Variation 6
Turning the thighs in:
Block between thighs

Effects
The inner rotation of the thighs broadens the pelvis and creates space in the lower abdomen. The broadening of the buttock bones makes the pose more stable. The block brings awareness to the inner thighs and clarifies the action of turning the thighs in. It also helps to activate the outer thighs.

Props
block

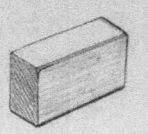

→ Sit in Dandāsana and use both hands to turn each front thigh from outside in ❶.

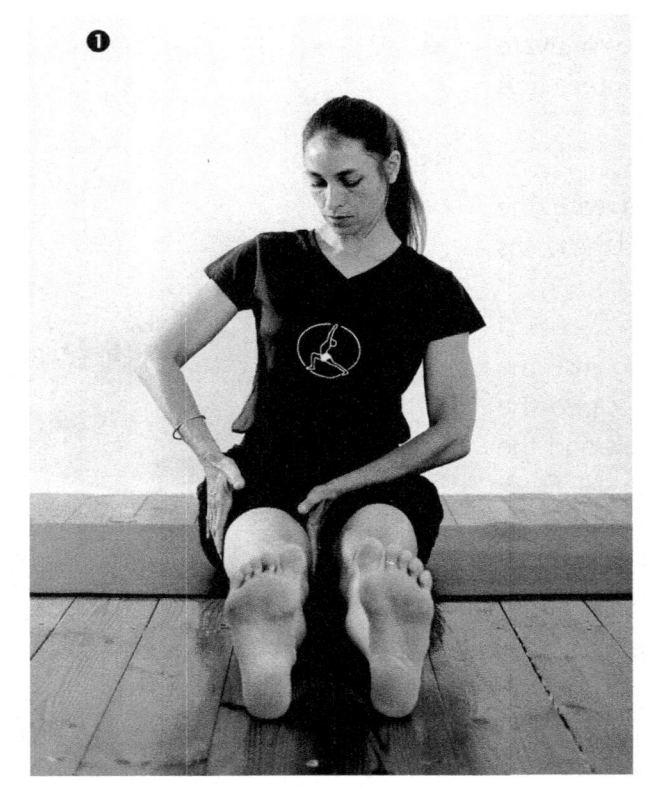

❶

> Place a block between the inner thighs.

> Keep turning the thighs inward; tighten the outer thighs to press against the block ❷.

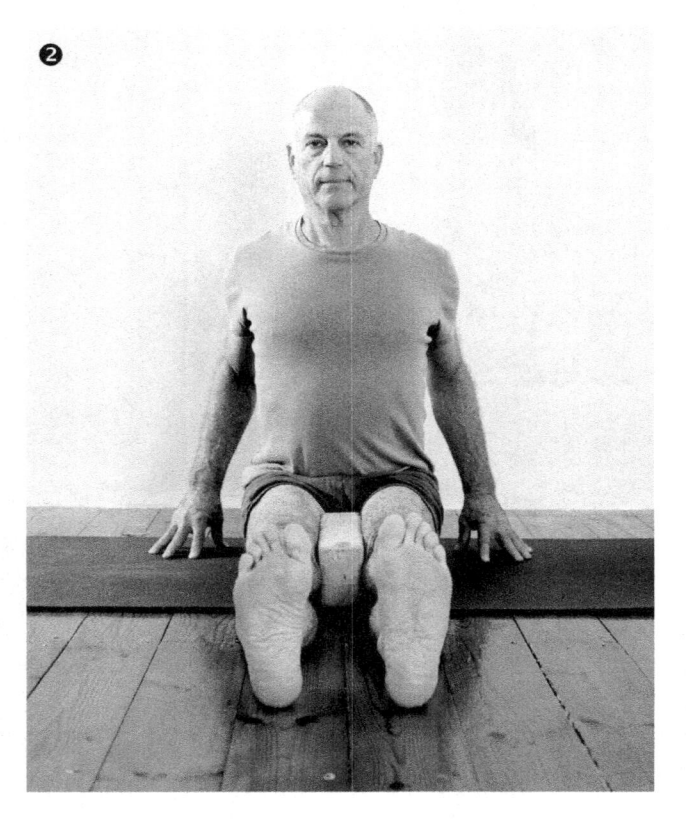

❷

Tips

✓ Turn the thighs until the front edges of the inner thighs are touching the block.

✓ Look at your legs and check that the midlines of the kneecaps and the front thighs are facing the ceiling. The two kneecaps should look identical.

✓ Press the legs down and check that the midlines of the back legs (the lines connecting the buttock bones with the back of the heels) are resting firmly on the floor.

Dandāsana

Variation 7
Stabilizing the legs: Tying belts around legs

Effects
This is a restorative variation of the pose. It can be very helpful in case of knee problems and stiff hamstrings. If you suffer from pain or tightness in the hamstrings or the back groins, it is recommended to start your practice by sitting in this pose for several minutes. This softens the muscles, increases circulation and prepares for more active work.

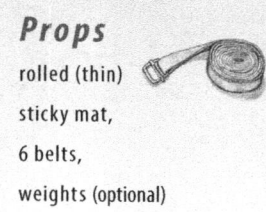

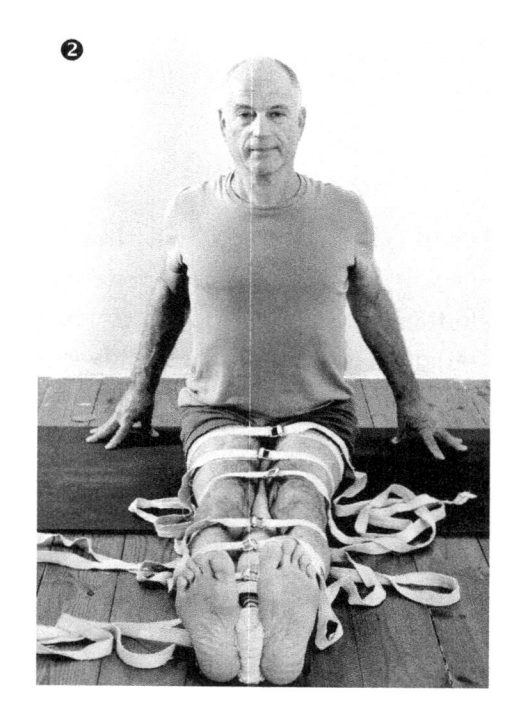

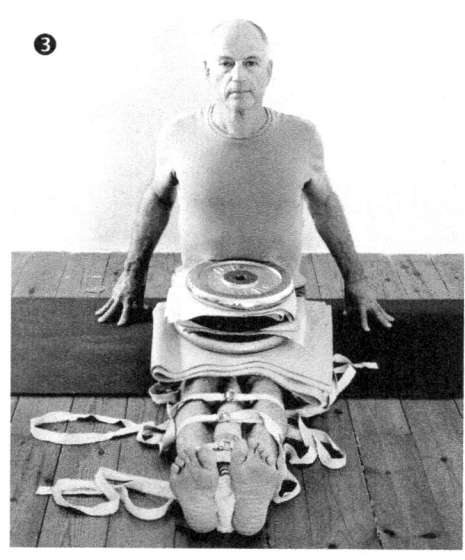

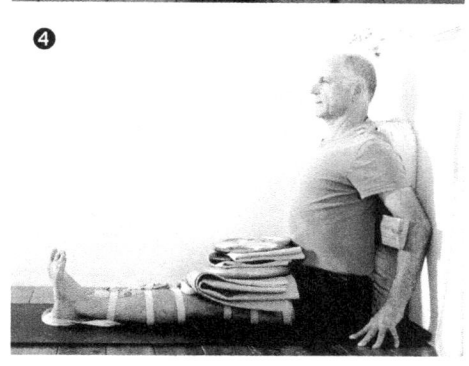

Props
rolled (thin) sticky mat,
6 belts,
weights (optional)

This variation requires several belts and optionally weights; if you do not have these at home, you may reduce the number of belts, or try it in your yoga center.

→ Sit in Dandāsana. Loop three of the belts around the thighs and the other three belts around the shins; place the belts in equal spacing with buckles in alternate directions (to ensure even pressure) but do not tighten them yet ❶.

› Roll a mat and insert it through the looped belts in between the legs. Hold the rolled mat in between the middle of the inner thighs and tighten the belts ❷.

Optional stage:

› Place weights (up to 50 Kgs. Or 110 pounds) on the thighs ❸.

Note:
Be careful not to place metal weights on the knees.

› Stay in the pose for 5 minutes or more.

Notes
✓ For comfort you can lean on a wall (or hold a belt wrapped around the feet – as in Variation 2 above.)

✓ To further open the chest, support the back with a bolster and a plank ❹.

✓ After exiting the pose, stand up slowly and take a few steps. Feel the effect on the legs and knees.

Props for Yoga / Chapter 2 / dandasana 11

Baddha Koṇāsana

About Baddha Koṇāsana and Upaviṣṭha Koṇāsana

Baddha Koṇāsana and Upaviṣṭha Koṇāsana are important poses for the internal organs of the reproductive system for both women and men. They create space in the pelvis and the lower abdomen and increase blood circulation in these regions. For women these poses are highly recommended during menstruation and pregnancy. Props can help develop the required flexibility in the hips and the groins.

> **CAUTIONS**
>
> Do not practice this āsana if you have a displaced or prolapsed uterus. If your knees are injured, do not practice this pose without the guidance of an experienced teacher.

Maintaining the Length of the Trunk

Baddha Koṇāsana

Variation 1
Lifting the pelvis to descend the knees: Sitting on a height

Effects
The hard surface of the block provides resistance to the buttocks; this helps to feel whether the weight is or is not distributed evenly on the buttocks. It also helps to extend the spine. Holding the feet draw them closer to the pelvis, to activate the back and open the chest.

Props
block or bolster,
belt (optional),
2 blankets (optional)

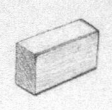

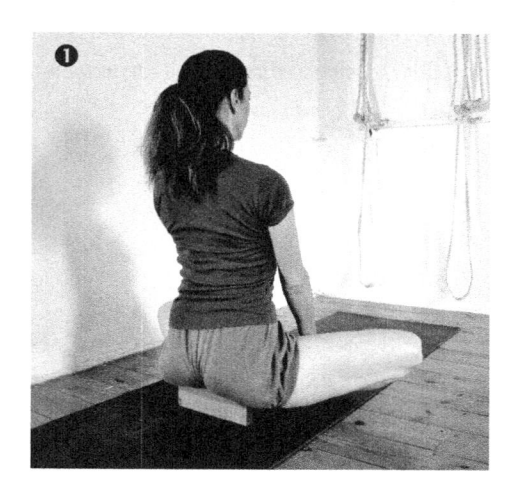

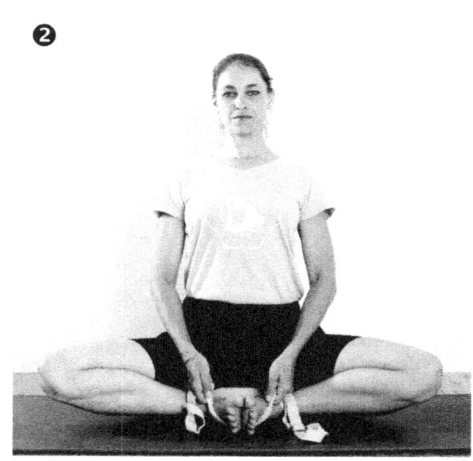

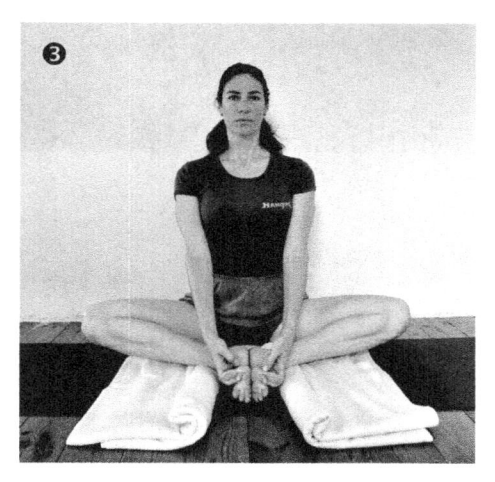

If when sitting in Baddha Koṇāsana the knees are much higher than the pelvis, then they cannot descend down and the back cannot extend up. In this case one needs to raise the buttocks on some support. We show a wooden block support here, but bolsters and blankets may also be used.

> Place a block flat on the floor and sit on it in Baddha Koṇāsana ❶.

> Hold the feet with both palms. If you do not reach the feet comfortably, use a belt ❷.

> Using the feet as an anchor, flex your arms and move the chest forward while rolling the shoulders back. Stay in the pose quietly for several minutes.

Note: To enhance the stretching of the inner thighs, roll two blankets and place them under the outer ankles ❸. This support lifts the ankles and shins and thus helps to open the groins and descend the thighs further.

Tips
Learn the symmetry of this pose: observe the sensation in the two buttock bones and check for evenness. Look at your thighs and knees and check their symmetry.

Props for Yoga / Chapter 2 / Baddha Konasana 13

Moving the Heels closer to the Pelvis

In Baddha Koṇāsana, the heels should eventually touch the pelvis and the knees should extend sideways and to the back.

Baddha Koṇāsana

Variation 2
Moving the heels to the pelvis: Bracing the shins and the thighs

Effects
The belts improve the opening of the groins while allowing the legs to relax. This variation creates widening of the lower abdomen, and hence it is particularly recommended for women during menstruation and pregnancy (and is beneficial for men, too).

Props
2 belts, blanket or block (optional)

→ Sit in Baddha Koṇāsana (support the buttocks according to your needs).

› On each leg, loop a belt around the root of the thigh and the ankle. To ease the belts' adjustment, tie them such that their loose ends point upward.

› Move the heels closer to the buttocks and tighten the belts to join each shin with its respective thigh.

Note: The belts can also be placed around the lower thighs, just above the knees, as shown for Padmāsana on page 67. This helps to stabilize the knees.

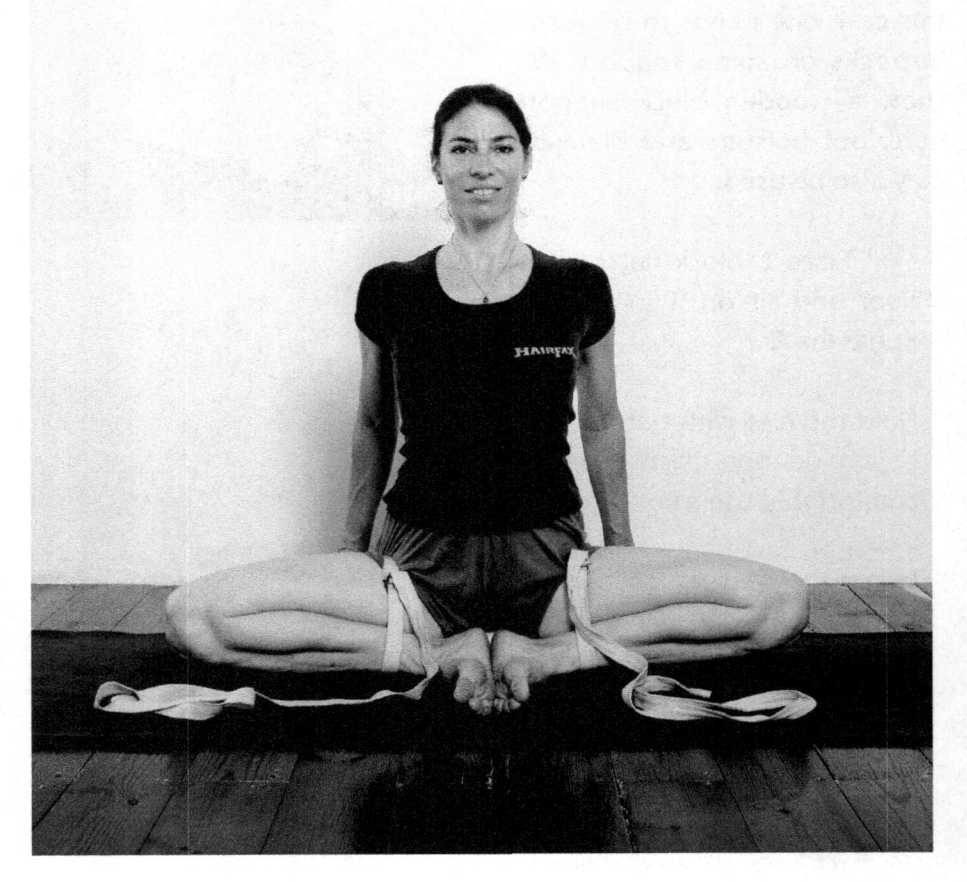

Applicability
Supta Baddha Koṇāsana

Baddha Koṇāsana

Variation 3
Moving the pelvis to the heels: Supporting the palms with blocks

Effects
This variation helps to extend the inner thighs and bring the pelvis forward. Entering the pose this way also opens the groins and moves the thighs and the knees further back.

Props
2 blocks, 3-folded blanket

⟶ Sit in Baddha Koṇāsana on the narrow side of the folded blanket, such that the heels touch the blanket. Initially the pelvis may be slightly away from the heels.

> Place a block on each side of the pelvis ❶.

> Push the blocks to lift the buttocks and move the pelvis forward; repeat this a few times until the pelvis touches (or comes close to) the heels. At the same time, keep the thighs rolling outward and backward ❷.

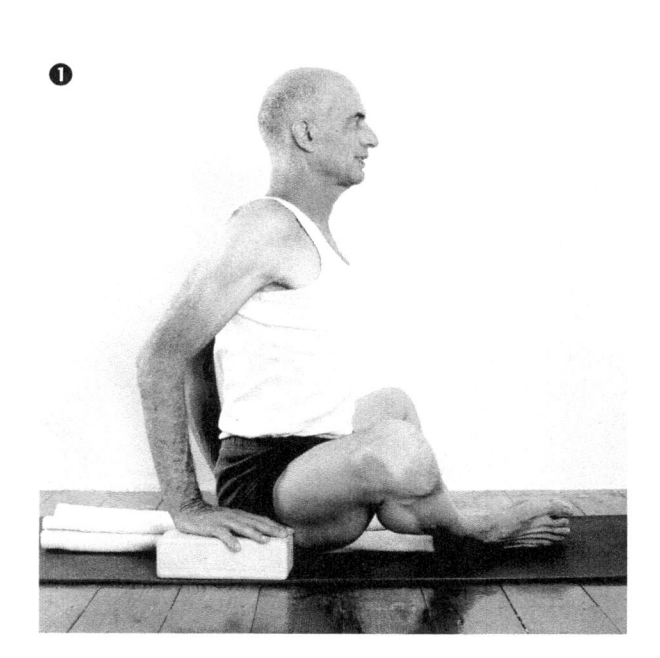

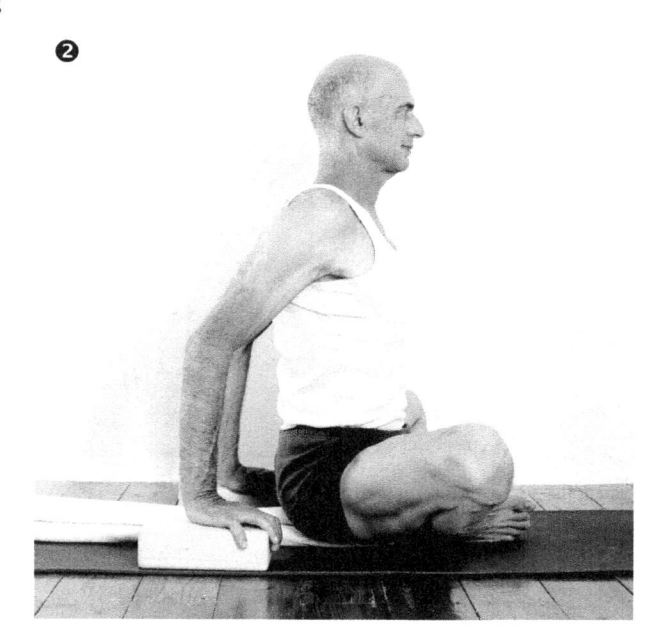

Increasing the opening of the thighs

Baddha Koṇāsana

Variation 4
Opening the thighs:
Using belts behind the knees

Effects
Pulling the belts extends the inner groins and thighs; it also creates space at the back of the knees.

Props
2 belts (or ropes), blanket or block (optional)

⟶ Take two belts and fold each in half.

▹ Sit in Baddha Koṇāsana with the folded belts inserted behind the knees. Hold the belts with straight arms and pull them sideways to broaden the inner groins and lengthen the inner thighs.

▹ You can change the direction of the pull to get different effects. For example, pulling the belts slightly backward rolls the thighs out and creates more opening in the inner knees.

Note: Two helpers (if available) can pull the belts for you; this is very pleasant as it allows the thighs to extend passively.

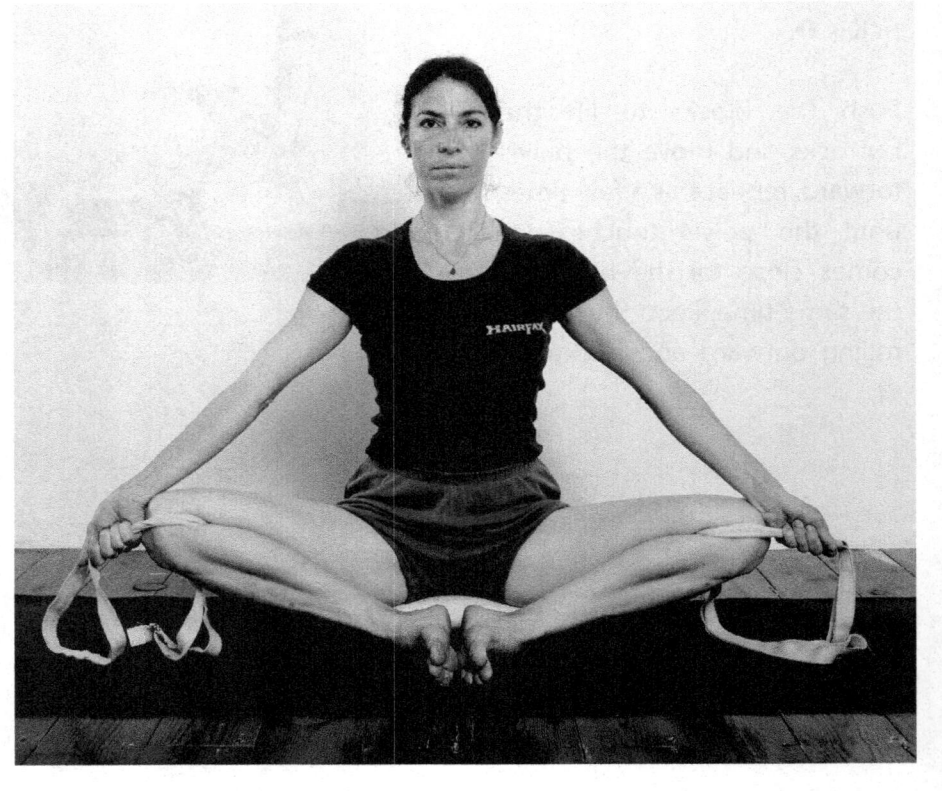

Tips

✓ If you have pain in the knees, use a doubled rope or something thick instead of the belts; this will create more space in the knee. In order to alleviate pain in the inner knee, pull (or ask the helpers to pull) the front end of the rope backward. This will create space in the inner knees.

Baddha Koṇāsana

Variation 5
Supporting the knees: Bracing the pelvis and the knees

Effects
The belts draw the femur bones into the hip sockets and create compactness in the pelvic girdle. This allows the opening of the groins and the extension of the spine. Working against the resistance of the belts can help open the thighs.

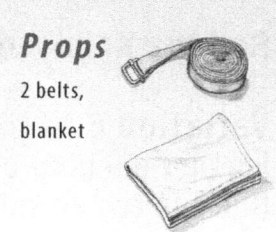

Props
2 belts, blanket

❶

> Sit in Baddha Koṇāsana on the mat or on a folded blanket.

> Loop two belts and place them loosely around the pelvis.

> Lower the belts down to the pelvis and position them around the knees, so as to hold each knee with the opposite hip ❶.

> Slightly lift the knees and tighten the belts, then release the knees down to stretch the belts.

> Roll the thighs backward. Move the outer thighs into the pelvis and open the inner thighs from the groins to the inner knees.

> A partner can help by pulling the belts while sitting in front of the practitioner and pressing his/her feet for stability ❷.

❷

Effects: The belts support the sacrum and ilium bones; this stabilizes the pelvic girdle. This effect is intensified by the partner's action.

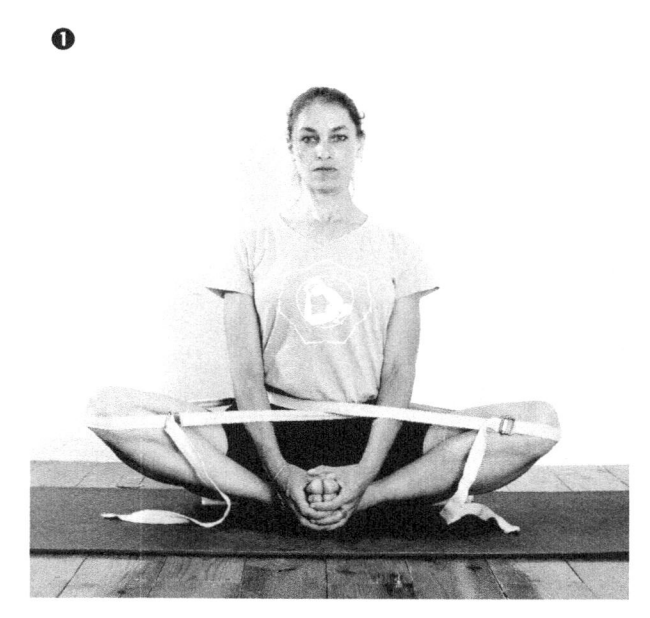

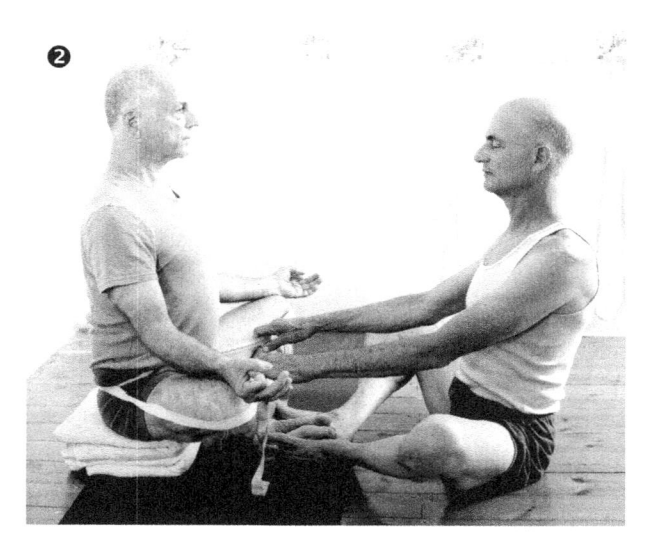

Baddha Koṇāsana

Variation 6
Further opening of the groins: Block between soles

Effects
The block helps to extend the thighs sideways and open the groins further; the knees go wider and further back moving the femur heads deeper into the hip sockets.

Props
block, blanket (optional)

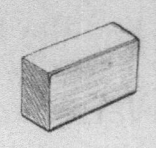

→ Sit in Baddha Koṇāsana on a folded blanket.

› Separate the feet and place a block between the soles.

› Press the heels against the block; move the inner thighs away from the pelvis and roll them outward.

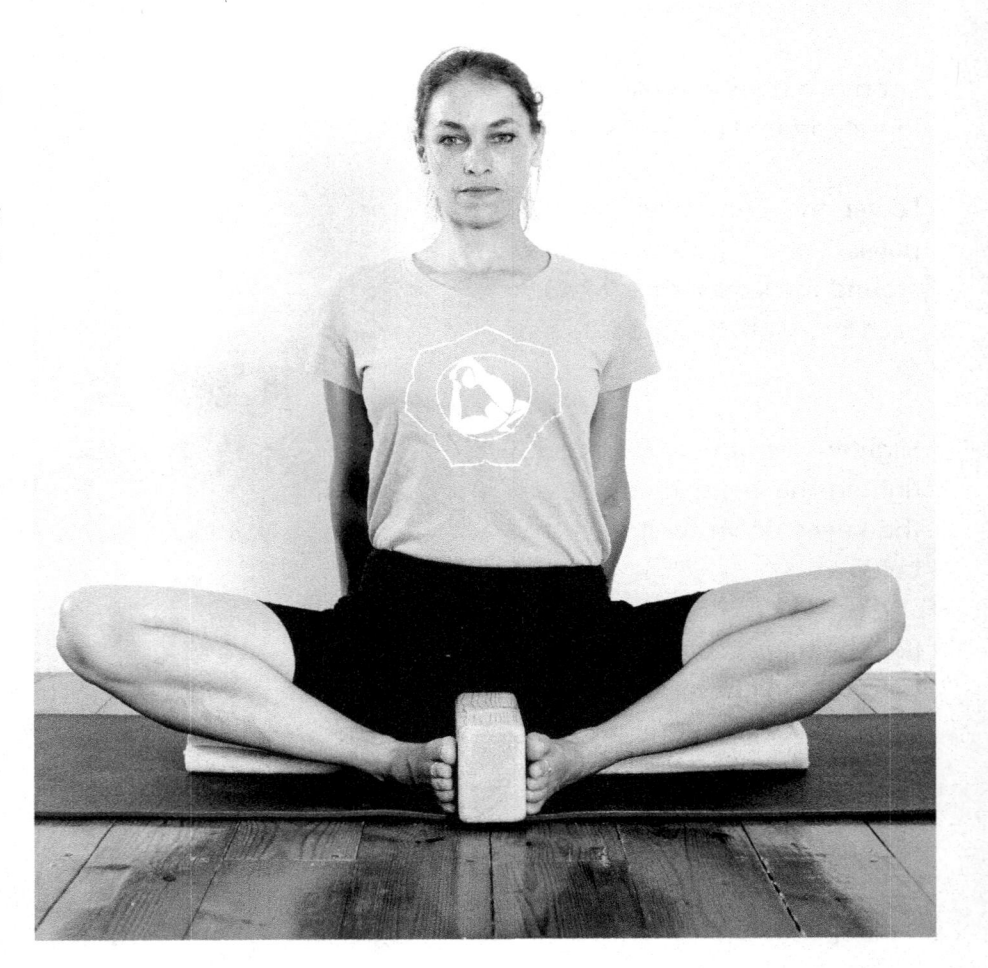

Restorative Baddha Koṇāsana

Baddha Koṇāsana

Variation 7
Supporting the back:
Using a chair

Effects
Entering the pose in this way help to keep the spine long and to release the groins. Once you are sitting, the chair supports the back and helps to maintain it erect and stable without effort.

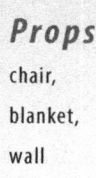

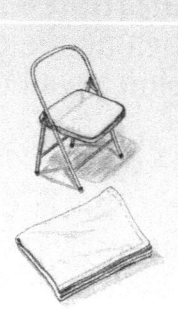

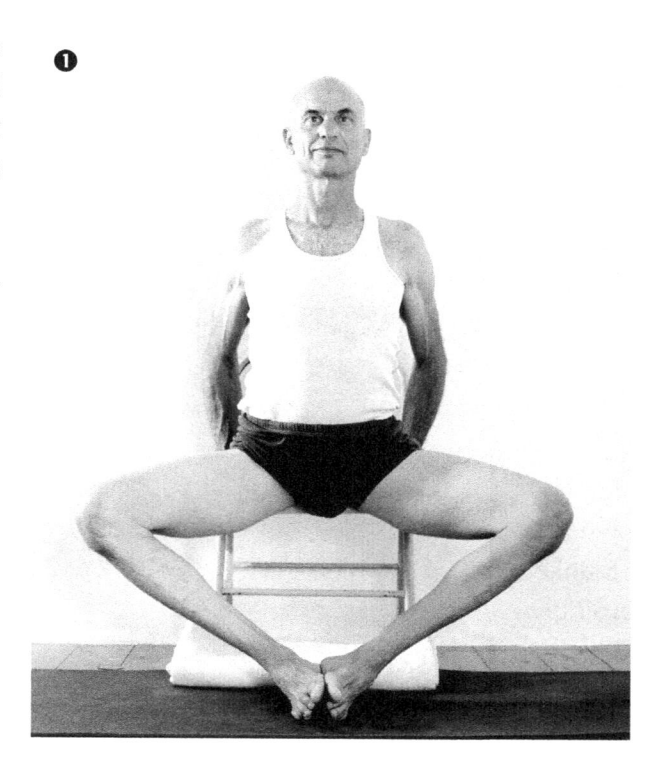

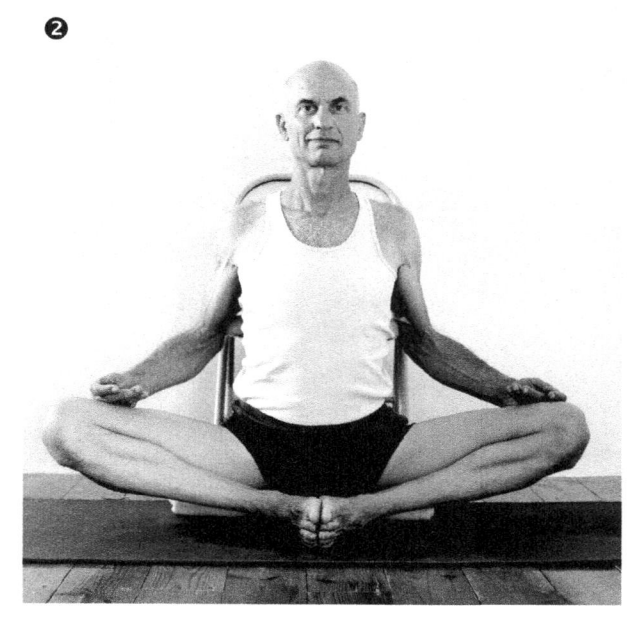

Props
chair,
blanket,
wall

→ Place a chair against the wall. If needed, place a folded blanket on the floor such that it extends slightly beyond the front edge of the chair.

> Sit on the chair and bring your feet together ❶.

> Move the hips slightly forward and then lower them down toward the floor. Move slowly, supporting the back by pushing the palms against the seat so as to maintain the length of the trunk.

> Finally, move the buttocks slightly back and sit on the blanket with the back supported against the front edge of the seat ❷.

Props for Yoga / Chapter 2 / Baddha Konasana

Baddha Koṇāsana

Variation 8
Opening the chest: Using a wall rope

Effects
The rope helps to open and lift the chest and to support the back.

Props
wall hook, rope (or belt), bolster + blanket (optional)

→ Sit in Baddha Koṇāsana in front of a wall rope; align your center with the hook.

› Insert your head and chest into the loop of the rope and place the rope against the bottom of the shoulder blades.

› Move backward until the rope is stretched and supports the back ❶.

› If the hook is too high for your needs, raise your seat (shown in ❷ by bolster and a folded blanket) and support the feet accordingly.

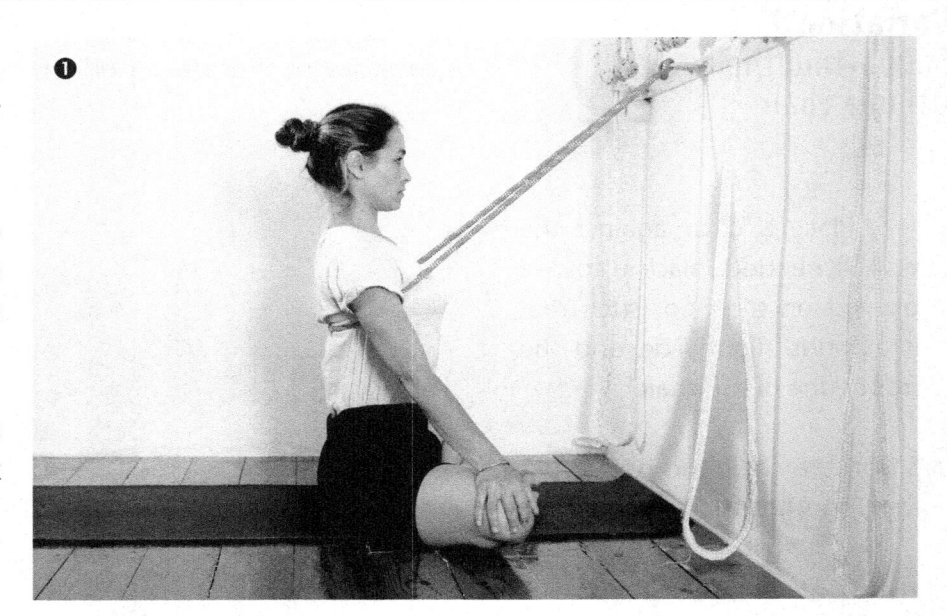

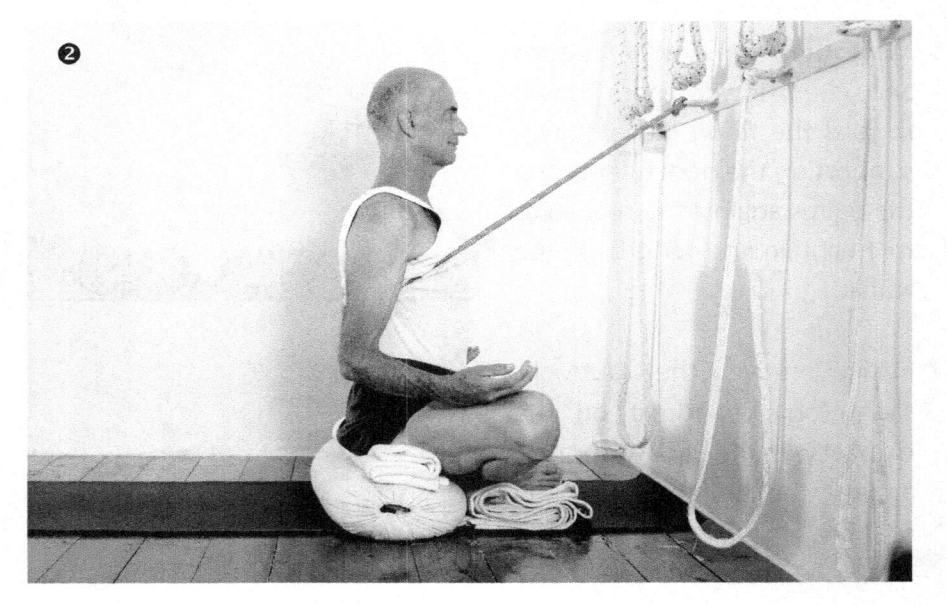

❶

❷

Advancing in the Pose

Baddha Koṇāsana

Variation 9
Preparing for Kandāsana:
Raising the feet

Effects
Raising the feet opens the inner thighs.

Props
bolster
or a folded blanket,
wall (optional)

This variation helps flexible people to open the groins and to extend the adductor muscles further. It can serve as a preparation for Kandāsana (LOY, Pl. 470).

→ Sit in Baddha Koṇāsana on a mat. You may support the back against the wall.

> Lift the feet and place them on a bolster or a folded blanket.

> Open the groins and lower the knees down.

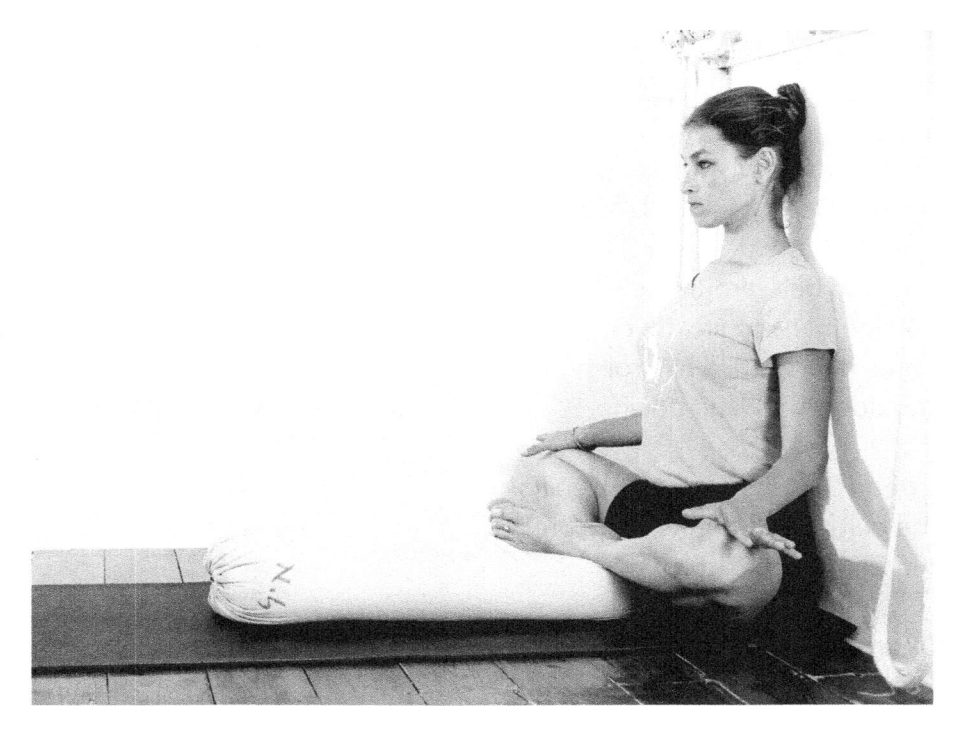

Upaviṣṭha Koṇāsana

Upaviṣṭha Koṇāsana

Variation 1
Stabilizing the back:
Holding belts

Effects
Pulling the belts activates the feet and legs. It also helps to hold the trunk upright and open the chest.

CAUTIONS
To protect the hamstrings muscles, always open the knees completely, extending them evenly on all sides. Do not allow the thighs to lift off the floor.

Props
2 belts,
blanket (optional)

→ Sit in Upaviṣṭha Koṇāsana on the mat or on a folded blanket.

› Loop a belt around each foot. Pull the belts to lift the chest and move it forward, while rolling the shoulders back and down.

› Extend the legs against the pull of the belts; open the feet and press the front thighs down.

You can also use the belts for Utthita Pārśva Upaviṣṭha Koṇāsana; to turn to the right side:

› Move the left hand forward and catch the belt of the right foot.

› Turn to the right and catch the belt of the left foot behind the back ❷.

› Now pull the belts; with exhalation move the right hand further back and turn more to the right side ❸.

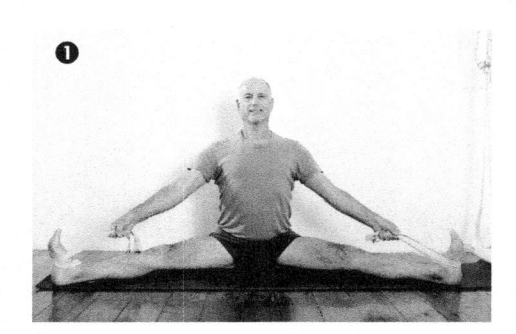

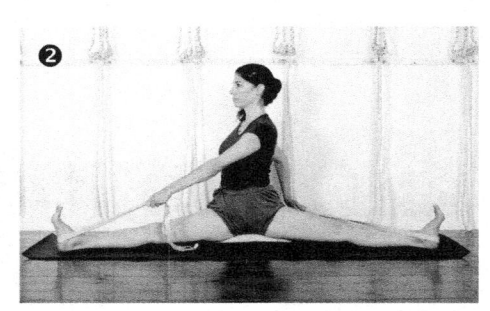

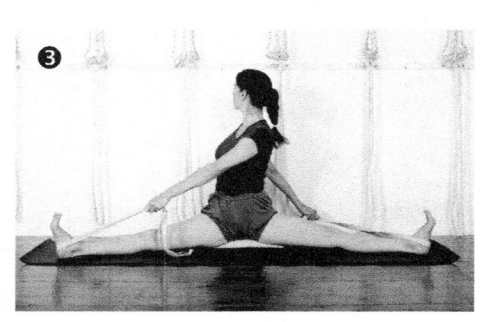

Upaviṣṭha Koṇāsana

Variation 2
Stabilizing the legs:
Bracing the pelvis and legs

Effects
The belts draw the femur bones into the hip sockets and create compactness in that area. The resistance of the belt helps to activate the legs and the feet.

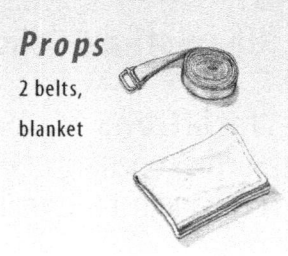

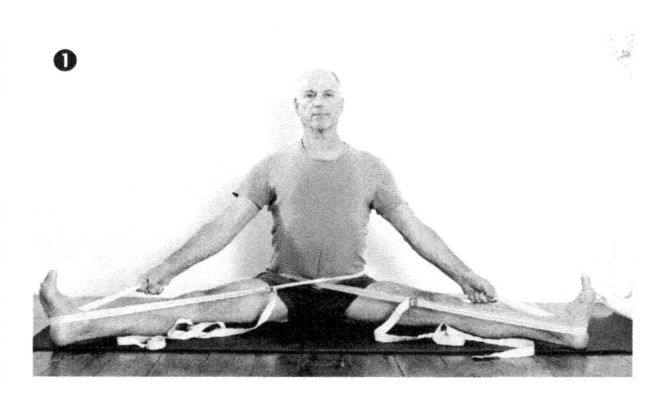

Props
2 belts, blanket

➤ Sit in Upaviṣṭha Koṇāsana on the mat or on a folded blanket.

❶

› Insert the head and trunk through the loops of two belts; lower the belts to the pelvis. Place one belt on the right heel, so as to form a loop from that heel to the left side of the pelvis. Form a similar loop from the left heel to the right side of the pelvis.

Note: If your legs are long, you will need long belts.

› Slightly bend the knees and tighten the belts, then straighten the legs against the resistance of the belts. Catch the belts.

› Extend the legs, open the feet and press the front thighs down. The midlines of the back legs should press the floor while the kneecaps and toes face directly up ❶.

› Tighten the outer thighs and pull them toward the pelvis; release the inner groins down to the floor and extend the inner thighs from the groins to the heels.

A partner sitting in front of the practitioner can pull the belts symmetrically to increase the effect while supporting the ankles of the practitioner using his/her feet ❷.

Effects: The pull intensifies the effects of this variation and helps to stabilize the sacrum against the pelvis.

Note: Two practitioners sitting face to face with their feet touching can help each other do this variation.

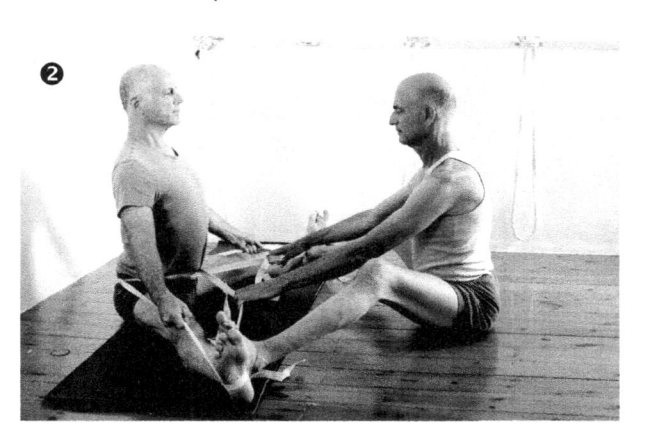

❷

Props for Yoga / Chapter 2 / Upavistha Konasana   23

Upaviṣṭha Koṇāsana

Variation 3
Further opening of the inner legs: Feet against the wall

Effects
The wall helps to activate and spread the legs further. The partner pushes the sacrum into the pelvis. This creates a tremendous space in the pelvis.

Props
wall, optional: ropes attached to the upper wall hooks

⟶ Sit in Upaviṣṭha Koṇāsana facing the wall with your inner feet against it.

› Support yourself by placing the palms on the floor behind the buttocks, lift the pelvis and move forward toward the wall, until there is a good stretch of the inner
› groins and inner thighs.

If wall hooks are available, then you can hold two upper ropes to pull yourself up ❶.

› A partner sitting behind you can push the sacrum into the pelvis ❷.

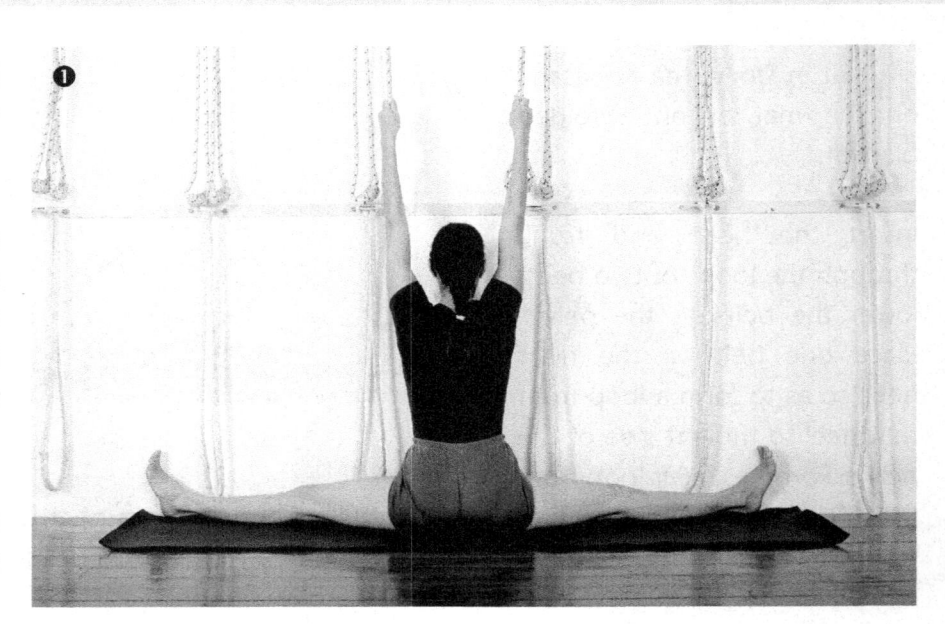

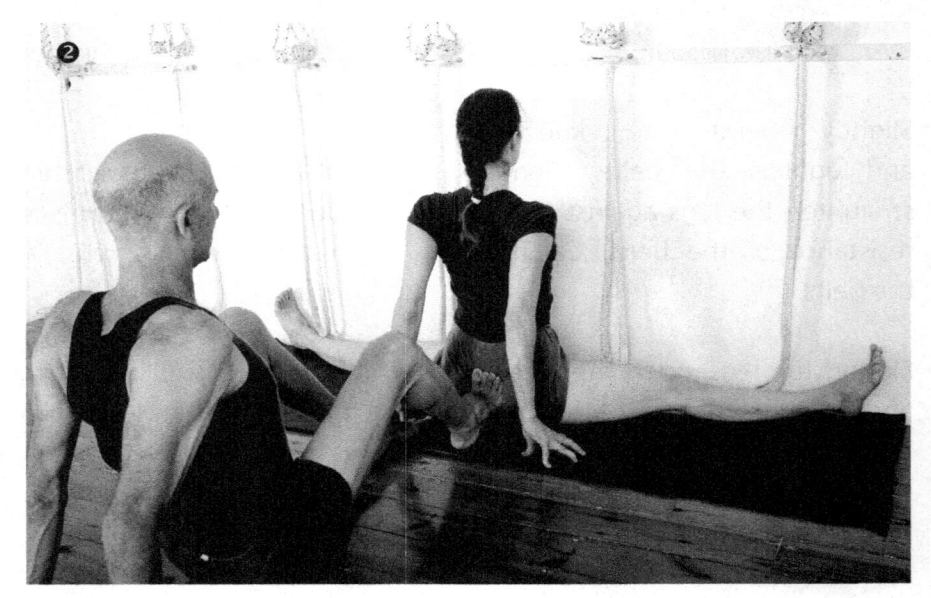

Tips
✓ Tip: Observe the inner space created in the pelvis and expand the breath there.

Upaviṣṭha Koṇāsana

Variation 4
Opening the backs of the legs: Heels on blocks

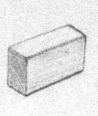

This is similar to Variation 4 of Daṇḍāsana.

> Sit in Upaviṣṭha Koṇāsana on a mat or on a folded blanket.

> Place a block under each heel. Extend the backs of the legs and Achilles tendons while pressing the backs of the heels firmly onto the blocks.

> Support the torso by pressing the palms on the floor. If the palms do not reach the floor firmly, place the finger tips on the floor, or place a block under each palm.

> Open the backs of the knees, pull the kneecaps toward the hip joints, and press the front thighs down.

> Use the arms to lift and open the chest; roll the shoulders back and down, and move the thoracic dorsal spine into the body.

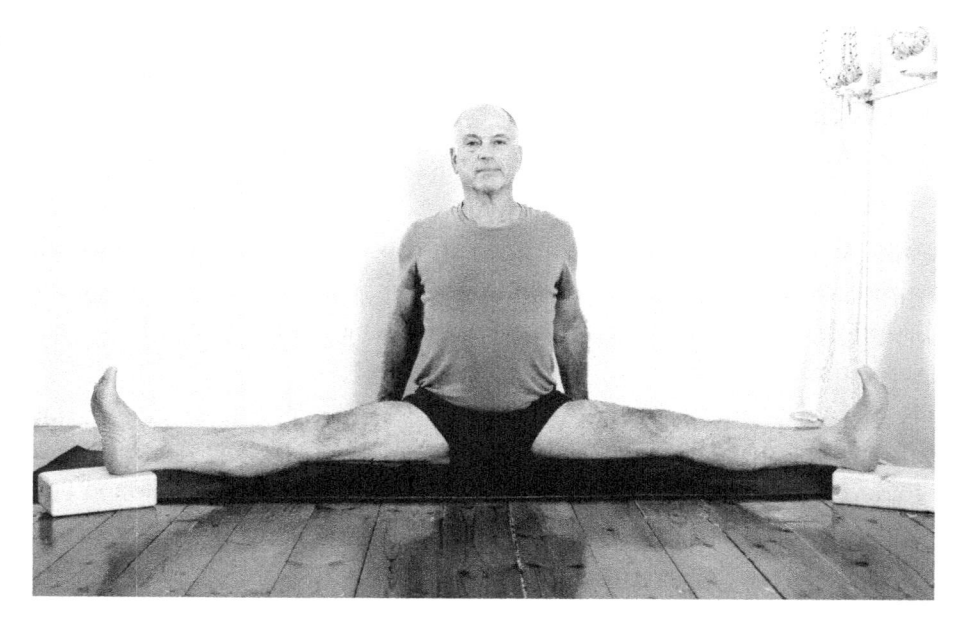

Effects
Lifting the heels allows the backs of the legs and knees to open and extend. The thigh muscles are exercised and developed.

Props
2 blocks,
Optional: blanket

Swastikāsana (Sukhāsana)

About Swastikāsana (Sukhāsana)

Swastikāsana (or Sukhāsana) is the main sitting pose for most people. It is a good substitute for Padmāsana when the latter cannot be achieved. In Swastikāsana, if the upright alignment of the torso cannot be achieved it is necessary to raise the seat from the floor.

Note about the names: By Swastikāsana we refer to the pose in which the legs are folded tightly and the outer edges of the feet are sharp. Sukhāsana ('the easy pose') is when the legs and the feet are relaxed in an 'easy' position.

There are many ways in which props can be used to provide stability and compactness, as well as for opening the chest and extending the trunk. We start with variations that help to adjust the pelvic area and continue with variations for the chest area. Most of the methods shown here are applicable to other sitting poses, and some of them can be combined. As usual, we encourage you to investigate and experiment with these options, and invent some of your own. Study these variations, feel the effects the props have on the pose, and then try to reconstruct the same effects without the props.

> **CAUTIONS**
>
> If your knees are sensitive, support them with a rolled blanket (see Variation 5).

Supporting the Buttocks

We show here various ways to arrange the support of the buttocks.

Swastikāsana

Variation 1
'Standard' Swastikāsana: Regular blanket support

Props
blanket

To do the pose when the right leg is bent first:

→ Sit in Dandāsana on a folded blanket; place the blanket under the buttock such that it also supports the upper back thighs.

› Use your hands to turn the tops of the thighs from outside in. This broadens the buttocks to create a wide base for the pose.

› Fold the right leg, and then fold the left leg such that the shins are crossed at their midpoints and the feet are under the knees.

› Press your finger tips on the floor to lift the buttocks slightly; release the groins and let the pelvis hang until it finds its vertical alignment. Slowly lower the buttocks until the heads of the buttock bones meet the blanket.

› Then place the palms on the knees and pull them back toward you, moving the sacrum in at the same time. Start with straight arms, then bend the elbows slightly and roll the backs of the arms (triceps) from outside in. Draw the bottom tips of the shoulder blades into the back chest and the inner shoulder blades toward the spine.

› Stretch the spine vertically up; open the chest by rolling the shoulders back and down while moving the shoulder blades in.

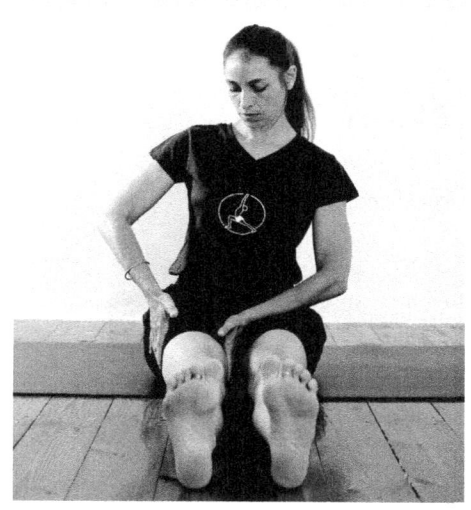

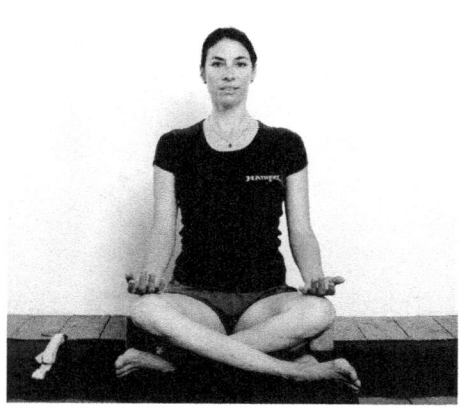

› Now release the arms and place them on the thighs with the elbows under the shoulders and palms facing up.

› Release any tension in the groin; let the thighs roll out. Relax the shins on the feet.

› Slightly pull in the skin of the outer foot of each leg and soften the ankles.

› Relax the face, eyes, inner ears, jaws, tongue, throat, shoulders, palms, abdomen, groins and feet.

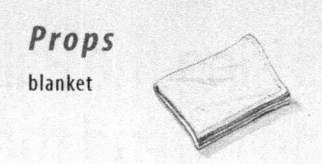

› Take long, soft inhalations to open the body; exhale softly and slowly to relax.

Tips

✓ Make sure to change the crossing of the legs every now and then (note the habitual tendency to cross the legs in the same order).

✓ If the groins are hard and the knees are higher than the groins, bring the feet a little closer to the body and spread the knees slightly more apart. You can also raise the seat by adding another blanket.

✓ Check which part of your buttocks touches the blanket. If the rear sides of the buttock bones take the main load then you will find it difficult to lift the spine from its root. This means that you need to raise the seat.

✓ Look forward and keep the eyeballs very soft. Do not gaze at any specific object, but mentally look into the body. Imagine you are looking from the back of the skull into a wide open field.

✓ Mentally observe the vertical central plumb-line of the pose from the crown of the head to the perineum. Make sure this imaginary line is absolutely vertical: not tilted or turned to the left or right, nor bend forward or backward. Arrange the body around this imaginary line.

Using the Palms to Extend the Trunk

In many cases the palms do not reach the floor fully in order to lift the pelvis effectively. Resting the palms on a raised surface helps this lifting action.

Swastikāsana

Variation 2a
Supporting the palms on a folded blanket

Effects
Pressing the palms down helps to extend the spine from the pelvis and to broaden the chest.

Props
blanket

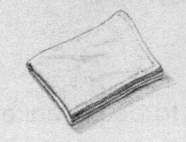

→ Create a long-and-narrow seat by a three-folded blanket.

▷ Sit in the center of the seat, place the palms on the folded blanket and press down to lift the chest.

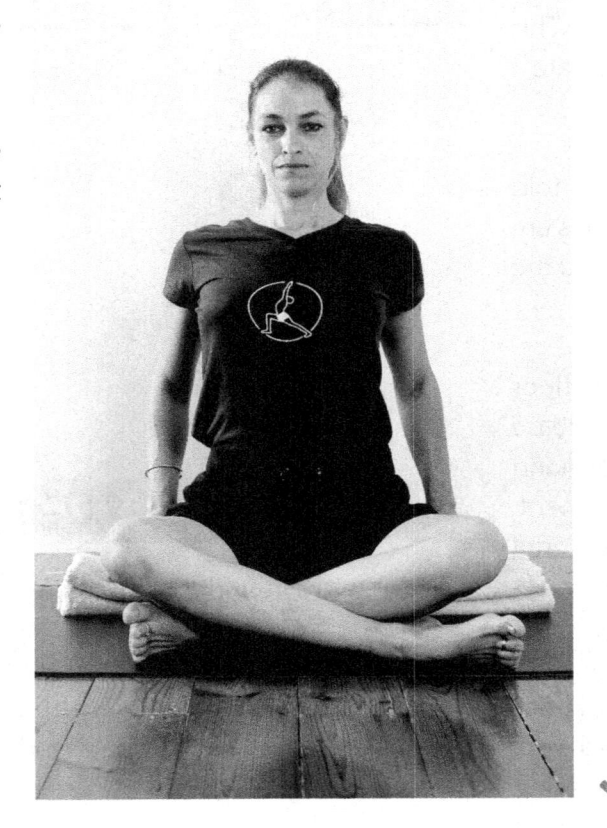

Tips

✓ Observe how the body weight is divided between the two buttock bones; check if one side feels lighter or narrower than the other.

✓ Look forward and note which eye has a sharper vision. Release the lighter buttock to get a more even feeling. Observe the impact of skeletal balance on the spine and on the sharpness of your eyes.

Swastikāsana

Variation 2b
Supporting the palms on blocks

Effects
When entering the pose as explained above, the pelvis can be lifted more easily. The arms help to extend the spine and lift and open the chest. Pressing the ring finger and the little finger gives access to the outer shoulders, while pressing the thumb and index fingers gives access to the inner shoulders and armpits.

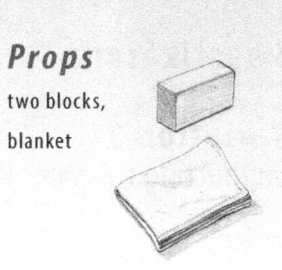

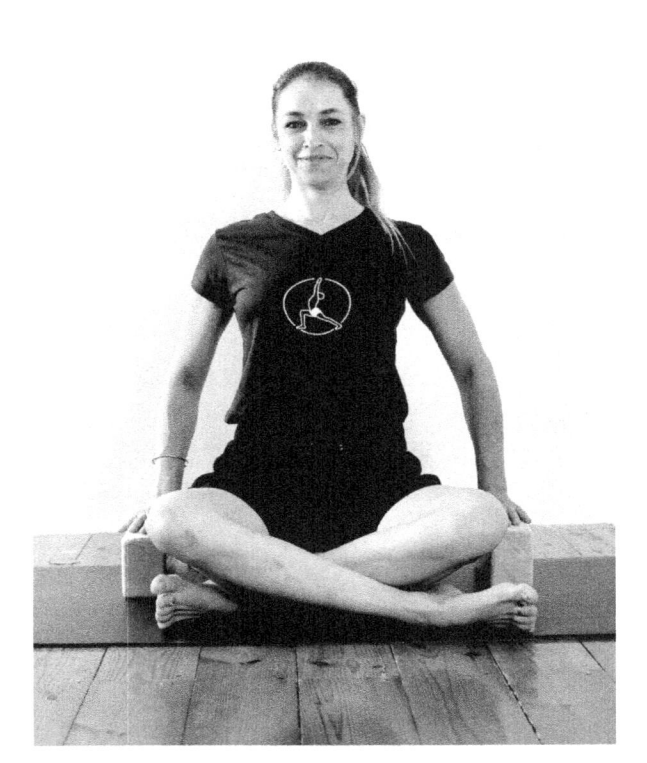

Props
two blocks, blanket

Blocks are especially useful, since you can place the entire palm and fingers on the hard surface. It clarifies the connection between the palms and the shoulders. Try the following:

→ Sit on a folded blanket in Swastikāsana with one block on each side of the seat.

> Place the palms on the blocks such that the middle fingers are pointing straight forward, marking the central axis of each hand.

> Lift slightly the thumbs and index fingers off the blocks and press the ring and little fingers down. Note the effect on the shoulders.

> Now lift the ring and little fingers and press the thumb and index fingers – observe what happens in the shoulders.

> Now press all five fingers observing the equal pressure of the outer and inner palms.

> Use the pressure to lift the sides of the trunk, without lifting the shoulders.

Tips
✓ Make sure the blocks are equidistant from the body and that the pressure of the palms on the blocks is equal.

Applicability
All sitting poses.

Props for Yoga / Chapter 2 / Swastikāsana 29

Swastikāsana

Variation 3
Supporting the shins with a blanket

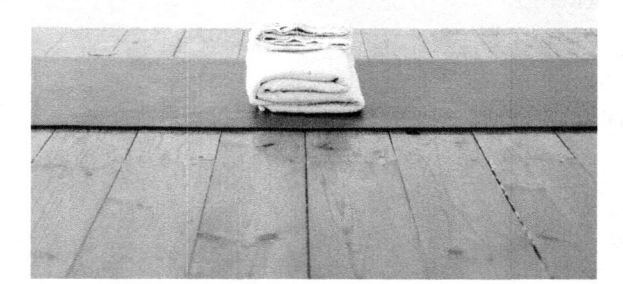

Effects
The support for the shins allows you to relax the legs and groins.

Props
blanket

→ Create a stepped seat by doubling one edge of a three-folded blanket ❶.

> Sit on the higher step. Rest the folded legs on the lower step ❷.

❶

❷

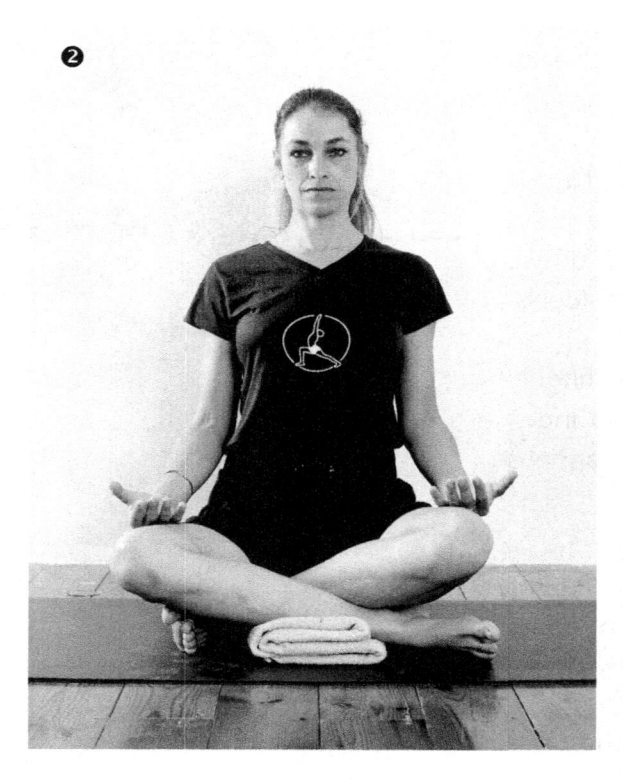

Applicability
Padmāsana

Swastikāsana

Variation 4
Spreading the buttock bones: Sitting on a rolled mat

Effects
The roll helps to widen the lower pelvic region and to support the root of the spine; it also supports the shins, which allows relaxation of the legs and groins.

Props
sticky mat

→ Roll a sticky mat.

> Center the rolled mat under the buttocks and sit on it.

> Make sure that the two buttock bones are supported symmetrically.

How to determine the desirable height of your sitting?

B.K.S. Iyengar writes:

> "In Tādāsana, space is created from the base of the pubis to the naval and the area there is kept flat. In sitting positions, simulate the Tādāsana stretch." (Light on Pranayama, ch.11, paragraph 21).

To get a better feel for Mr. Iyengar's words, do the following experiment:

> Stand in Tādāsana and extend the spine, then use your thumb and middle or ring finger to measure the distance between the pubic bone and the navel.

> Keep that distance between the fingers and sit down. Now compare the distance you measured in Tādāsana with the current distance between the pubic bone and the navel. If you find a considerable shortening of the measurement you took, then you probably need a higher support for the buttocks.

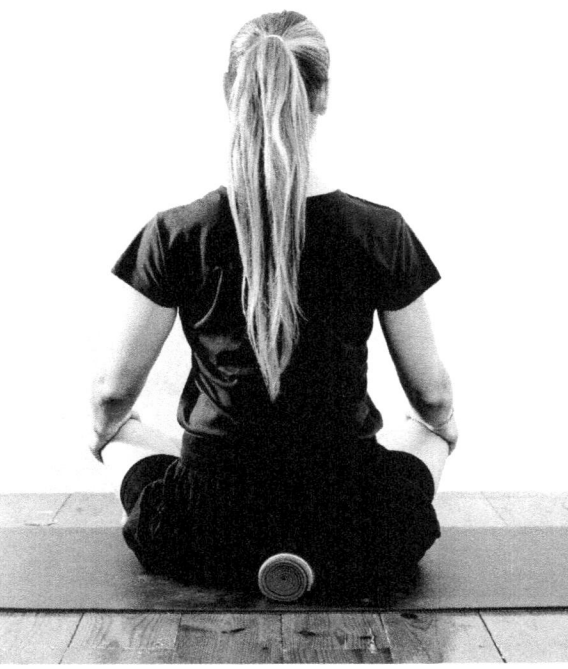

Note
A rolled blanket may be substituted for the rolled mat

Applicability
all sitting poses except for Vajrāsana.

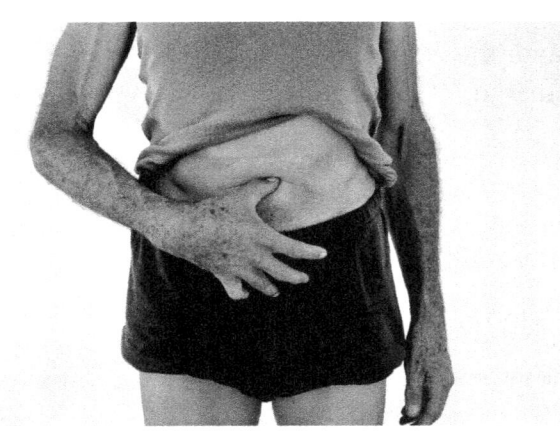

Swastikāsana

Variation 5
Arrangement for long sittings: Using a high support

Effects
The higher seat, coupled with shin support and the hands position releases tension from the limbs, relaxes the front groins and enables the spine to extend from its base without effort. The knee and hand supports enable the limbs to relax.

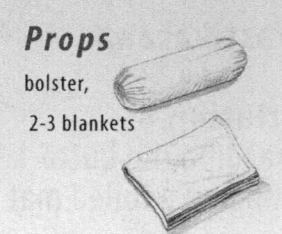

Props
bolster, 2-3 blankets

When sitting in Swastikāsana, the top of the folded knees should be about leveled with the front groins. When you raise your seat considerably, the knees tend to drop and pull the lumbar spine forward. This fatigues the back and groins during an extended sitting. Here is a way to support the knees for a long and comfortable sitting:

→ Sit on a bolster (if the bolster is too soft, place a folded blanket on top).

> Roll a blanket and tuck it between the shins and the feet.

> Make sure you sit on the heads of the buttock bones, and the lift sacrum and pubic bone up vertically from the base.

> Make sure that the two knees are at the same level and well supported.

> Another way to support the knees is to brace them with a belt.

> Some people will find it comfortable to place another three-fold blanket on top of the thighs and rest the palms on it (see Variation 15 on page 43).

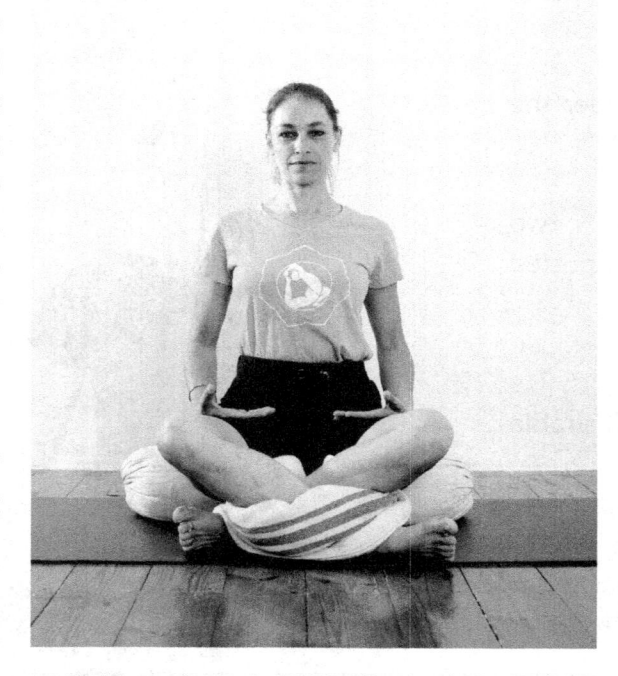

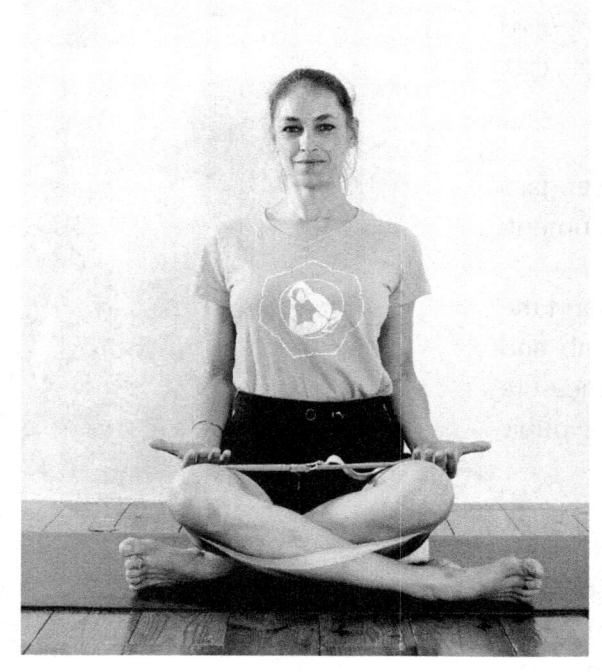

Applicability
Vīrāsana

Swastikāsana

Variation 6
Sensitizing the buttocks area: Sitting on a block

Effects
The wooden surface creates a different feeling. You will experience a stronger earth element and a better lift in the trunk. The feeling in the buttock bones is much sharper, and you can better sense the weight on each buttock.

Props
block

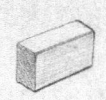

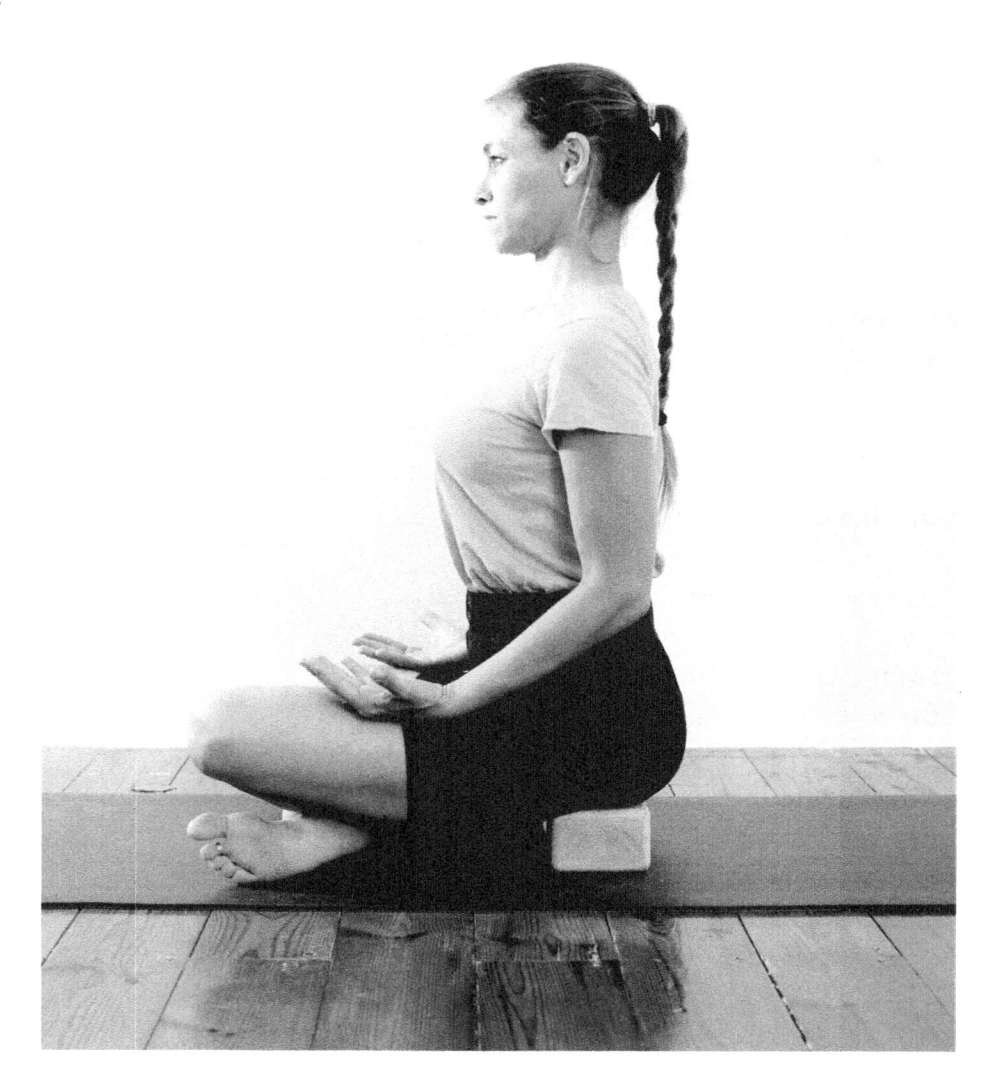

Unlike a bolster or blankets, a wooden block does not allow the buttocks to sink.

Tip
- Learn to balance the weight evenly on both buttocks.

Applicability
all sitting poses except for Padmāsana, in which a block would be too high.

Swastikāsana

Variation 7
Bracing the legs

Effects
The belts create stability and comfort (sthirata & sukhata). They provide 'borders' for the pose; they support the knees and sacrum and help to draw the femurs (thigh bones) deeply into the hip joints. When the pelvis is thus stabilized, the lower abdomen becomes soft and quiet. The combination of external compactness with internal broadening is very soothing and healthy for the inner organs.

Creating compactness in the pelvis prevents the spine from sagging and keeps the pose stable and alert. The two actions needed are:

Moving the heads of the femurs (thigh bones) into the sockets of the hip joints

Moving the sacrum forward into the pelvis.

We show first how it can be done with one belt and then two ways of using two belts.

Using one belt

➡ Loop a belt around the sacral band and the knees.

▷ Lift the knees slightly and tighten the belt.

▷ Now release the knees to stretch the belt. Make sure the femur bones are moving into the hip joints.

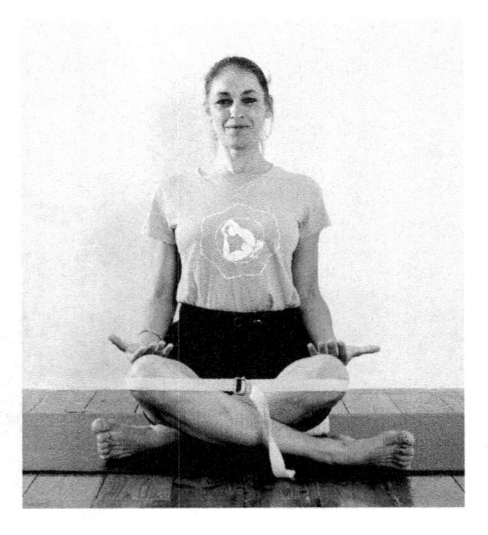

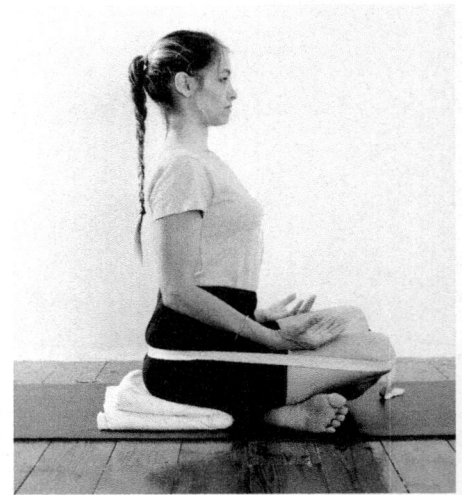

Applicability
Padmāsana, Vīrāsana.

Props
1-2 belts

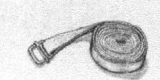

Using two crossed belts

→ Brace each leg with a separate belt.

› Lift the knees slightly and tighten the belts until you feel compactness, evenness and stability. Then release the knees.

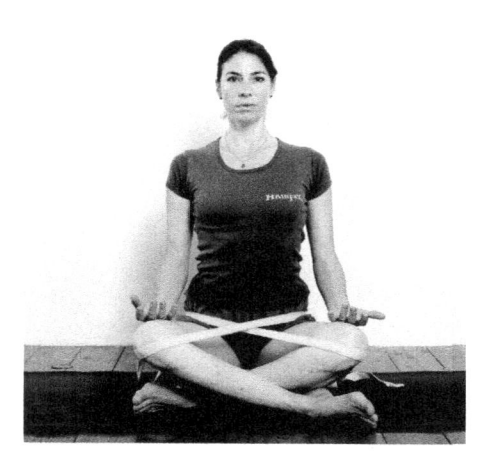

Applicability
Padmāsana, Baddha Koṇāsana.

Using Two joined belts

→ Open one belt and loop it in the second belt.

› Place the crossing of the belts on the sacral band and brace the knees.

› Adjust the belts such that buckles are close to the knees

› Slightly lift the knees and tighten the belts, then release the knees.

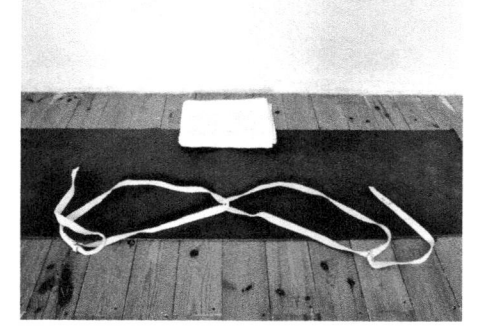

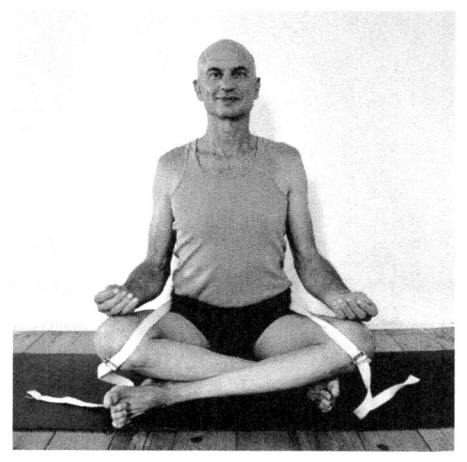

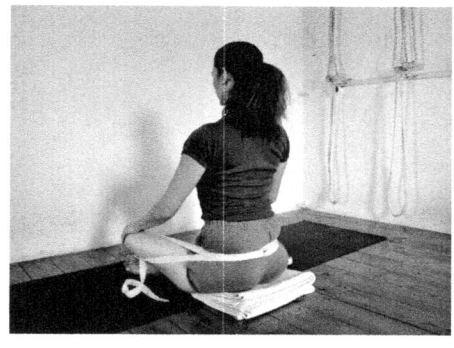

Tips
Soften the abdomen and observe the breathing in this area.

Props for Yoga / Chapter 2 / Swastikāsana

Swastikāsana

Variation 8
Compacting the base: Bracing the pelvis with a belt

Effects
The belt creates compactness in the pelvis which, in turn, helps to lengthen the spine upward and to soften the abdomen.

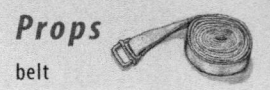

Props
belt

⟶ Stand in Tādāsana, bend the knees slightly and tie a belt around the pelvis girdle.

> The belt should be at the level of the hip joints (bracing the two greater trochanters of the femurs).

> Tighten the belt with one hand while using the other hand to move the belt in the other direction toward the buckle (see Variation 5 of Tādāsana).

> Then sit down.

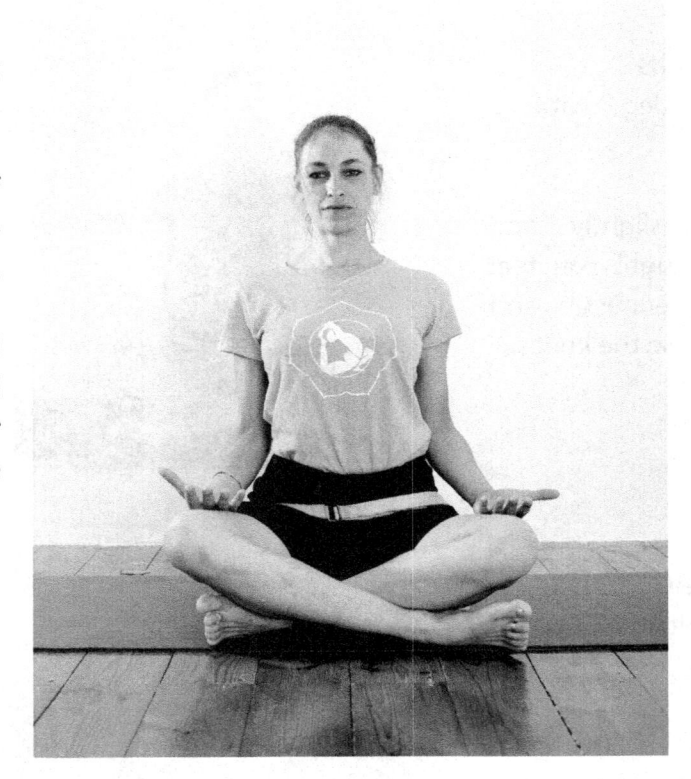

Tips
✓ Sit with the belt in this way for a while and observe the effects. Then loosen the belt and observe again. What has changed in the experience of the pose? Articulate these differences.

Applicability
All sitting and standing āsana. A belt can be used this way during an entire practice session.

Swastikāsana

Variation 9
Moving the sacrum in: Block between sacrum and wall

Effects
The support of the block stabilizes the sacrum, and hence the entire spine. It induces quietness and draws the attention to the pelvic area. The pelvis is the abode of Apāna Vāyu – the downward moving energy whose abode is the pelvis and lower abdomen. Hence this variation is useful for learning Apānic breathing.

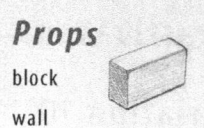

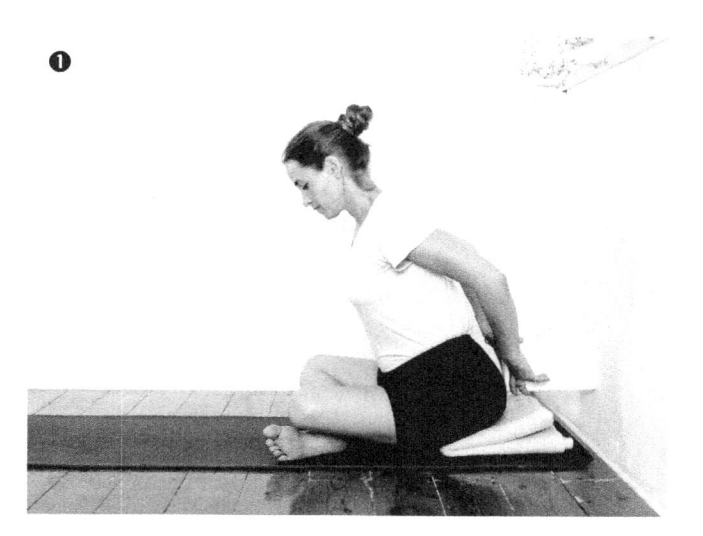

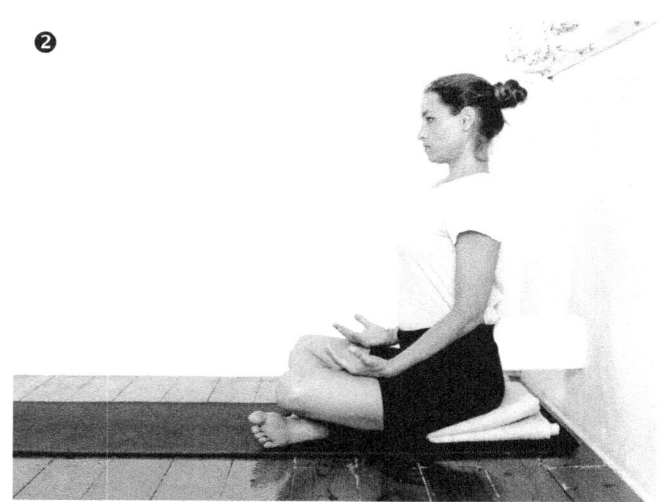

Props
block
wall

▶ Sit with your back to the wall, one block-length away from the wall.

▶ Lean slightly forward and insert the block from above, in between the wall and the sacrum ❶. Gently move the block down, ironing the sacral skin downward, until the block is centered against the sacrum.

▶ Sit upright. Make sure the block is held between the wall and the sacrum with a light pressure.

▶ Roll the shoulders back and sit straight ❷.

❶

❷

Applicability
All sitting poses, Tādāsana, Utthita Hasta Pādāsana.

Swastikāsana

Variation 10
Stabilizing the base:
Pulling the shins

Effects
Pulling the shins is another way to create a framework for the pose. The sacrum can be moved in against this pull.

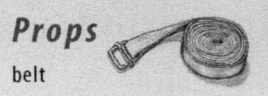

Props
belt

→ Sit in Swastikāsana. Hook a belt around the crossing of the shins and pull it towards you.

› Move the sacrum in against this pull.

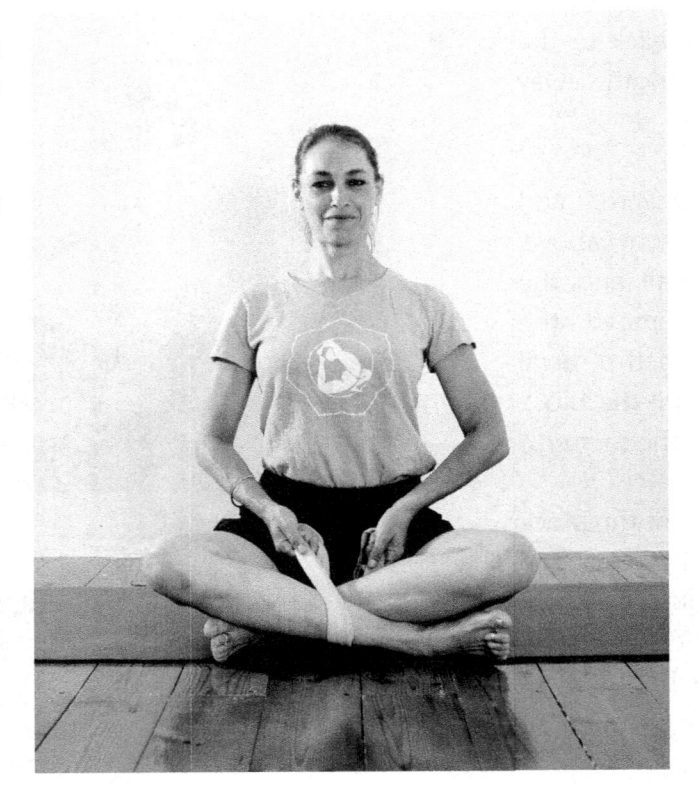

Applicability
Padmāsana. In Baddha Koṇāsana the belt can be hooked under the feet.

Opening the Upper Body

We now turn our attention to the upper body. By opening the upper body we refer to actions like lifting the rib cage; drawing in the thoracic vertebrae and the shoulder blades; rolling the shoulders back and down, and so on. These actions take time to learn and props can be very helpful.

Swastikāsana

Variation 11
Supporting the chest:
A block between wall and back

Effects
The support of the block stabilizes the thorax and helps to open the rib cage. It is a good way to practice Pranayama.

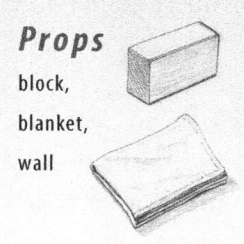

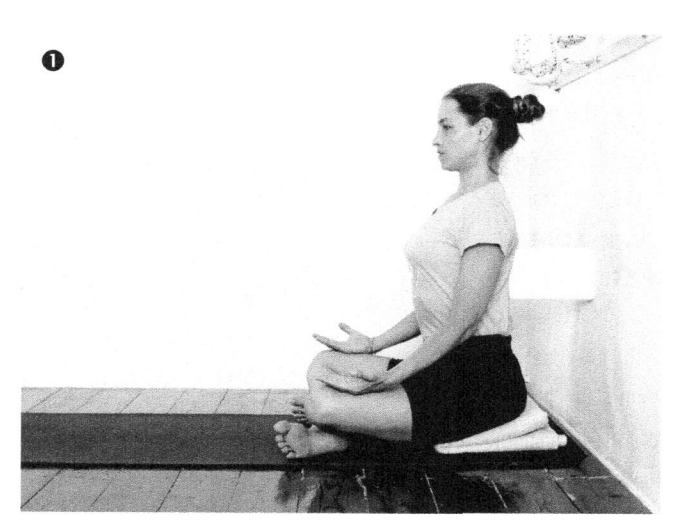

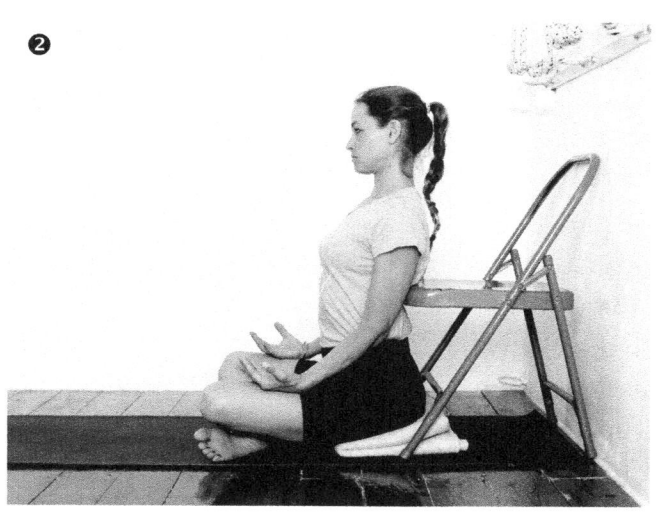

Props
block,
blanket,
wall

This is similar to Variation 9, but here the block is placed to support the chest (two blocks can be used to combine both).

⟶ Sit with your back to the wall, one block-length away from the wall.

› Lean slightly forward and insert the block to support the middle of the spine.

› Sit upright. Make sure the block is held between the wall and the thoracic vertebrae with a slight pressure.

› Roll the shoulders back and sit straight ❶.

› It is also possible to support the back with a chair placed against a wall ❷.

Applicability
all sitting poses, Tādāsana.

Props for Yoga / Chapter 2 / Swastikāsana 39

Swastikāsana

Variation 12
Aligning the spine:
Sitting against an external corner

Effects
The corner enables you to sense accurately the position of the vertebrae and to align them. The plank supports the thoracic spine and thus opens the chest.

Props
a protruding wall edge, plank (optional)

→ Sit with your spine against the vertical edge formed by the meeting of two walls (or against a corner of a column).

> Center the sacrum symmetrically on this edge, and then do the same with the occiput (back of the skull). Align the vertebrae one above the other between these two ends and feel their contact with the vertical edge ❶.

> *Note:* Due to the natural curvature of the spine, the lumbar vertebrae and the neck vertebra should not touch the corner, but should extend up in proximity to it.

> Now you can lean slightly forward and place a plank between the chest and wall.

> You can either position the elbows behind the plank to lean on it (as in ❷), or in front of the plank. In the second case, push the elbows gently against the plank to coil the side ribs forward and up.

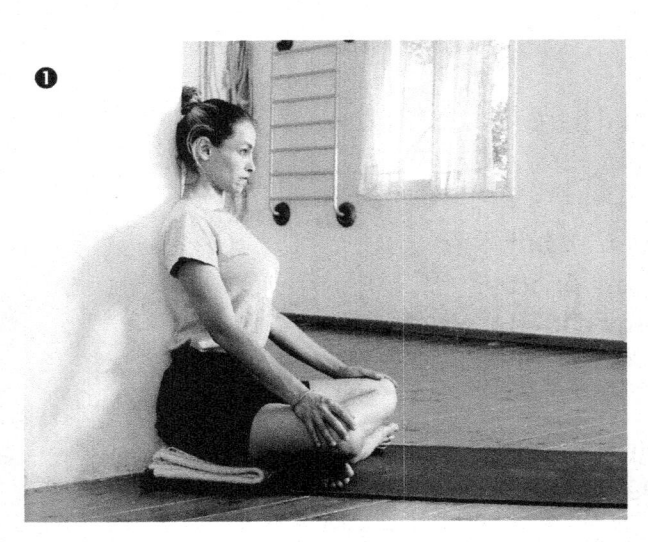

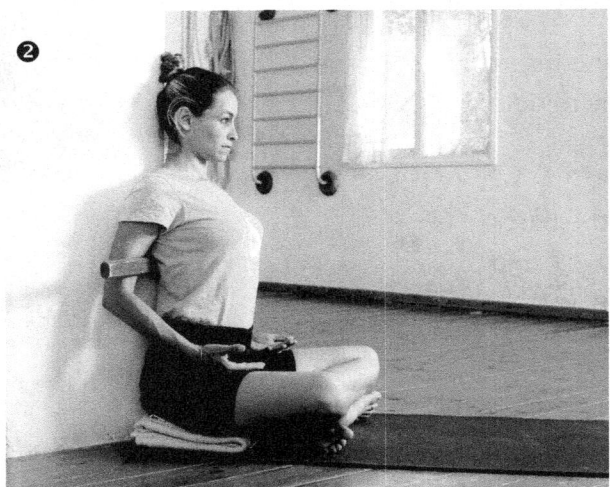

Applicability
most of the sitting poses.

Swastikāsana

Variation 13
Supporting the back: Using a hooked rope

Effects
The chest is stabilized in an optimal position while the front ribs are lifted without exerting the back muscles.

Props
a wall hook, rope (or belt)

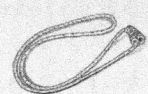

This is similar to Variation 8 of Baddha Koṇāsana.

→ Sit in front of a wall hook (a firm door handle can do the job just as well).

› Tie a rope to the wall hook and wrap it around your trunk just below the chest.

› Adjust the length and the position of the rope such that when you lean back your sacrum is vertical, the back muscles are supported and the chest is well opened.

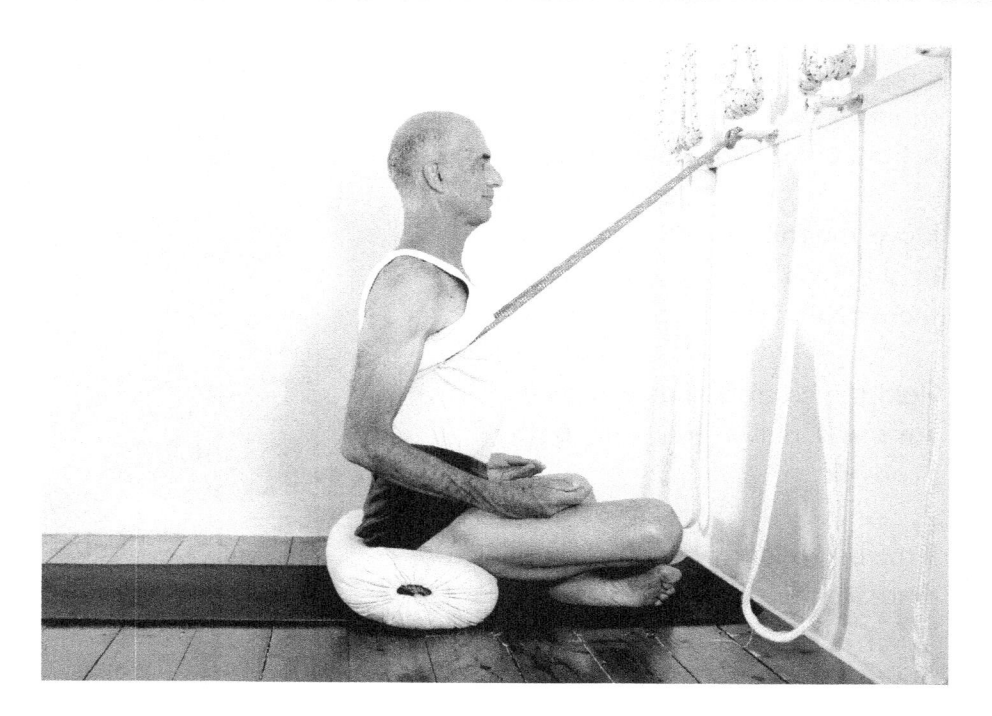

Applicability
all sitting poses.

Swastikāsana

Variation 14
Rolling the shoulders back: Crossed "shoulder jacket"

Effects
Pulling the belt helps to roll the shoulders back and to move the shoulder blades down and towards the spine. This stabilizes the back and opens the chest. It brings awareness to the (invisible) back body.

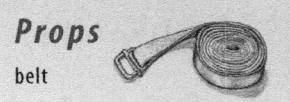

Props
belt

→ Place an open belt on the shoulder girdle, such that it rests in front of the shoulder tops.

> Move the loose ends of the belt under the front arm pits and cross them behind your back.

> Hold the crossed ends with bent arms and pull evenly with both hands ❶.

> If the belt is long enough you can embrace the outer elbows ❷.

> Another option is to place the belt across the shoulder blades, pass the loose ends forward under the armpits and then roll them back over the shoulders and cross them behind the back ❸.

Note: this variation may require a long belt.

> Stay in the pose for a few minutes allowing the breath to fill the entire chest cavity; then, without changing the shape of the chest, slowly release the belt and hold the pose.

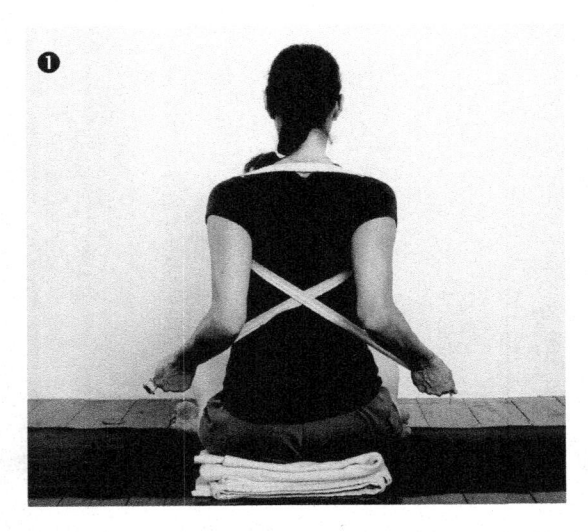

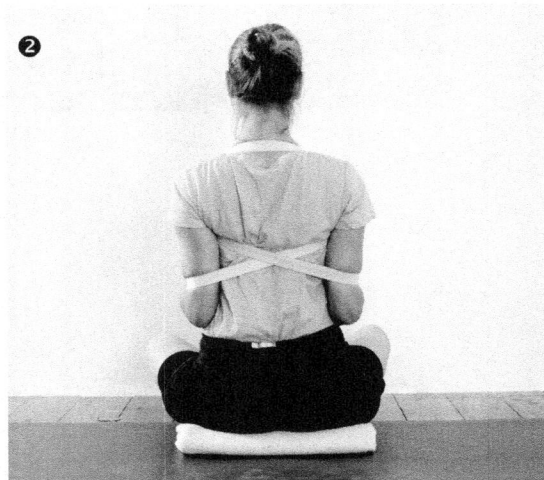

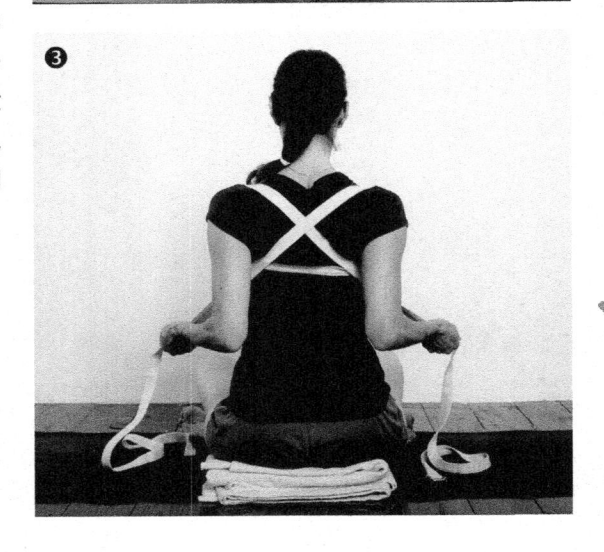

Tips
✓ Beware not to compress the spine or allow the lumbar spine to move forward.

Applicability
all sitting poses and Tādāsana.

42 Props for Yoga / Chapter 2 / Swastikāsana

Swastikāsana

Variation 15
Stabilizing & resting the arms: Belt on elbows

Effects
The resistance of the belt clarifies the actions of the arms, shoulders and shoulder blades; it brings awareness to the (invisible) back body. The belt and the support for the palms help to keep the arms passive.

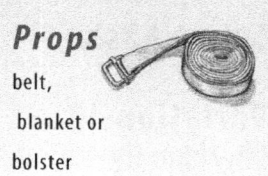

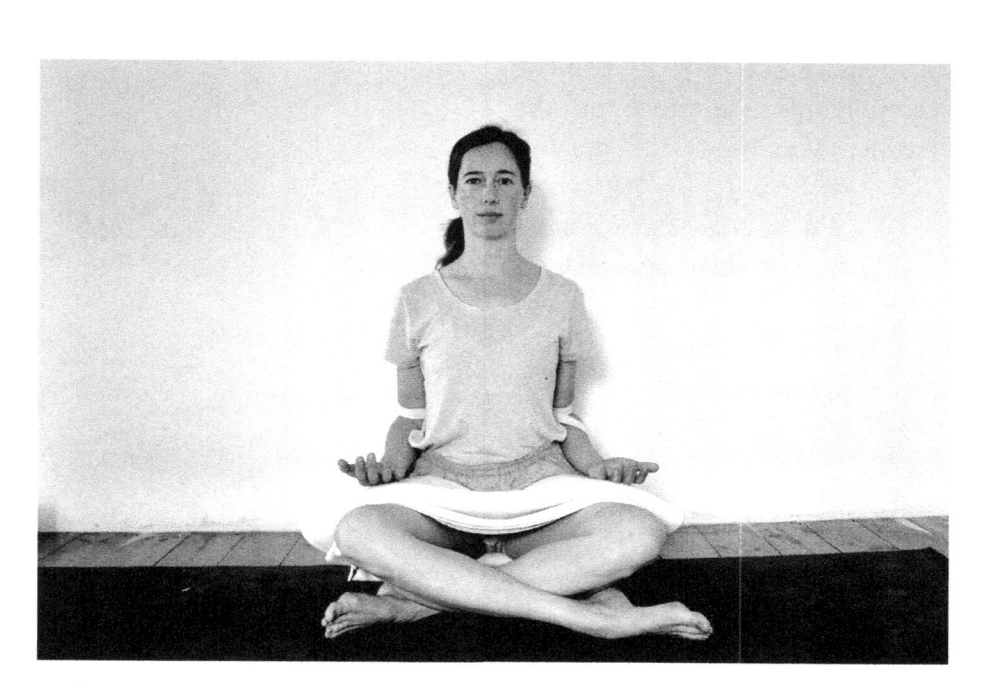

Props
belt,
blanket or
bolster

In sitting poses, one has to surrender the organs of action (*karmendrias*), this however is not easy since these organs are the core of our activity. In the sitting poses the legs are folded, but the arms are free to move and may remain active. Stabilizing the elbows and resting the hands help to pacify the arms.

In this variation the use of the belt is similar to its use in Sālamba Sarvāngāsana.

→ Sit in Swastikāsana and place a bolster or a folded blanket on your lap. Loop a belt to shoulder width.

› Insert your hands into the loop behind your back and then rest the palms on the blanket.

› Extend the inner arms down and gently work the elbows against the belt, as if you want to stretch it.

Tips

✓ Adjust the height of the support for the palms such that the forearms are parallel to the floor.

✓ Roll the back of the upper arms (triceps) inward and move the dorsal spine and shoulder blades in.

Applicability
all sitting poses and Tādāsana.

Swastikāsana

Variation 16
Checking the upright alignment: A block on top of the head

Effects
the weight of the block sensitizes the crown of the head and clarifies its location with respect to the spine. Even the slightest tilt will cause the block to slide. This is a good indication for the vertical alignment and helps to develop balance and stability.

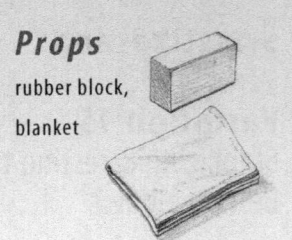

Props
rubber block, blanket

⟶ Sit erect on a blanket; carefully place a block on the crown of your head.

> *Note:* Rubber block is preferable, in case the block slips from the head!

› Gently extend the spine up as if to push the block higher.

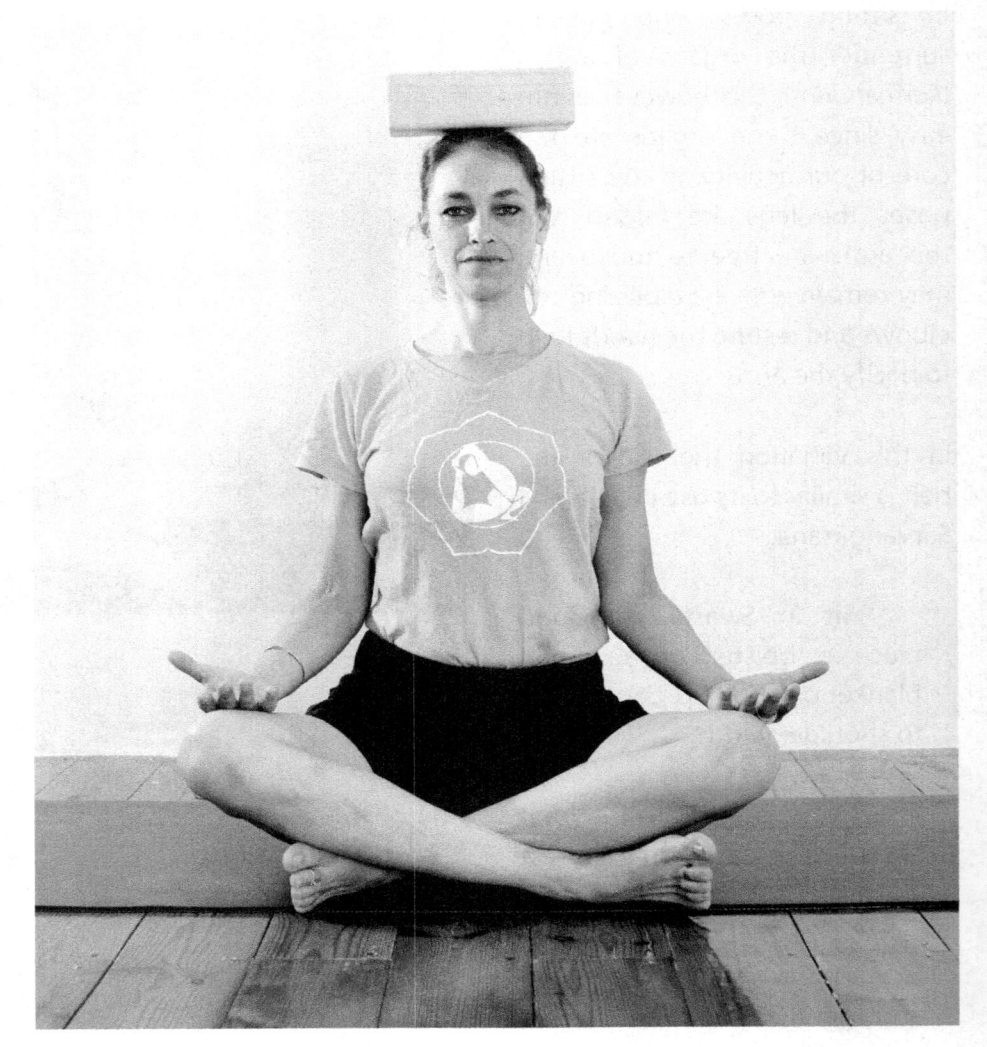

Tips
- ✓ Learn the sensation of a perfectly erect and balanced torso, with a centered vertical axis.
- ✓ Learn to keep corrective movements to a minimum without dropping the block!

Applicability
all sitting poses and Tādāsana

Swastikāsana

Variation 17
Sensitizing the chest:
A belt around the chest

Effects
The belt helps to feel the movement of the ribs and the change in the volume of the chest cavity during the breathing cycle. It draws the attention inward. In the second (upper) position, the belt helps to move the shoulder blades to their correct place.

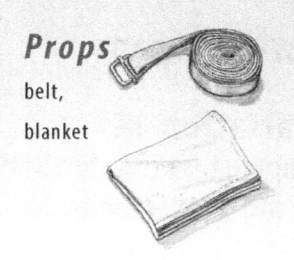

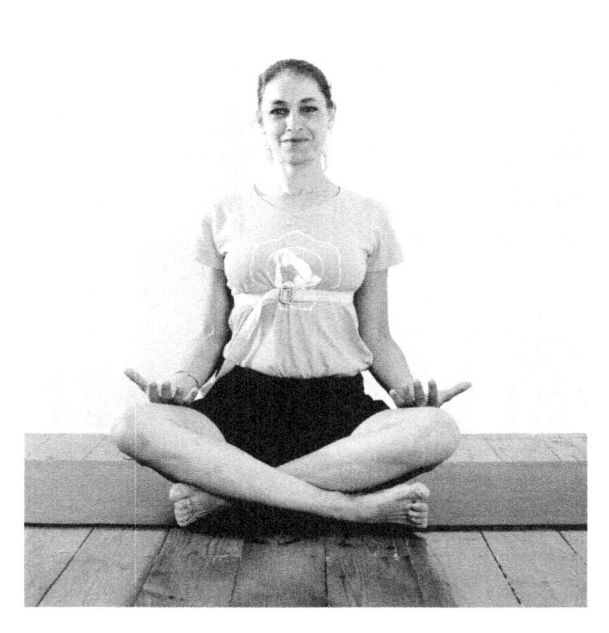

Props
belt,
blanket

A belt sharpen the awareness of the movement of the ribs during the breathing cycle. This is very helpful for Pranayama practice.

> Wrap a belt around the torso, just below the chest. Tighten it moderately, so as to permit expansion of the lower ribs during deep breathing.

> Close your eyes; take a slow, deep inhalation. As the chest expands, observe how the skin of the front chest rubs against the belt.

> Move the belt up and tighten it around the top of the chest.

Of course, you may try to combine the two exercises, using two belts. But it is advisable to start with one belt.

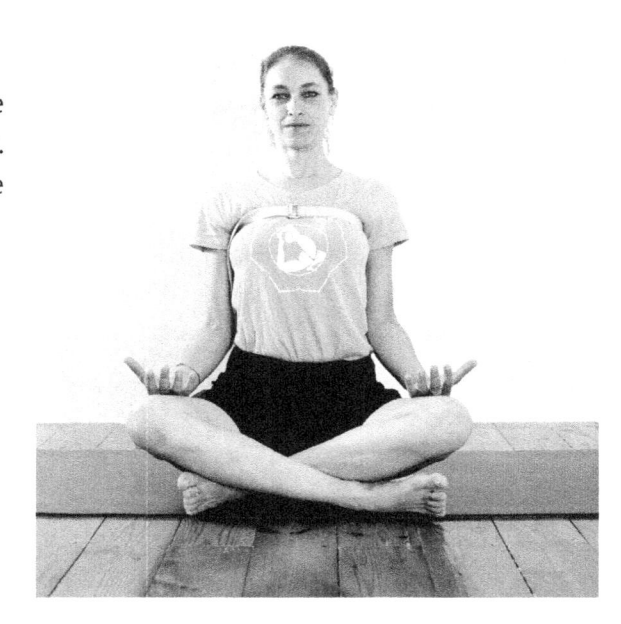

Applicability
In essence, all poses can be done with a belt around the top chest.

Props for Yoga / Chapter 2 / Swastikāsana

Swastikāsana

Variation 18
Supporting the chin in Pranayama:
Using a rolled belt

Effects
The chin support relieves strain from the neck. It helps to stabilize and balance the head. Personally I prefer the rolled belt, because the bandage is too wide to fit in the collar bones cavity.

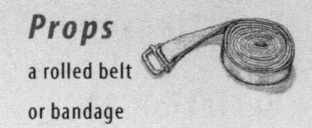

Props
a rolled belt or bandage

Swastikāsana is instrumental for sitting Pranayama, in which a chin lock (Jālandhara Bandha) is required. If the chin does not reach the top of the chest comfortably, it can be supported by a rolled belt or bandage.

→ Do Jālandhara Bandha and measure the gap between the chin and the notch between the collar bones.

› Roll a belt sufficiently to fill that gap.

› Lift the chest, place the roll in between the two collar bones and lower the chin until it rests on the support and keeps it in place.

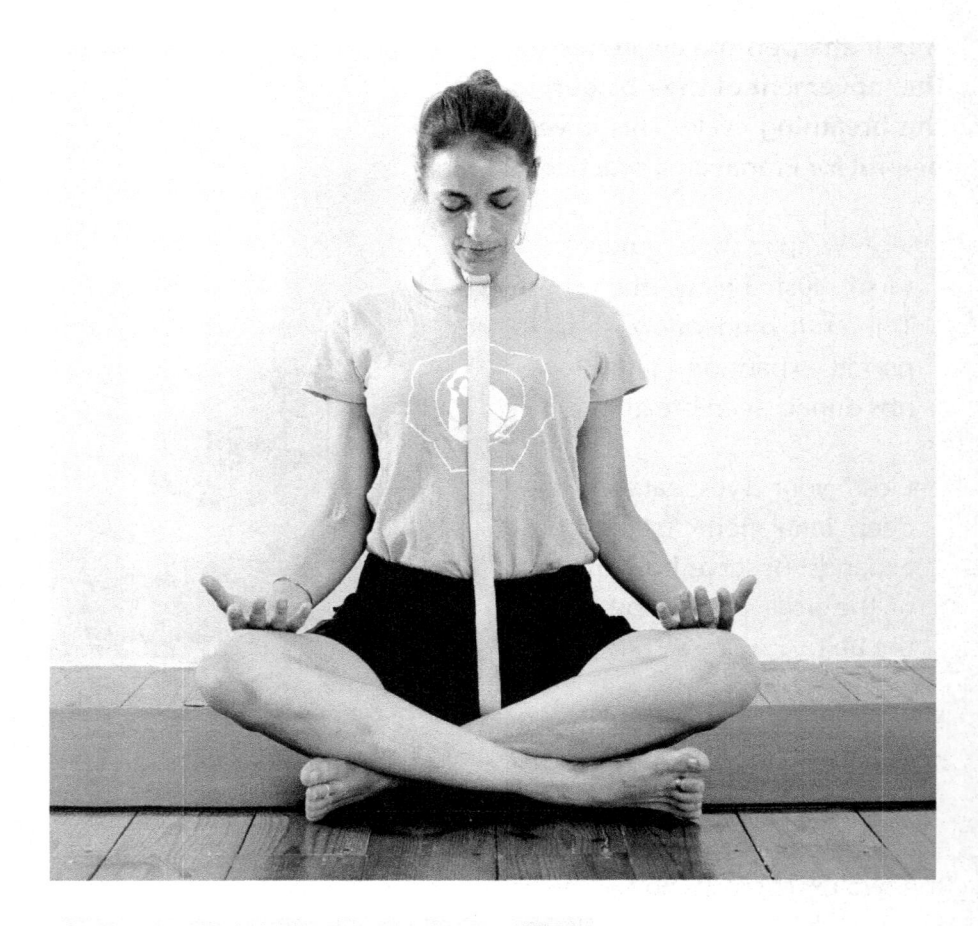

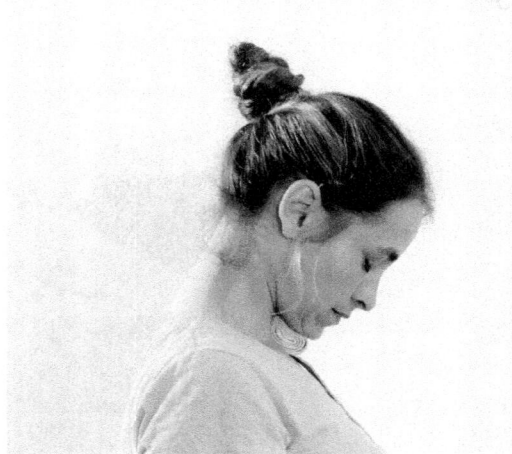

Applicability
all Pranayama sitting poses.

Vajrāsana

About Vajrāsana and Vīrāsana

In Swastikāsana, Padmāsana and Baddha Koṇāsana the thighs are rolled out. Here, in Vajrāsana (and Vīrāsana) the thighs are rolled inward, and the knees brought together.

> *Note:* Vajrāsana is not included in *Light on Yoga*; however it is a good preparation for Vīrāsana since it prepares the knees and ankles for Vīrāsana.

> ⚠ **CAUTION**
>
> If your ankles are injured use a support for the shins as shown in Variation 3 of this pose.

Vajrāsana

Variation 1
Joining the ankles and knees: Using belts

Effects

This pose (along with Vīrāsana) develops the arches of the feet and relieves pain caused by heel spurs. The ligaments of the ankles and the knees are extended. The belts ensure that these joints are properly aligned. The blanket at the back of the knees extends the ligaments of the knees and creates space for the folding action; hence this variation is a boon for healthy knees. The belts keep the legs joined without effort so the pose can be held for a long time; it is soothing and quieting for the mind.

Props

2 belts, 3 blankets

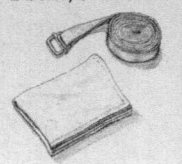

In Vajrāsana the knees and ankles should be joined; we use two belts to keep them in contact:

→ Sit in the center of the mat (if it is the thin type, fold it to make it softer).

› Loop a belt around the top of the knees; center the buckle between the two knees to make it accessible after entering the pose.

› Loop another belt around the ankles, fasten it to join the ankles loosely; center the buckle behind the ankles, facing the floor, to make it accessible after entering the pose ❶.

› Kneel and then bend forward to lift the hips and thighs. Slide a folded blanket over the shins until it enters into the backs of the knees ❷.

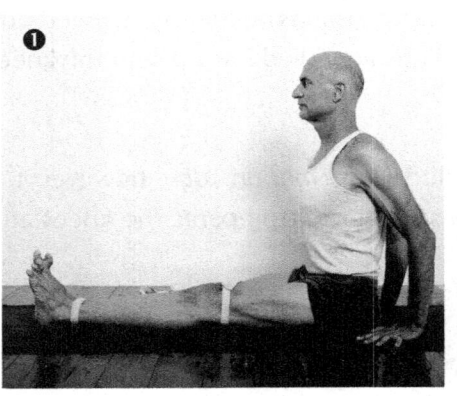

› Now extend the feet backward and sit on the heels. Spread the metatarsals evenly on the floor.

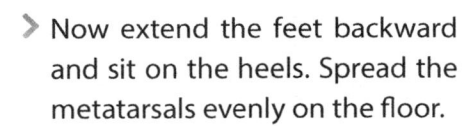

› In each foot, the centerline of the metatarsals (top side of the foot) should be pressed to the floor such that the nails of all the five toes (including the small one) touch the floor. Join the big toes and spread the other toes sideways.

› Rest the back of your palms on the thighs. For longer stays place a folded blanket on the thighs in order to raise the palm support.

› Sit straight, roll the shoulders back and open the chest. Relax the face, eyes and jaws and look forward with a soft gaze ❸.

Note: You can add another folded blanket under the buttocks to keep the lower spine erect and make the pose more comfortable.

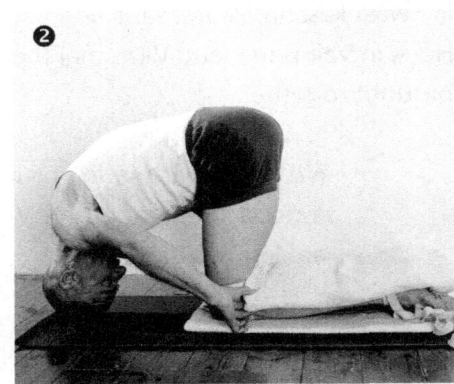

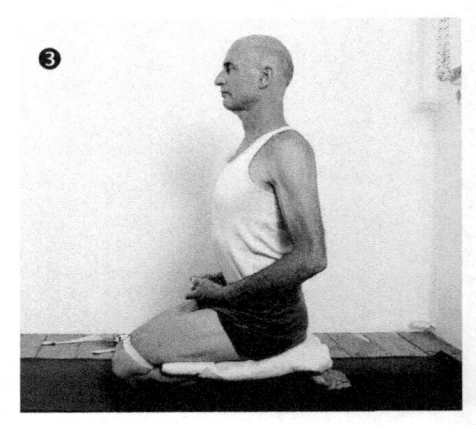

Tips

✓ Adjust the belts so that the two legs are aligned and in contact, but without pressure. The lower belt should keep the inner and outer ankles parallel to each other.

Vajrāsana

Variation 2
Improving feet flexibility: Stretching the toes inward

Effects
This variation stretches the feet thus improving the flexibility of the ankles, tarsals, metatarsals and toes. It is important for people with flat feet and for those suffering from heel spurs. It improves the circulation to the feet.

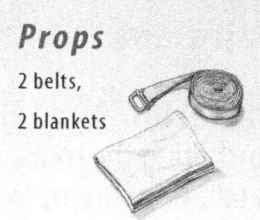

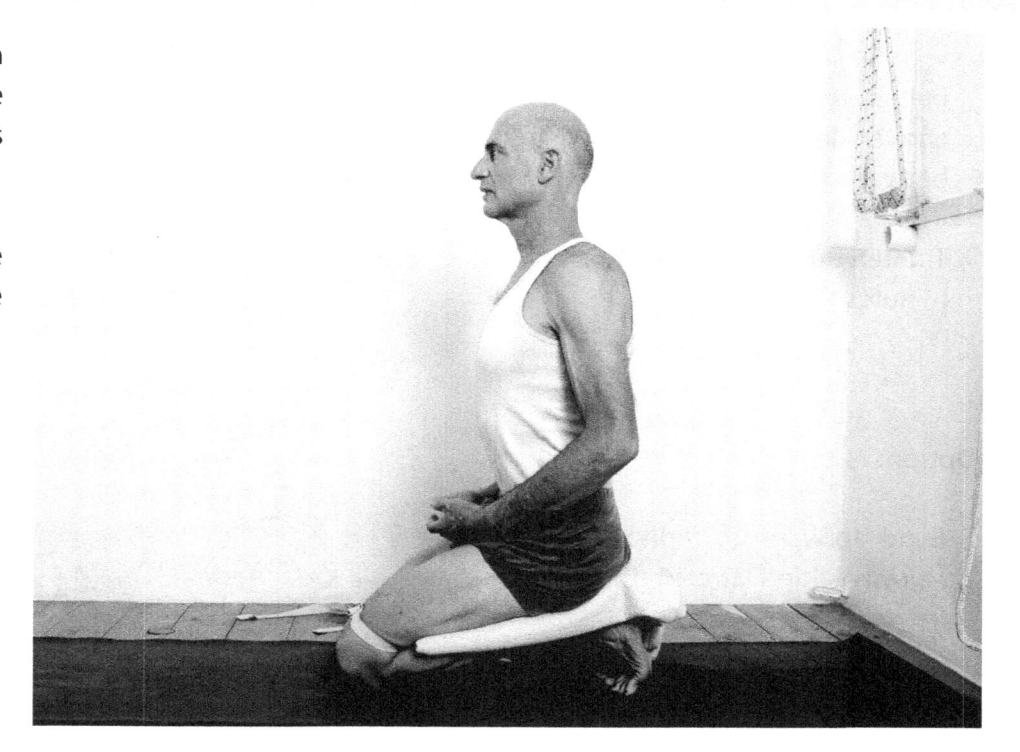

Props
2 belts,
2 blankets

> After sitting in Vajrāsana for a few minutes raise the pelvis and draw the toes forward (towards the knees).

> Sit on the heels when the feet are flexed forward (ankle dorsiflexion).

Tips
✓ You may experience pain or pressure on the toes and feet – learn to bear this pain patiently for a few moments. With practice the flexibility of the feet will improve and the pain will decrease.

Vajrāsana

Variation 3
Anchoring the roots of the legs:
A belt from groins to ankles

Effects
Bracing the groins creates firmness and grounding and improves the knees' flexibility.

Props
belt

→ Sit in Vajrāsana and loop a belt around the top of the thighs and ankles. Keep the buckle in between the legs.

> Tighten the belt and sit for several minutes ❶.

Option:

> Bend forward to Adho Mukha Vajrāsana and stretch the arms forward ❷.

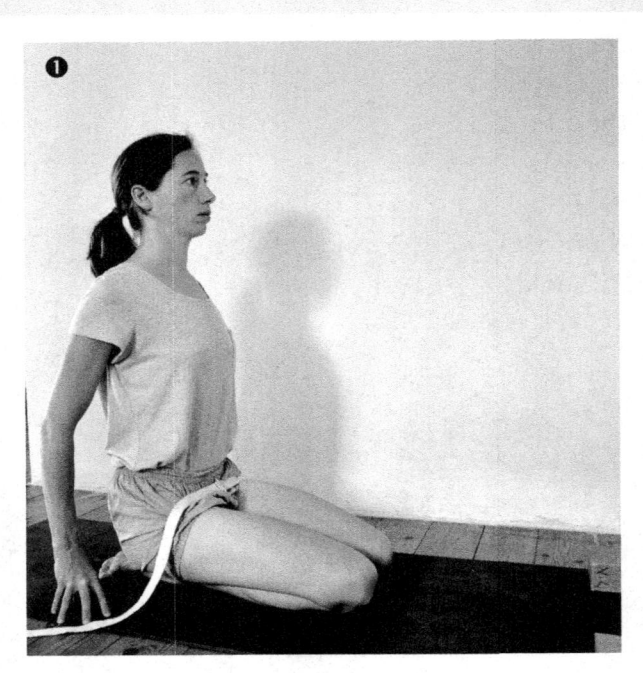

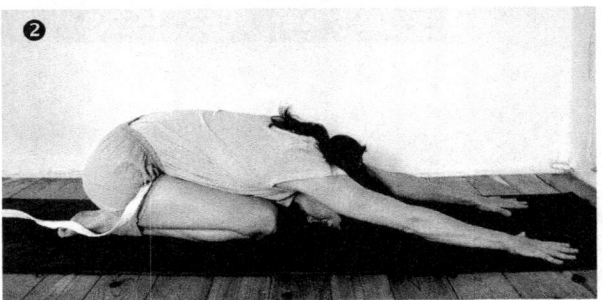

Tips
✓ The forward stretch in Adho Mukha Vajrāsana with the belt opens and releases the lower back.

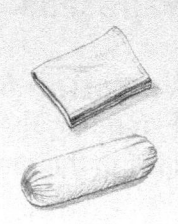

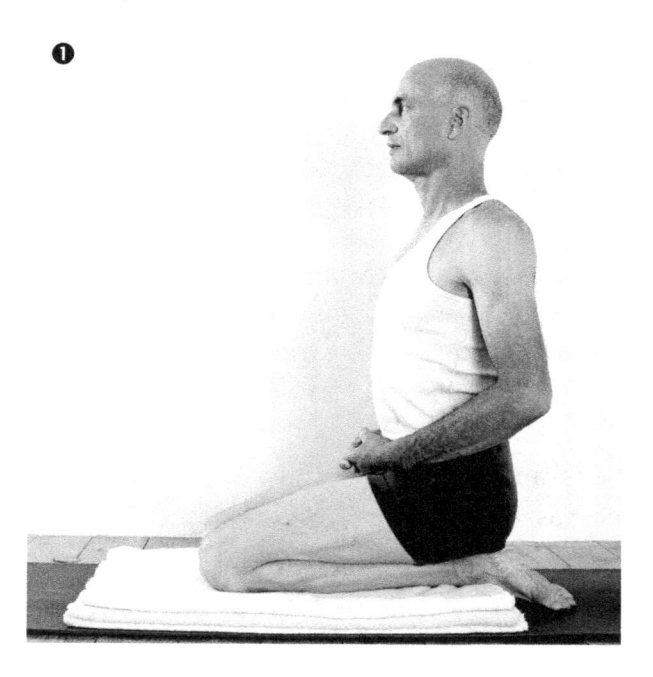

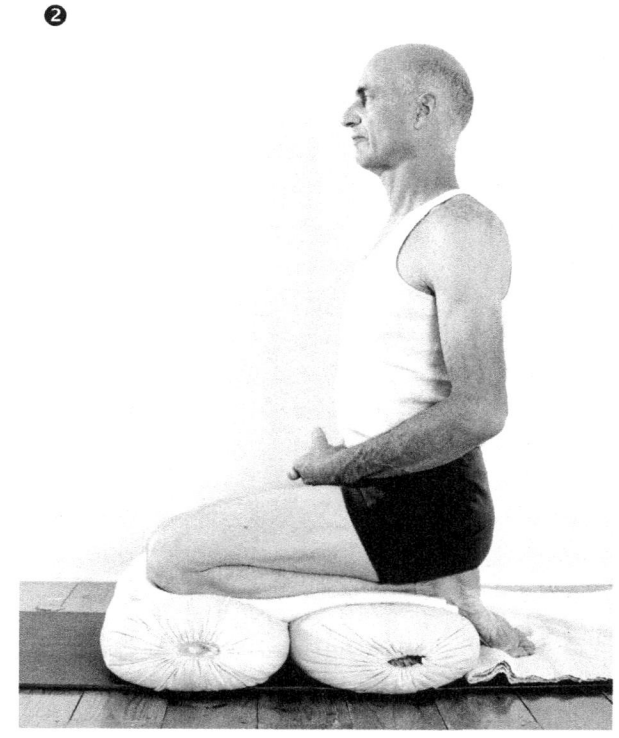

Vajrāsana

Variation 4
Doing the pose when the ankles are stiff: Adding support for the shins

Effects
Raising the shins and knees above the level of the feet reduces the stretch of the ankles and makes it bearable for people with stiff front ankles. Try performing the āsana first with blankets; if the stretch is still unbearable switch to the bolsters. Gradually replace the bolsters with blankets, and then reduce the number of blankets, until you can sit on the flat mat.

Props
3-4 blankets
or
2 bolsters
+ blanket

For some people sitting on the heels may create excessive and painful stretch of the front ankles (due to limited plantar flexion); in this case the extension of the ankles should be controlled.

> Use 2-3 folded blankets to create a platform with a stepped edge.

> Sit in Vajrāsana such that the shin bones and front ankles rest on the platform, the metatarsals are on its stepped edge and the toes are on the floor ❶.

> If the stretch of the front ankles is still unbearable, use 2 bolsters for the platform instead of the blankets ❷.

Applicability
Vīrāsana

Vajrāsana

Variation 5
Extending the ankles: Lifting the metatarsals

Effects
The front ankles get a good stretch.

Props
blanket

This variation is, in a sense, opposite to the previous one – it is intended to create more flexibility and extension (increase the plantar flexion of the ankle).

⟶ Sit in Vajrāsana such that the ankles rest on the floor but the toes and metatarsal are raised on a folded blanket.

› You can still use the belts and blanket behind the knees as in Variation 1.

› Spread the toes on the folded blanket.

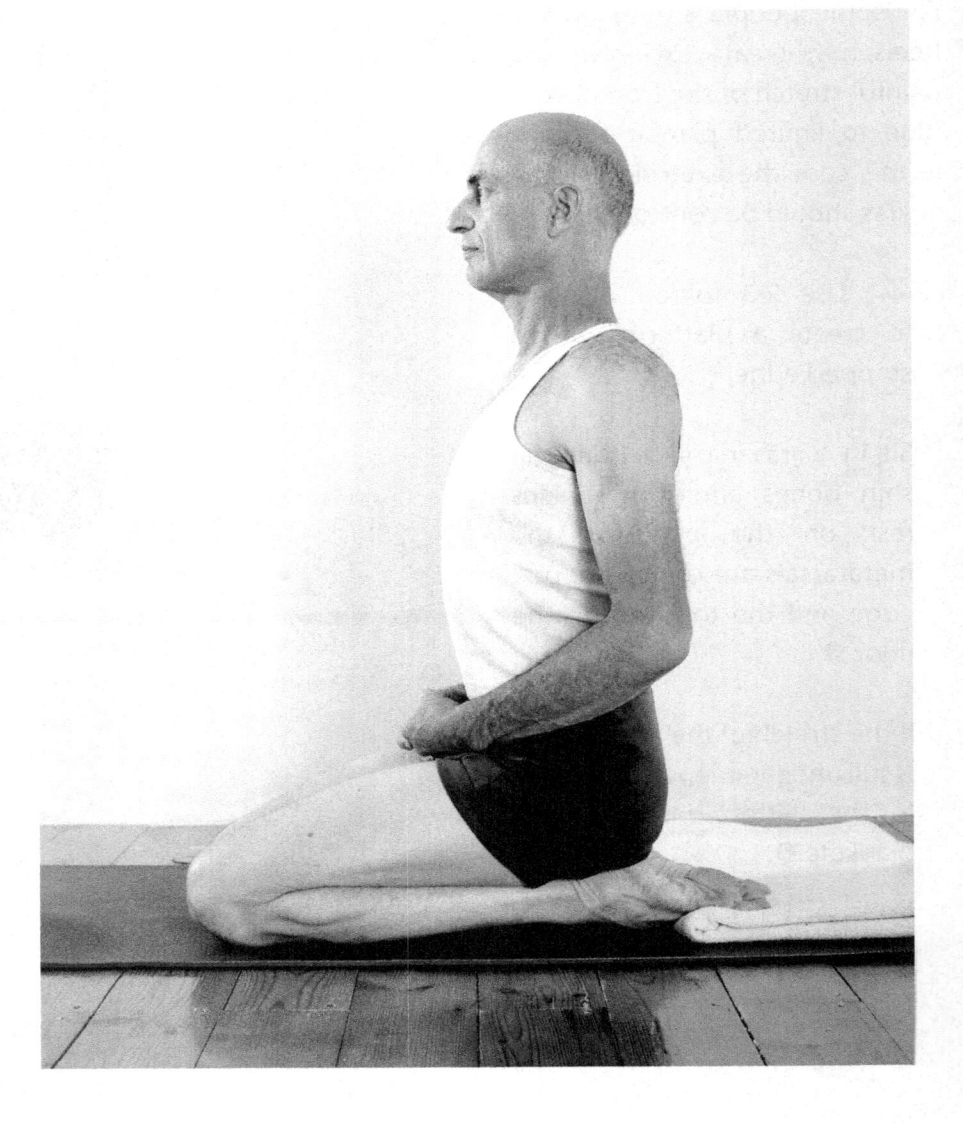

Applicability
Vīrāsana

Vīrāsana

About Vīrāsana

Vīrāsana is a symmetrical sitting pose in which the spine can be held upright with ease. It improves the flexibility and health of the knees and ankles. Many people who find it difficult to fold the legs in Swastikāsana or Padmāsana can sit comfortably in Vīrāsana. However, the base of the pose is narrow, making it prone to sideway tilts, especially in long sittings with eyes closed.

> ⚠ **CAUTION**
>
> If the ligaments of your knees are injured, use a bolster to support your seat, or do Vajrāsana Variation 1 (see above) instead of Vīrāsana

Vīrāsana

Variation 1
Spreading the calves from the thighs:
Entering into Vīrāsana

Props
folded blanket or a block

→ Kneel with joined knees while keeping the feet spread apart.

> Place the sitting support in between the spread feet.

> As you lower the buttocks, use both hands to separate the calf muscle from the thigh: Starting with the right leg, grip the top of the calf muscle with the right hand, iron it toward the heel and then rotate it outward. At the same time, grip the back of the right thigh with the fingers of the left hand and rotate it inward ❶.

> Arrange the left leg in a similar fashion.

> Sit down gradually; keep the knees joined and lower the thighs symmetrically in between the shins.

Note: be sensitive to your body. If the pain in the knees and/or the feet becomes excessive do not force the pose. Rise on your knees and add height to your seat. Over time, if you practice this pose regularly, you will be able to reduce the height.

> Adjust the ankles and feet such that the inner and outer ankles are equally extended (see that the inner ankle is not shortened) and the feet are extended back, in line with the shins.

> Spread the toes and make sure that the small toes are also touching the floor ❷.

> Release the skin of the knees by gently pulling the skin from under the bottom of the knee to the top of the knee. Turn each knee from inside out. The inner and outer knee should be at the same height.

> Sit on the heads of the buttock bones. Extend the spine upward, open the chest and look forward ❸.

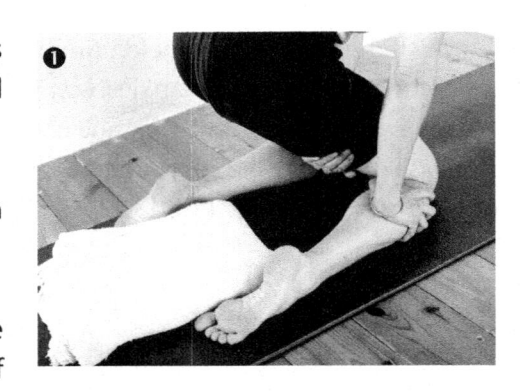

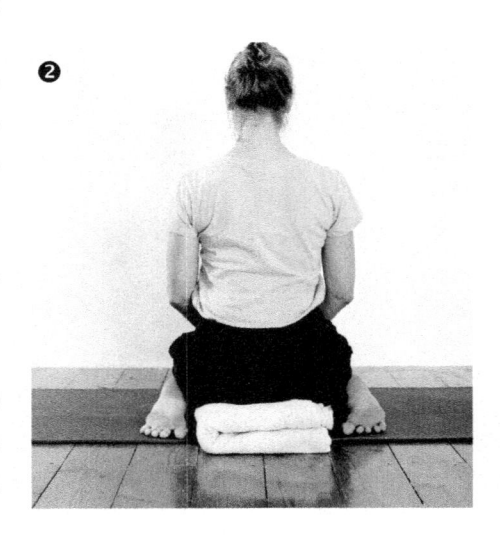

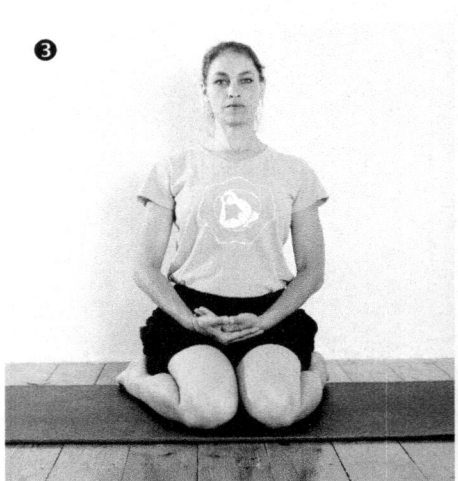

Tips
✓ If the sacrum is leaned back and does not extend up, increase the under-buttocks support.

Vīrāsana

Variation 2
Compacting the base: Strapping the legs

Effects
The belt keeps the legs together without effort and stabilizes the pose by creating compactness at the base.

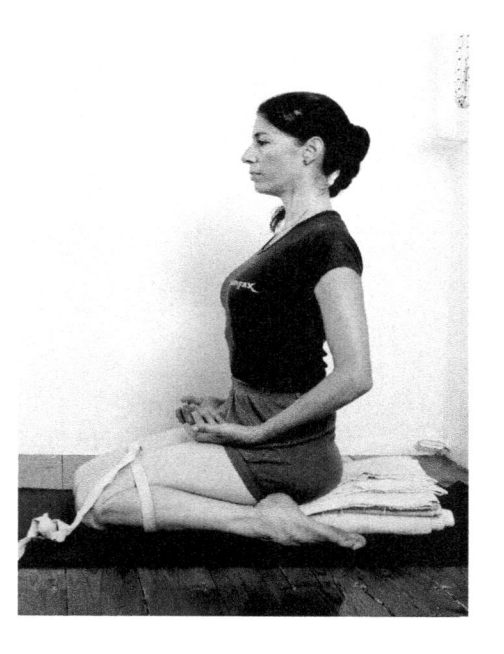

Props
bolster or a folded blanket, 1 or 2 belts, weight (optional)

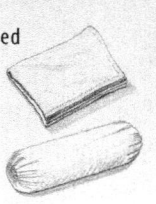

Vīrāsana may be used for Pranayama or meditation. A belt can help keep the knees and thighs joined and create compactness.

→ Sit in Vīrāsana, lift the knees slightly and insert both knees through a belt loop.

> Turn the thighs out, until the centers of the front thighs are facing directly up. Turn the shins out to move the outer shin bones and outer sides of the feet toward the floor.

> It is also possible to place weights (up to 30 Kgs or 65 pounds) on the thighs (not shown).

Effects: The weight increases the earth element of the pose thus creating stability and quietness. It also improves the movement of the knees.

Tips

✓ The belt can be positioned at various locations to get different effects. You can also use more than one belt to combine effects. For example, use one belt around the lower thighs and another around the upper thighs.

✓ When using two belts, the higher belt stabilizes the root of the thighs - thus allowing the lower abdomen to release - while the lower belt keeps the knees together.

Applicability
Supta Vīrāsana

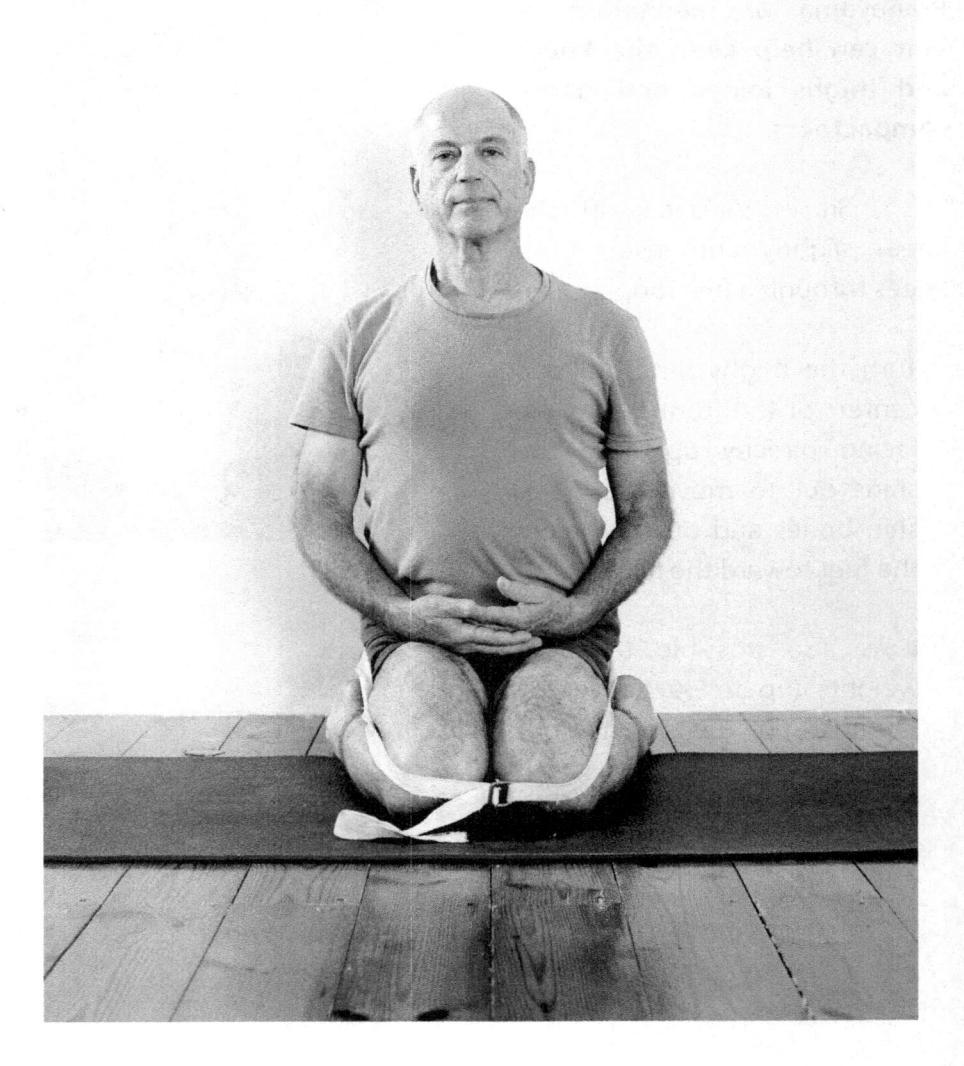

Vīrāsana

Variation 3
Compacting the base:
Strapping the pelvis and knees

Effects
The horizontal belt around the pelvis and knees creates a framework for the base of the pose. The support for the sacral band helps to extend and stabilize the spine without effort.

Props
bolster or a folded blanket, 2 belts

This is another way to support the pose for long sittings:

→ Enter the pose sitting on a suitable support.

› Loop a belt around the pelvis and the knees; slightly bend forward until the sacrum is moving forward, then tighten the belt and sit up.

› The belt should support the sacral band from behind and the knees from the front.

Vīrāsana

Variation 4
Supporting the hands in Vīrāsana: Bolster on thighs

Props
bolster,
2 belts

Placing the hands on the thighs in Vīrāsana may cause the shoulders to roll forward thus limiting the broadening of the chest. To get a better support for the hands, place a bolster on top of the thighs. This is especially helpful during long stays in the pose.

> After you are seated, place a bolster across the thighs and place the back of your palms on it. Adjust the arm position such that the elbows are directly under the shoulders and level with the palms.

> Place the hands on the bolster, palms facing up at shoulder width.

> Roll the biceps and the inner shoulders outward, extend the spine up, broaden the chest and softly look forward, or close the eyes.

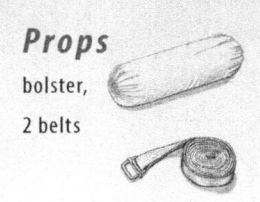

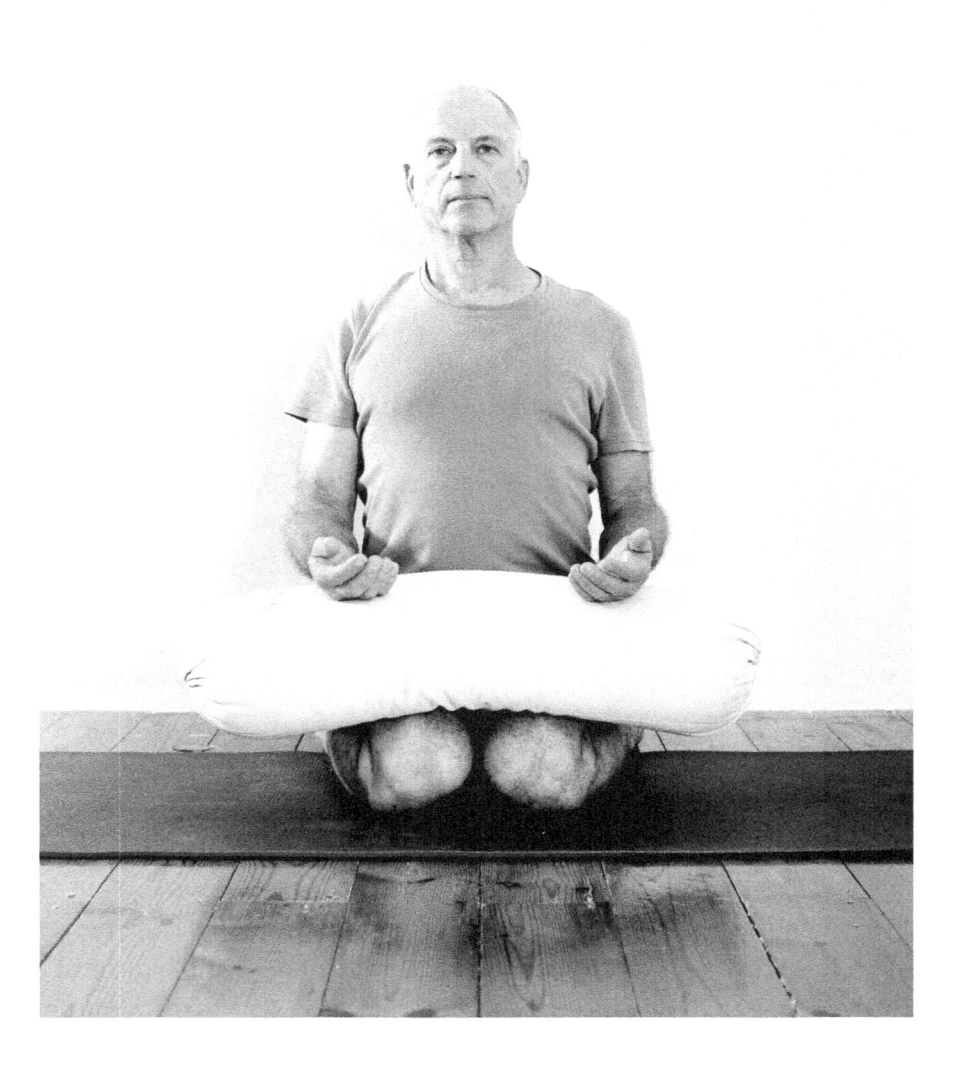

Padmāsana
About Padmāsana

Padmāsana, or the Lotus pose, is the classical "royal" yoga pose. Who does not aspire to sit in Padmāsana and look like the Buddha or one of the ancient Yogis? Indeed, when properly done, this pose brings about both stability (*sthirata*) and comfort (*sukhata*). When describing the sitting posture most suitable for Pranayama, B.K.S Iyengar writes:

> *"Although a number of postures are in use, in my experience Padmāsana is the king of them all for the practice of pranayama or meditation (dhyāna). It is the key to success in both cases. In it, all the four areas of the body mentioned above (the lower limbs, the torso, the arms and the neck and head) are evenly balanced and the brain rests correctly and evenly on the spinal column, giving psychosomatic equilibrium. The spinal cord passes through the spinal column. In Padmāsana, the adjustment and alignment of the spinal column and the ridges on either side move uniformly, rhythmically and simultaneously. The prāṇic energy flows evenly, with proper distribution throughout the body. In Siddhāsana the top part of the spine is more stretched than its other parts, while in Vīrāsana it is the lumbar spine that is more stretched. Some of these postures may be more comfortable, but for accuracy and efficacy Padmāsana is the best of them all. In Padmāsana the thighs are lower than the groins; the lower abdomen is kept stretched, with maximum space between the pubis and the diaphragm, enabling the lungs to expand fully. For those using Padmāsana, particular attention should be paid to the three important joints of the lower body – the hips, knees and ankles – which have to move effortlessly."* (Chapter 11, paragraphs 13-15).

Padmāsana is indeed a wonderful pose; but, at the same time, it brings greater potential for knee injuries. When it comes to Padmāsana, the proverb "Haste is from the Devil" is very appropriate. Ankles, knees and hips must all be properly prepared to avoid injuries which may take years to recover from.

While the hip is a ball-and-socket joint, the knee is a hinge joint. A ball-and-socket joint allows movement in all directions while a hinge allows movement in one plane only. The movement that enables the interlocking of the legs in Padmāsana must start from external rotation of the hip joint. If the thigh bone rotates sufficiently, the foot is automatically positioned above the opposite thigh, and can be placed at the root of that thigh without creating undue pressure on the knee or the ankle ❶.

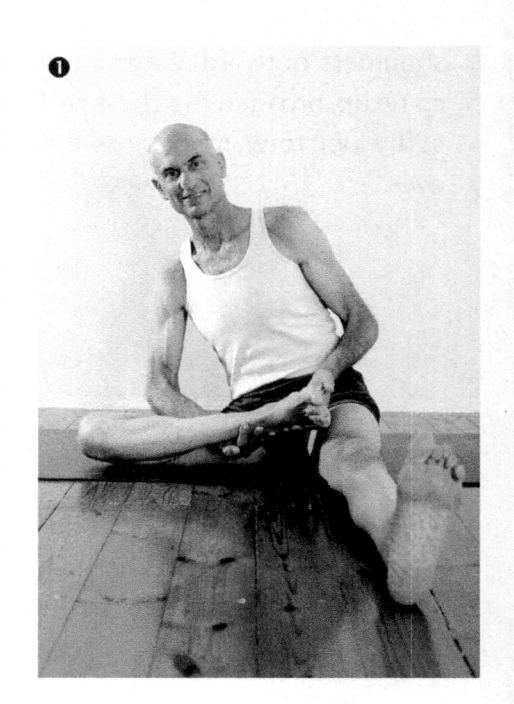

> **CAUTIONS**
>
> Do not practice this pose if your knees or ankles are injured.

However, if there is not enough movement in the hip joint ❷, and you try to force the pose, then you are inviting injury at the knee or the ankle.

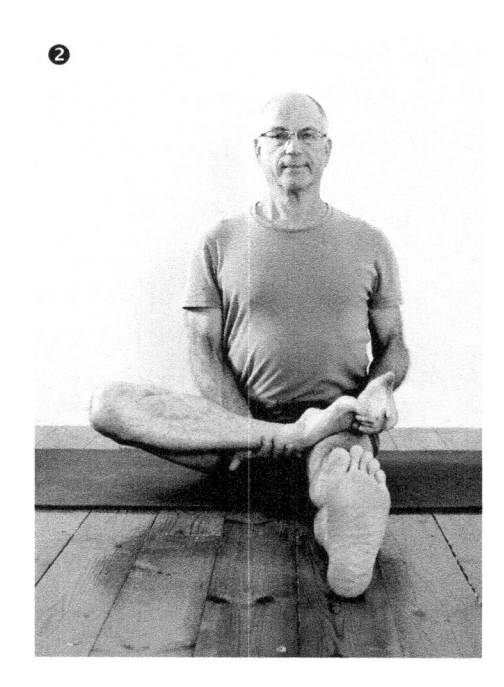

❷

A Preparation Sequence for Padmāsana

We show here a sequence that can be used as a preparation for Padmāsana. It represents a gradual and safe way to work towards the full pose. Moreover, it is an effective warm-up sequence even for those who have already mastered the pose. If Padmāsana is currently not within your reach, you may do this sequence, or parts of it, for several months (or years) before attempting the full pose. Remember that pain within the knees or around the knees indicates that something is wrong; it is not the kind of pain you should bear; it is a harmful pain. Whenever you experience such a pain, stop and change what you do or ask a knowledgeable teacher how to proceed. Work towards this pose not only with persistence but also with patience, sensitivity and caution.

Padmāsana

1
Adho Mukha Swastikāsana

Effects
This preparation lengthens the buttock muscles and creates movement in the hip joints. When doing with the right leg folded first, the left buttock gets a stronger stretch.

Props
optional blanket

⟶ Sit in Dandāsana and fold the right leg, then the left leg, to Swastikāsana.

› Bend forward; stretch the arms forward and place the forehead on the floor, or on a folded blanket. Stay in the pose for a few minutes.

› Come up to Swastikāsana.

› Change the folding of the legs and repeat the pose for the same duration.

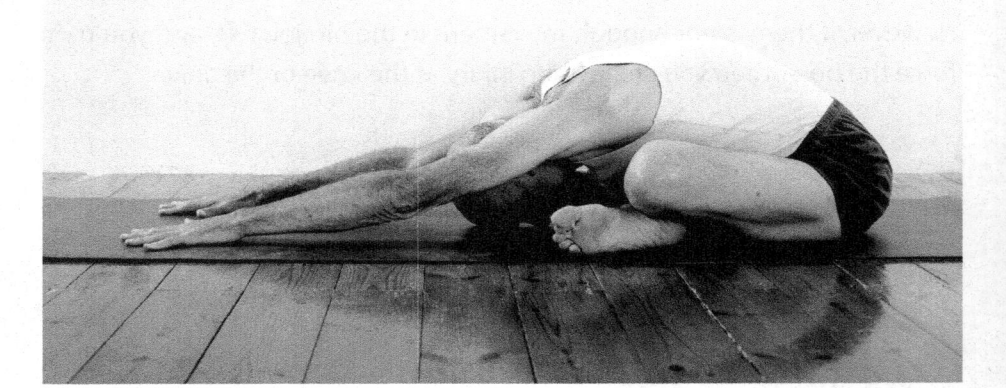

Padmāsana

2
Baddha Koṇāsana
& Adho Mukha Baddha Koṇāsana

Effects
This variation flexes the hip joint and elongates the adductor muscles.

Props
(Optional):
column,
block,
bolster

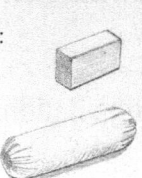

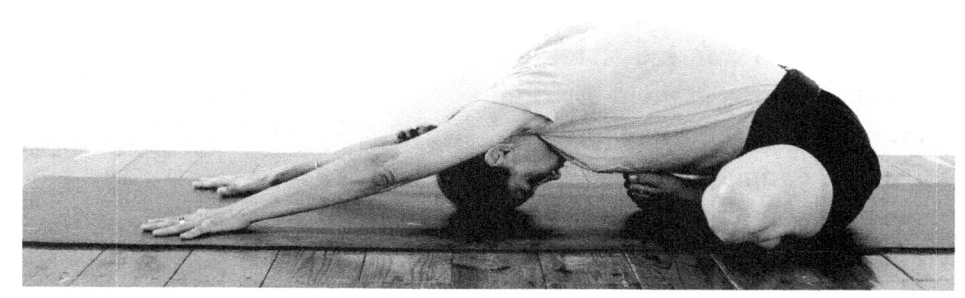

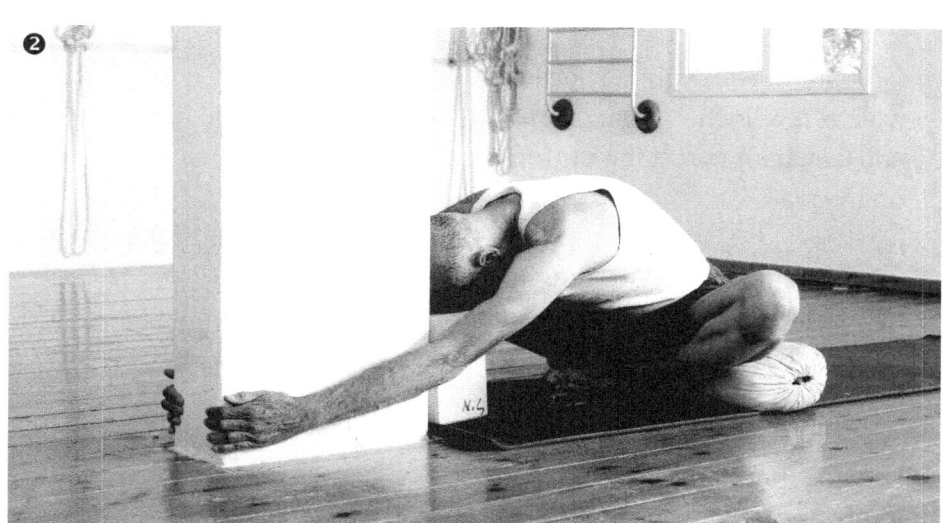

→ Sit in Baddha Koṇāsana. Roll the thighs out and draw the knees backward and down toward the floor.

› After staying for a while, bend forward. Place the forehead on the floor ❶.

› If bending forward is difficult, do the pose in front of a column (or a table leg, or a low wall hook); hold the column with both hands symmetrically and pull yourself forward.

› Place your head on the floor or on a suitable support (folded blanket, block or a chair) ❷.

Props for Yoga / Chapter 2 / Padmāsana 61

Padmāsana

3
Ardha Baddha Padmottānāsana

Effects

In the standing position, gravity pulls the knee of the bent leg away from the hip joint, creating more space in the hip and knee joints. The thigh becomes free to rotate from its root rather than from the knee or ankle.

Props

wall

Ardha Baddha Padmottānāsana (see LOY Pl. 52) is a standing pose in which one leg is folded in Padmāsana and held by the corresponding hand. To prepare for sitting Padmāsana, the pose is done here standing against a wall, without bending forward. To do the preparation on the right leg:

> Stand with your back to the wall, a few inches away from it, and lean back to rest the buttocks on the wall.

> Bend the right leg. With the right hand catch the outer ankle and with the left hand catch the outer foot ❶.

> Use the hands to roll the right thigh and ankle outward, while lifting the foot and placing it as high as you can on the left thigh.

> Release the right knee down toward the floor and backward toward the wall ❷.

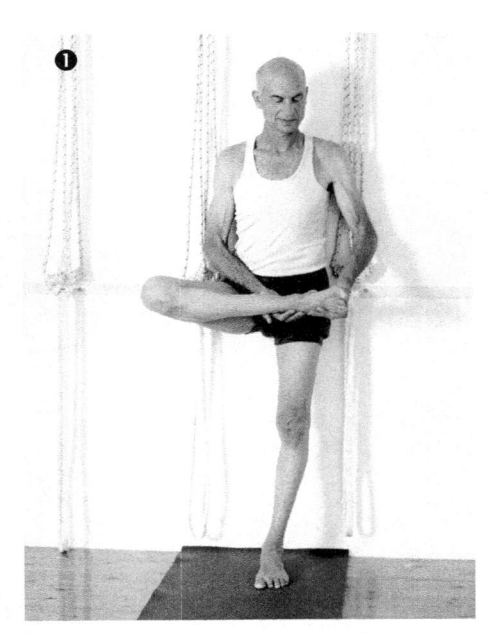

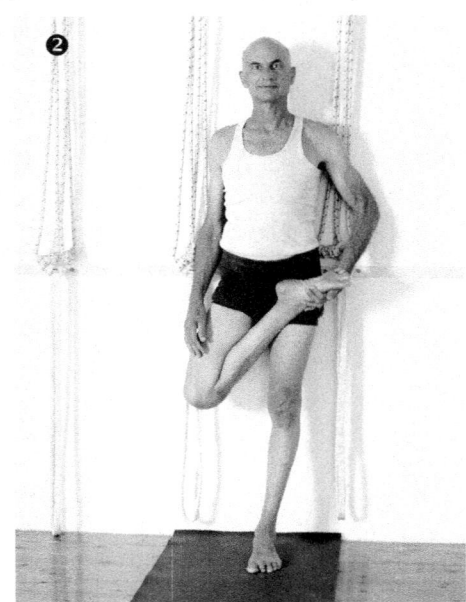

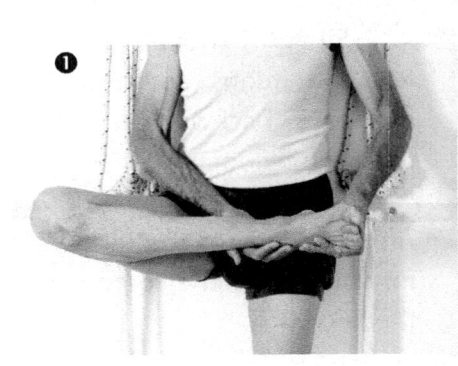

Tips

✓ When folding the leg hold the outer ankle and move it into position by turning the leg gently from the hip joint, as if serving an offering.

Padmāsana

4 Akunchanāsana

Effects

This is a good way to create length in the muscles and ligaments around the hip joint including the gluteus muscles, bringing more flexibility and rotation of the thigh at the hip joint.

Props

wall,
belt,
bolster
(optional)

This is the second movement shown in *Light on Yoga* for Supta Pādāṅguṣṭhāsana (LOY Pl. 286). To do the pose on the right leg:

→ Lie on the back with your feet against the wall.

› Loop a belt around the right foot and catch the belt with the right hand. Your right leg is bent and turned out.

› Move the right elbow backward, behind the head and rotate the right thigh outward.

› Catch the right foot with the left hand or hug it with the left inner elbow and draw it closer to you so that the right shin moves toward the top chest and the foot moves toward the left shoulder.

› Keep the shin at 90° relative to the thigh and move it so it is parallel to your upper chest.

› Keep the left leg well extended, foot pushing against the wall and thigh pressed down to the floor.

› If possible, look forward above the right shin, toward the left leg ❶.

› ❷ shows the pose done on the left side.

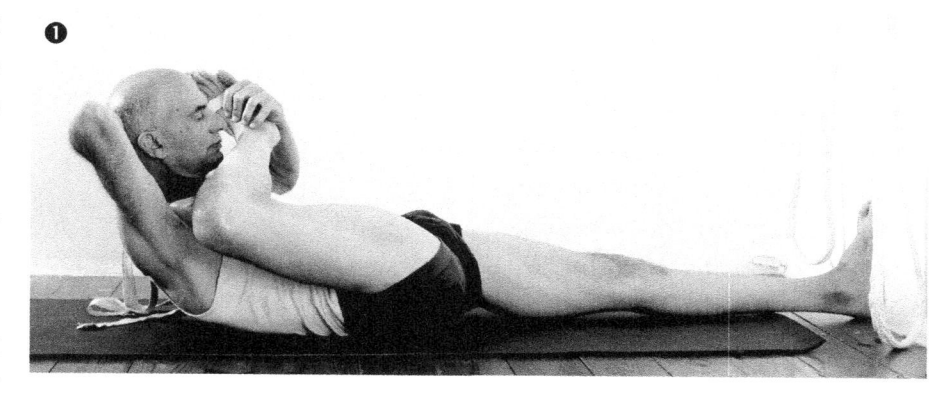

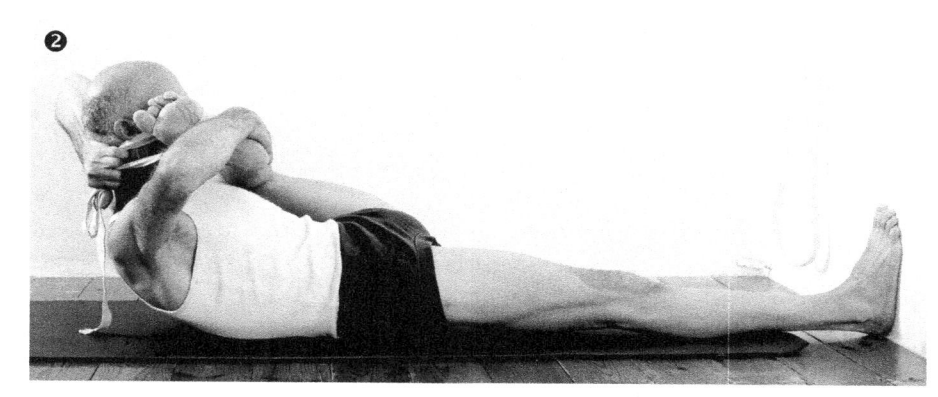

Notes

An easier variation to work on this movement (of the hip joint) is when the other leg is bent and the foot placed on the floor (instead of stretching the leg on the floor).

A bolster or two can be placed to support the upper/middle back.

Tips

✓ Draw the head of the femur into its socket and move the leg from the hip joint.

✓ Open the right foot and keep extending the inner ankle and the inner foot. As you pull the foot closer to your trunk, move the knee away from it.

✓ Keep the length of the right side of your trunk and the forward orientation of the chest. Keep the head straight and in line with the spine.

Padmāsana

5
Sitting Akunchanāsana

Effects
Similar to the previous variation, but here gravity pulls the trunk down; hence this variation is more intense.

Props
bolster, blanket (optional)

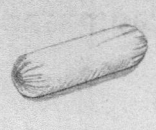

Akunchanāsana can also be done in prone, sitting or standing positions (see below.) The movement of the hip is the same in all cases: the thigh is turned out from the hip and the foot is moved toward the opposite shoulder. We will show these three variations here; but in regular practice you can select one or two of them.

To do the pose on the right leg:

⟶ Put a bolster widthwise on the mat and if necessary, a blanket to support the outer right knee.

› Bend the right leg and place the right buttock on the bolster and the foot in front of the bolster, in line with the left shoulder. The right shin should be parallel to the chest. Keep an angle of 90° between the shin and thigh.

› Extend the left leg backward and lift the front thigh.

› In order to keep the trunk parallel to the wall in front of you, rotate the trunk from left to right. Move the left hip forward until it is in line with the right one.

› Support the trunk with the hands, lift the chest and look forward.

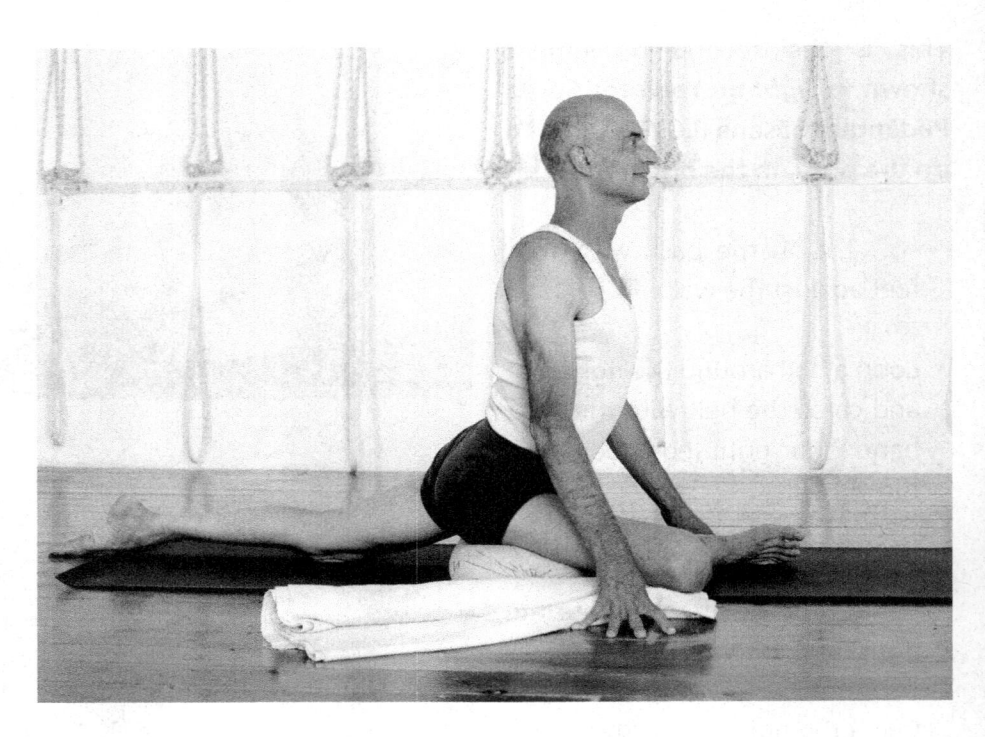

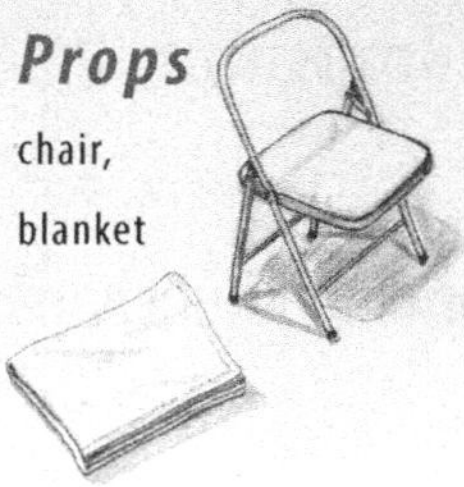

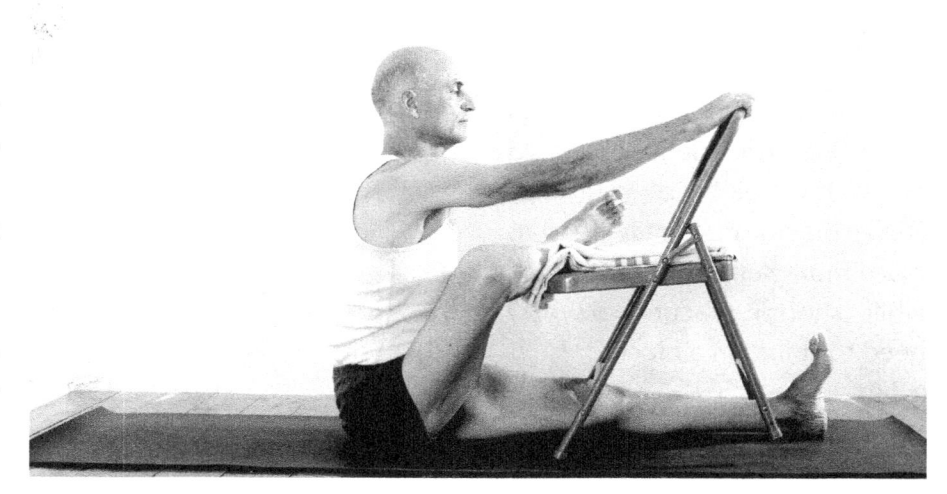

Padmāsana

6
Akunchanāsana with chair supporting the leg

Effects
The chair takes some load off the hip-joint and enables a gentle workout of the muscles around it.

Props
chair, blanket

To do the pose on the right leg:

→ Place a blanket on the chair for cushioning. Sit in front of the chair and place the right shin on the seat, such that the right foot is close to the left shoulder.

> *Note:* You may need to sit on some height in order to place the shin on the seat.

› Hold the chair and pull it to lift the back and move the trunk forward, toward the chair.

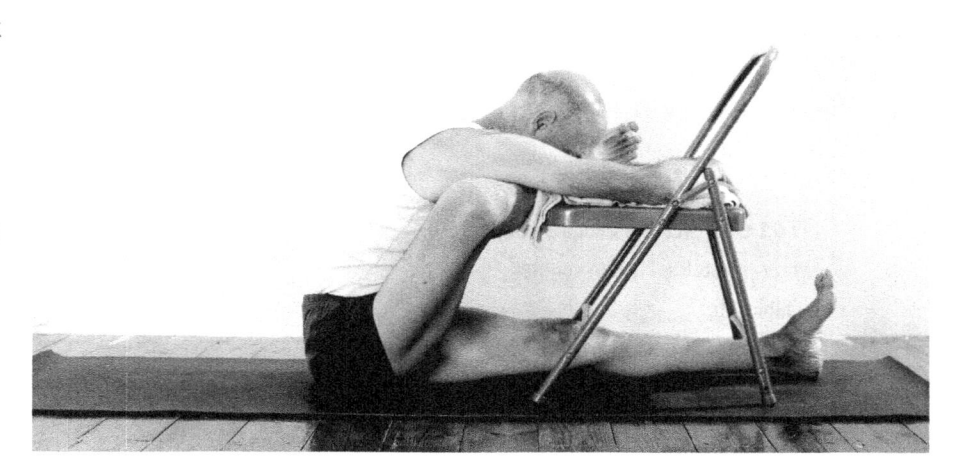

› If possible lean forward and bring the chest closer to the shin.

Padmāsana

7
Standing Akunchanāsana

Effects

In lying down Akunchanāsana (as in No. 4 above) the muscles of the hips are stretched, but there is less rotational movement in the thigh, and the pull may put pressure on the inner knee. In this variation lifting the leg creates the required external rotation of the femur.

Props

high stool, blanket

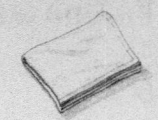

To do the pose on the right leg:

→ Place a blanket on the stool for cushioning. The stool should be at the height of your hips (Taller practitioners may need to place more support on the stool, while shorter practitioners may need to stand on a block).

> Stand in front of the stool and place the right shin on its seat, such that the right foot is aligned with left shoulder.

> Press the hands against the stool and lift the chest.

> *Note:* Instead of a high stool you can use the kitchen counter, a table, etc.

> Now lie over the right leg, bringing the top chest closer to the right shin.

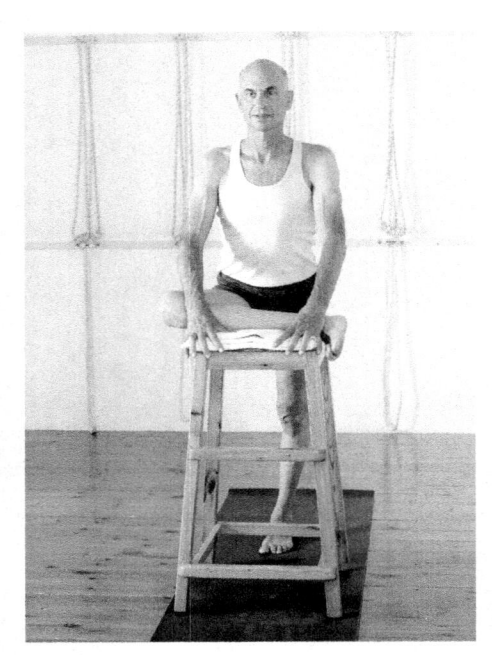

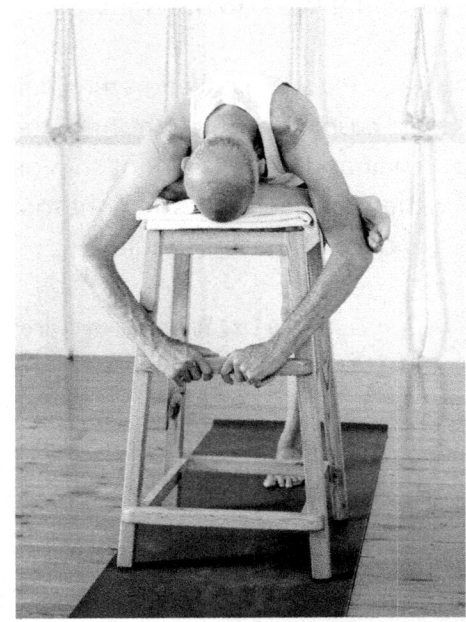

Padmāsana

8
Supta Ardha Padmāsana
(or Ardha Matsyāsana)

Effects

In lying down, there is no weight on the hip and the buttock; thus the thigh has greater freedom to move. This is a very gentle way to move the leg into half Padmāsana.

Props

2 belts; optional bolster or two

We show how to stabilize the knee by fastening a belt around it. This option is recommended, in cases of knee is sensitivity, since it secures the knee and prevents unhealthy movement. To do the pose on the right leg:

> Lie on the back; bend the right leg at the knee, such that the back of the thigh folds exactly in line with the calf muscle, then fasten a belt just below the knee to prevent sideways movement of the shin ❶.

> Roll the thigh outward from the hip. Use your hands to intensify the rolling action of the buttock and the thigh.

> Now place a belt around the right ankle and pull it towards you. Pull slightly stronger with the left hand (which pulls the outer ankle). This will roll the ankle and the shin from inside out ❷.

> Slide the foot along the left thigh as high as you can.

Note: The leg should rotate from the hip-joint. Do not pull the foot strongly as this may harm your knee! Avoid any unpleasant sensation in the knee.

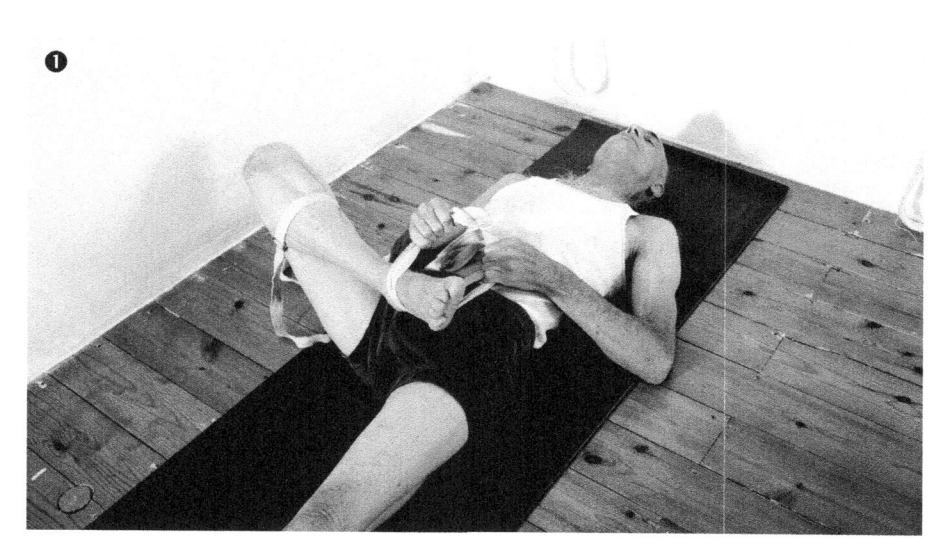

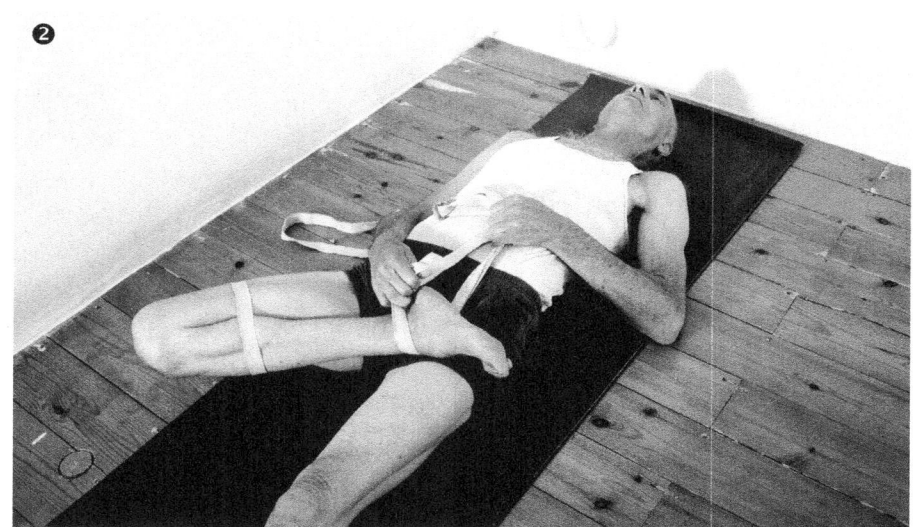

> Now let the right knee descend towards the floor.

Note: If you cannot rotate the thigh and bring the foot over the opposite thigh, then you are not ready for the pose. In this case, continue to work on the previous preparations.

Padmāsana

9
Matsyāsana
(or Supta Padmāsana)

Props
2-3 belts,
2-3 bolsters
(optional)

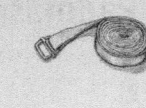

After repeating the previous variation (Ardha Matsyāsana) several times on each leg, and making sure that the knees are descending close enough to the floor, you can proceed to the full pose. We are showing the simple variation of Matsyāsana where the back is flat on the floor (see LOY Pl. 114). To do the pose with the right leg first:

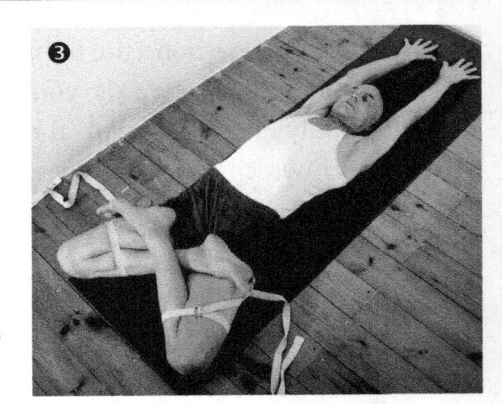

→ Bend the right leg to Ardha Padmāsana as in the previous variation.

> Bend the left leg (you can now tie another belt around the left knee). Roll the left thigh out as before and move the foot above the inner right knee ❶. If the left foot can be placed above the right knee, on the thigh, then gently draw it toward the right groin.

⚠ **CAUTION** If the left foot is lower than the right knee, do not force it over the right thigh. Instead, support the thighs with bolsters, and continue to work patiently on lowering both knees down.

> After interlocking the legs in Padmāsana, release the knees down. Stretch the arms over the head and rest in the pose.

> If the knees do not descend or there is pressure, or soreness, support the thighs with two or three bolsters and relax the knees onto the bolsters ❷.

> Once you get more freedom, draw the knees closer to one another and press them down toward the floor ❸.

> Another belt can be looped around the two knees. Tighten this belt gently from the left to the right to draw the knees closer to one another (not shown).

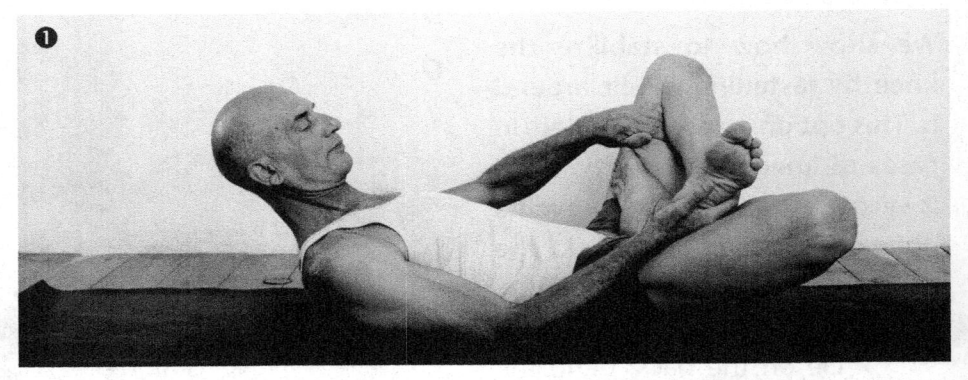

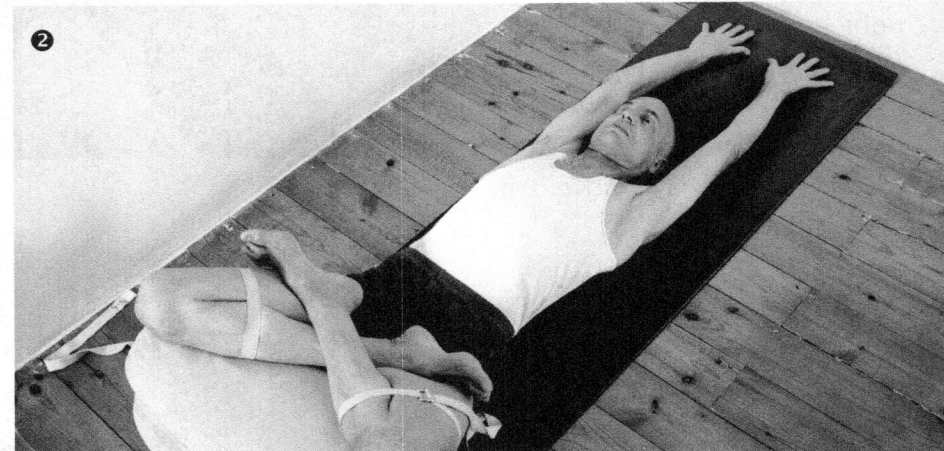

Padmāsana

10
From Ardha Padmāsana to full Padmāsana

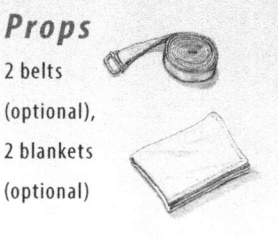

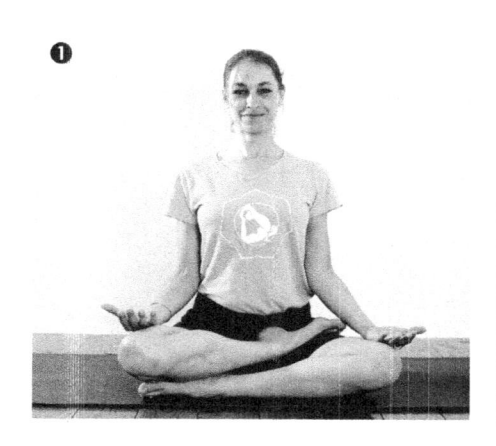

Props
2 belts (optional),
2 blankets (optional)

❶ ❷ ❸

Here too, belts can be used to stabilize the knees (see the previous variations). To do the pose with the right leg bent first:

▶ Sit and bend the right leg. With the right hand catch the inner thigh close to the knee, and with the left hand catch the outer ankle.

▷ Roll the right thigh outward; roll the right ankle outward as you bring the leg closer and place the foot on the top of the left thigh.

▷ Now bend the left leg and place the left foot under the right knee; this is Ardha Padmāsana ❶.

✓ *Note:* If needed, support the right knee with a folded blanket.

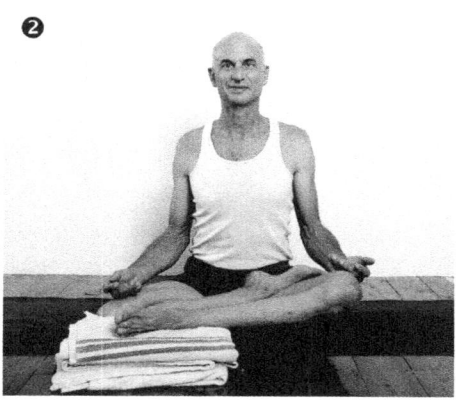

After doing this several times on each leg you can proceed to the full pose:

▶ Sit in Ardha Padmāsana with the right foot on the root of the left thigh.

▷ Bend the left leg and hold it the same way you held the right leg. Roll the left thigh outward and move the foot closer to the right knee.

▷ Now, if the right knee is on the floor and you can easily lift the left foot above it, then you can slide the foot all the way to the root of the right thigh.

CAUTION If the right knee is higher than the left foot – do not proceed to full Padmāsana yet. Place the left foot on a folded blanket in front of the right knee and release the right knee down, as shown in ❷.

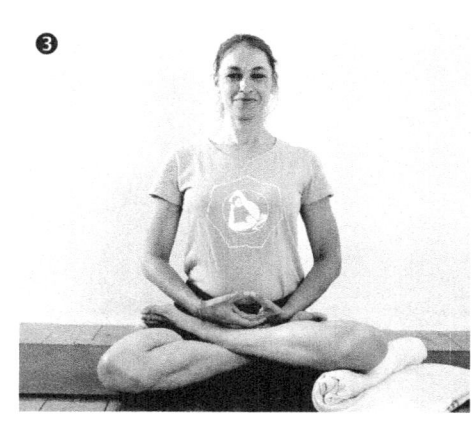

▷ Once both feet rest on the upper thighs of the opposite legs, draw the knees closer.

▷ To make the pose more comfortable and stable support the left knee with a rolled blanket and place a thin blanket under the buttocks.

▷ Keep the spine erect and stay quietly in the pose, holding your hands in a Mudra of your choice ❸.

Tips

✓ When moving the foot over the right thigh, slide it in a circular movement near the floor, without lifting the left knee. Keep rolling the left thigh outward; this enables the foot to lift above the right thigh.

Chapter 3
Surrendering to Mother Earth: Forward Extensions
(Paśchima Pratana Sthiti)

About the Forward Bends

Forward bends stretch the long muscles of the body in the legs and back, and massage the abdominal organs. They flex the pelvic joints, improve circulation in the pelvic region and promote health in the reproductive and digestive systems. They are especially useful for women since they regulate menstrual flow. Psychologically, these are cooling and relaxing āsanas. While back bends are dynamic in nature and done to open and energize the heart center, forward bends are done to cool and pacify the brain. If you suffer from sorrow or depression – practice back bends, if you feel *Rājasic* (irritated, overactive, short tempered) – practice forward bends.

Ultimately, one can stay for prolonged periods (3-10 minutes) in a forward bend keeping the spine well extended and the forehead resting on the shin (or shins); at that stage, the breath becomes effortless, and quietness, passivity, inwardness and humbleness are induced.

In *The Hero's Contemplation*, Pisano writes:

"In forward extensions, abandoning the head towards the knee and beyond symbolizes surrender and capitulation of all strategies. Frontal brain perception dies away and makes way for the humility of the earth. One is crowned by one's own vacuity."[6]

Note:

For each variation we indicate the minimum required props. Use additional support in the following cases:

If your lumbar spine area sinks when sitting in Dandāsana - use folded blankets or other support to raise the seat

If your palms do not reach the feet when bending forward - use a belt to grasp the feet

If your forehead does not reach the legs in the final position - support it with additional blankets as necessary.

[6] See page 292

[7] Geeta S. Iyengar, *Yoga in Action - Preliminary Course*, p. 73

According to Geeta S. Iyengar[7], forward bends:
- Bring the brain and the heart to a restful state
- Soothe the nerves and calm the mind
- Stimulate the digestive system and help in dealing with acidity, flatulence and vomiting
- Promote health in the adrenal glands, gonads and ovaries
- Moderate or temper:
    - High blood pressure
    - Hypertension
    - Anxiety
    - Short temper
    - Headaches
    - Insomnia
    - Myopia and glaucoma
    - Fatigue
    - Weakness
    - Low fever.

The effect of forward bends on the heart was explained by B.K.S. Iyengar. He said that in our case, the heart is vertical and is positioned anterior to the spine, while for four-legged animals, the heart is horizontal and positioned under the spine. The horizontal orientation of the heart allows it to relax. In forward bends, we position our spine and heart in horizontal orientation, closer to earth, and this has positive effects on the heart and the blood pressure.

Adho Mukha Vīrāsana

About Adho Mukha Vīrāsana

Adho Mukha Vīrāsana is a 'soft' forward bend which allows anybody, even people with tight hamstrings, to experience the soothing effect of forward bending. Placing the forehead on the floor relaxes the brain and internalizes the mind; hence this pose is often taken as the very first pose in a class – it allows for a few moments of being with ourselves quietly to feel the body and breath. In this pose we learn to use the arms in order to stretch the entire trunk forward. The arms in Adho Mukha Vīrāsana work much like they do in Adho Mukha Śvānāsana, but with less weight-bearing; hence this pose is a good preparation for Adho Mukha Śvānāsana.

The pose shown in *Light on Yoga* (Pl. 92) is part of the Vīrāsana cycle in which the knees are joined and the buttocks are resting on the floor, between the heels; however, as preparation in the beginning of the practice, or for relaxation after back bends (or other strenuous poses), Adho Mukha Vīrāsana is usually done with spread knees. Most of the variations we present are therefore with spread knees; we will also include one variation of the classic pose (as shown in *Light on Yoga*).

Depending on your purpose, the pose can be done with the big toes touching and the buttocks resting on the heels ❶, or with the feet parallel and the buttocks resting on the floor in between the heels ❷. The first option is more relaxing since the flexion of the knees and the extension of the ankles is lessened. If, however, you wish to get more movement in these joints, do the second option.

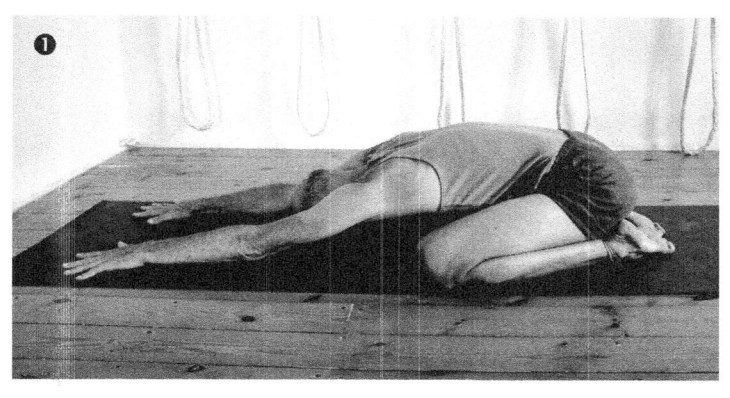

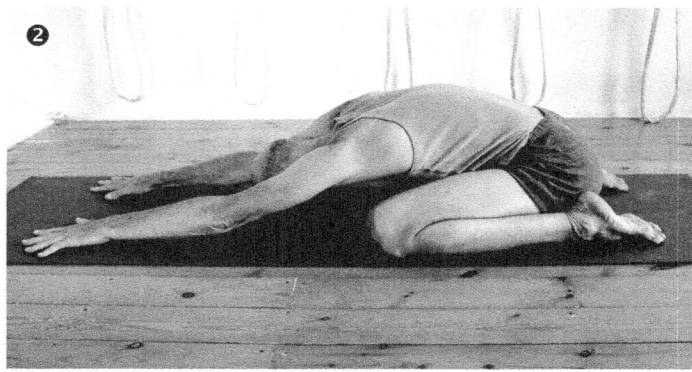

Adho Mukha Vīrāsana

Variation 1
Anchoring the pelvis:
Partner pulls back with a rope

Effects
The rope stabilizes the pelvis and the hip joints, providing a firm anchoring for the trunk to stretch forward. The weight of the hands on the practitioner's back brings awareness to the stiffer parts, releases the muscles and creates space in the back ribs.

Props
rope, partner

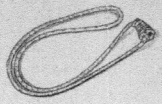

> Practitioner: Sit in Vīrāsana and place a rope across the front groins, such that the ends of the rope project outward on each side of the pelvis.

> Partner: Sit or stand behind the practitioner, hold the two ends of the rope with hands close to the practitioner's body, and pull back to stabilize the practitioner's pelvis.

> Practitioner: Bend forward to Adho Mukha Vīrāsana and extend the trunk forward.

> Partner: Place the palms on the practitioner's sacral band, and gently lean to press the sacrum in to lower the pelvis down (not shown).

> ⚠ **CAUTION** The last step of applying pressure on the practitioner's back should be done with sensitivity. Start by placing your hands without applying pressure; gradually increase the weight on the practitioner's back, in tune with her/his response.

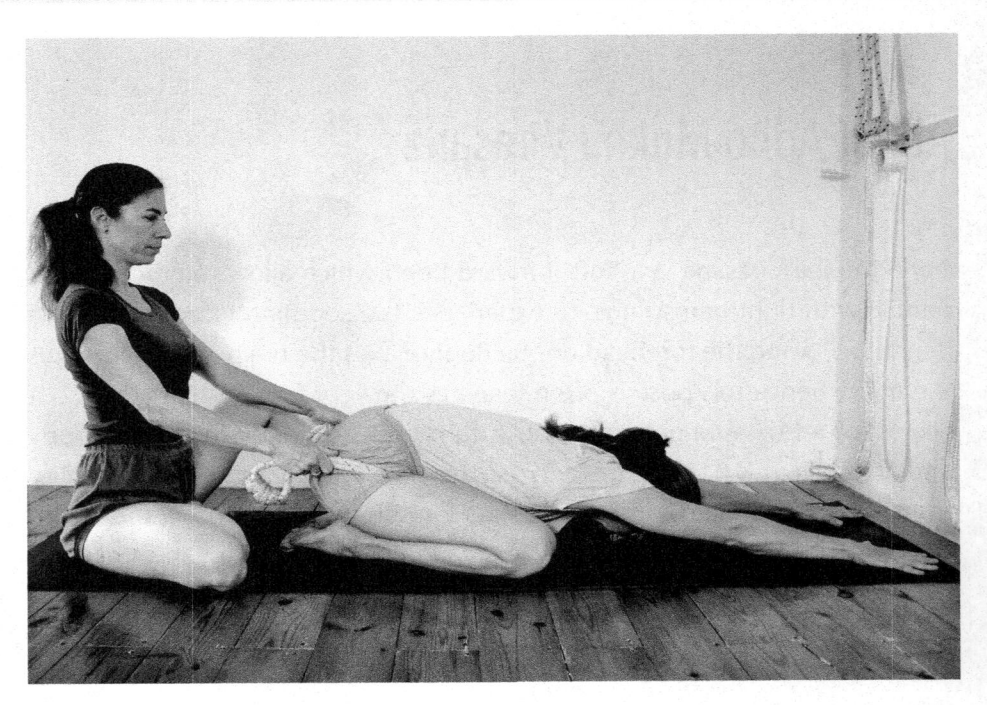

Adho Mukha Vīrāsana

Variation 2
Stretching forward: Anchoring the legs and palms on blocks

Effects

Tying the legs anchors the pelvis in place and moves the buttocks down (much like the help of the partner in the previous variation). Supporting the palms helps to broaden the chest, extend the trunk forward while lowering the torso to the floor.

Props

2 wooden blocks,
2 belts,
blanket (optional)

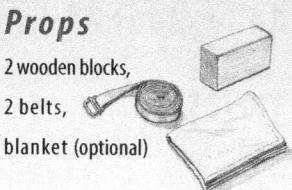

→ Place the blocks in front of you.

> Sit on the heels and spread the knees. Loop a belt around each top thigh and ankle. Tighten the belts to move the top thighs down ❶.

> Bend forward, place the palms on the blocks and stretch forward, sliding the blocks to stretch forward (it is better not to position the blocks on the sticky mat) ❷.

> Raise the head and look forward; extend the arms forward from the armpits and turn the arms inward (triceps rolling towards the floor and then the face). Press the blocks while broadening the chest and lowering the middle of the back toward the floor.

> If the head does not reach the floor with comfort, place a folded blanket to support the head and rest the forehead on it ❸.

Note: An inverted chair can be used to support the arms; in this case a bolster and/or several folded blankets are needed to support the forehead (See Variation 6 on page 79).

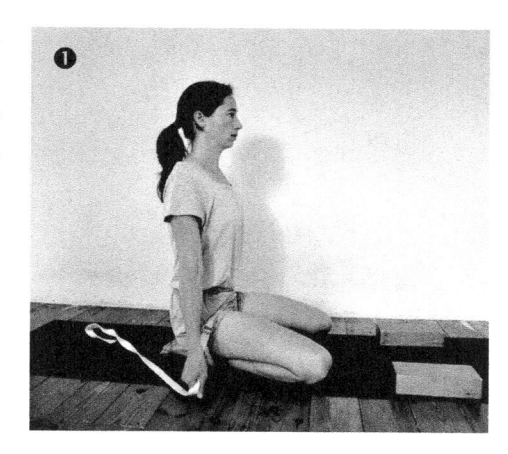

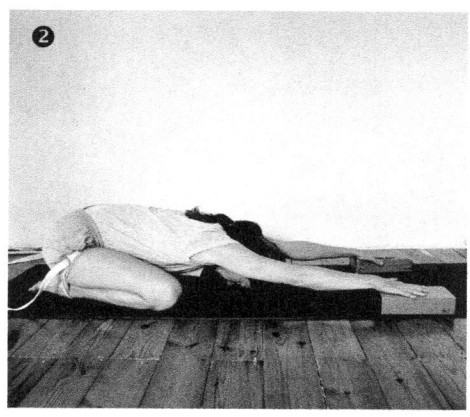

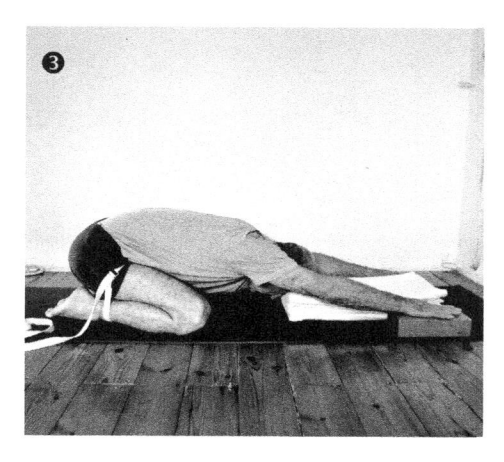

Tips

✓ The centers of the shinbones should touch the floor. Avoid spreading the knees too wide as this may roll the shins inward too much and harden the groins.

✓ For complete relaxation of the brain the lower forehead (the eyebrow line) should be supported. If it does not reach the floor, support the forehead with blankets, bolster or chair.

Adho Mukha Vīrāsana

Variation 3
Stretching forward:
Partner extends the trunk forward

Effects
This is a very good passive stretch for the spine and trunk. One can feel how the trunk is extended while keeping the muscles of the back soft.

Props
partner

⟶ Instruction for the helping partner:

> After the practitioner enters Adho Mukha Vīrāsana, ask him/her to slightly lift the trunk; Put your thumbs on the front groins of the practitioner to hold the pelvis in place.

> *Note:* In some cases inserting the thumbs in the front groin of the practitioner is not enough and in order to stabilize her/his pelvis you will need to place your palms on her/his sacral band.

> Ask the practitioner to catch your ankle and then move the foot back with raised heel. Move the leg back until the practitioner's trunk is stretched well; then increase the stretch by lowering your heel towards the floor.

> *Option:* Walk your palms on the practitioner's back to soften and flatten it.

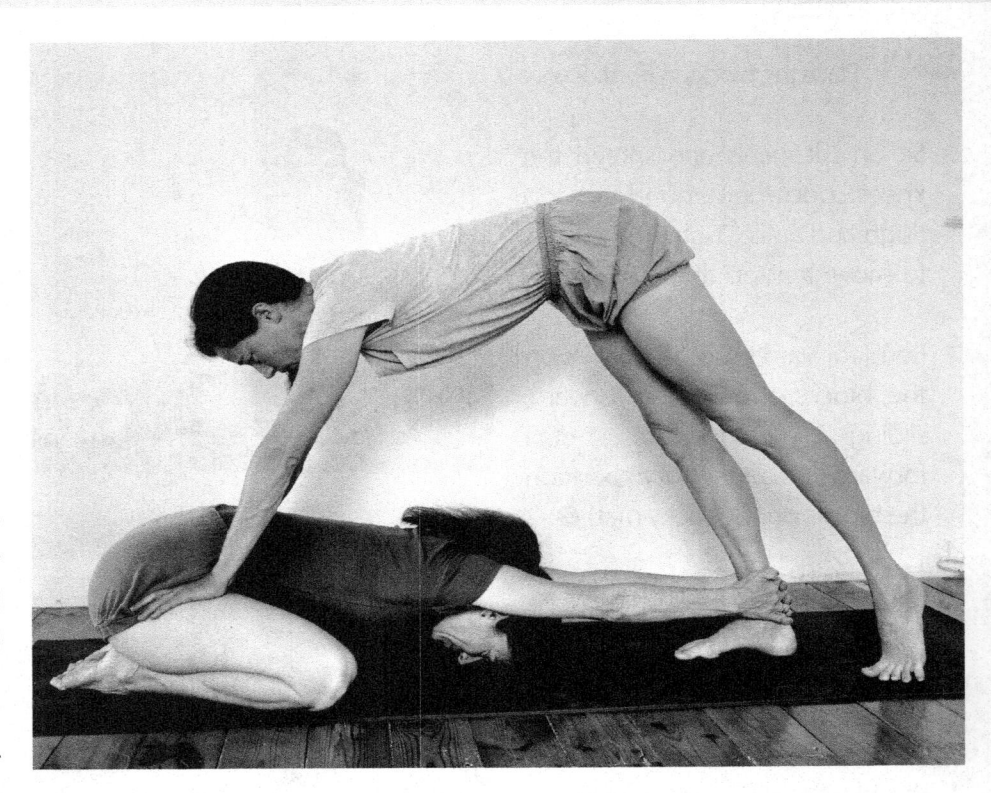

Adho Mukha Vīrāsana

Variation 4
Overcoming stiffness in the ankles: Raising the shins

Effects
The platform enables people with stiff ankles to do the pose and to gradually increase their flexibility. The bolster is usually needed because of the extra height of the legs.

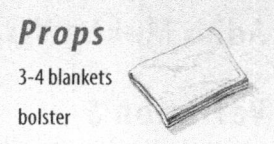

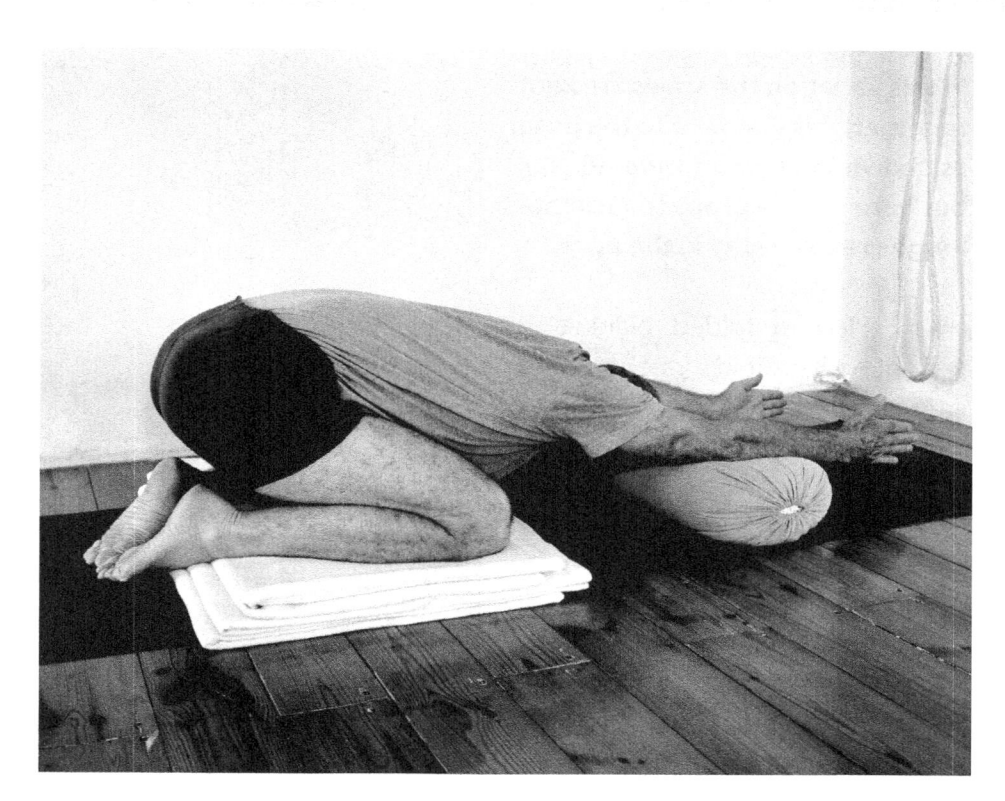

Props
3-4 blankets
bolster

In some cases the ankles do not extend well and sitting on the heels or between the heels is painful. In this cases use blankets under the shins, as shown in Vajrāsana Variation 4 (see page 51).

> Make a platform of 3 to 4 blankets. Place the blankets in a stepwise fashion. Place a bolster widthwise in front of the platform.

> Sit on the platform in Vīrāsana with the ankles on the stepped edge of the platform and the toes extending beyond it.

> Bend forward and place the forehead and elbows on the bolster.

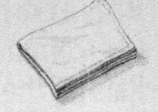

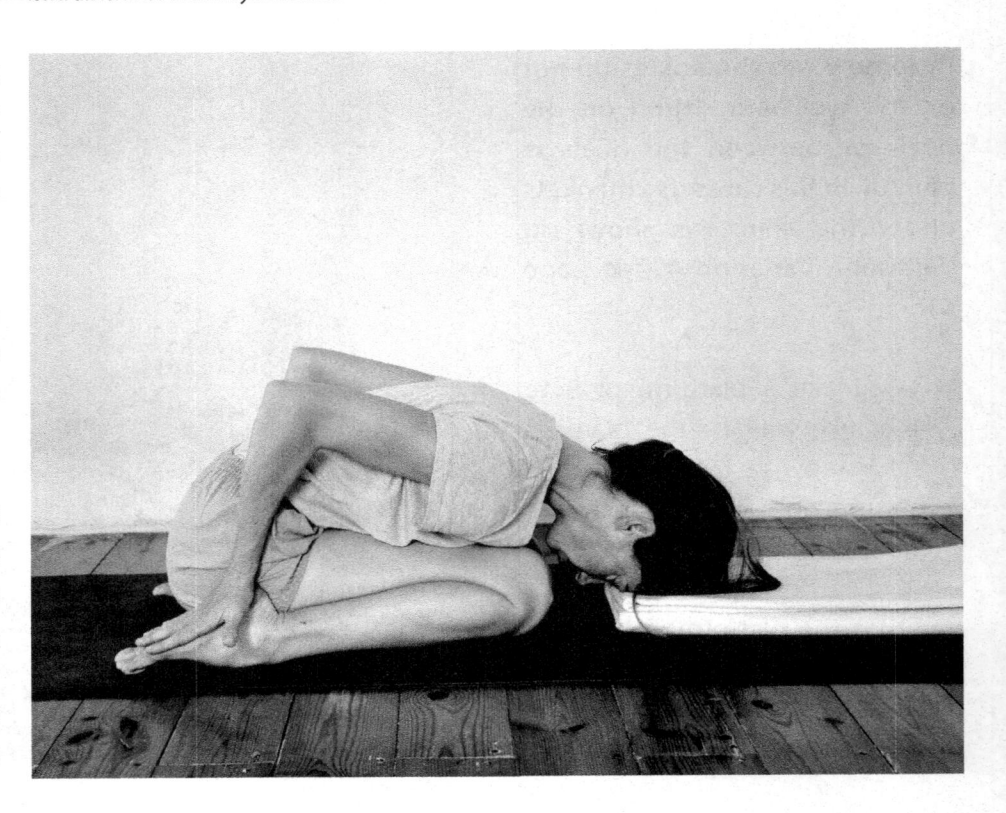

Adho Mukha Vīrāsana

Variation 5
Stretching the sacral band:
Keeping the knees together

Effects
Doing the pose with spread knees is more relaxing and allows the abdominal organs to widen; however, when the knees are kept together the sacral band is stretched and the abdominal organs are squeezed which stimulates the digestive system. Supporting the forehead enables one to enjoy these benefits even if one is not able to lower the forehead all the way to the floor.

Props
blanket or bolster

In this variation the knees are kept together; this is similar to the pose as shown in *Light on Yoga* (Pl. 92), but here we use props to facilitate longer, relaxed stay in the pose.

⟶ Place a folded blanket in front of you. Sit in Vīrāsana, knees together, buttocks in between the heels.

› Bend forward and place the forehead on the blanket. Stretch your arms forward to extend the trunk.

› Soften the groins and allow the thighs and buttocks to recede down to toward the floor.

› Then lower the head down and place the palms on the feet as in *Light on Yoga*.

Note: If a folded blanket is too low for your head to rest comfortably, use a higher support like a bolster.

Adho Mukha Vīrāsana

Variation 6
Restorative Adho Mukha Vīrāsana: Supporting the body

Effects
Supporting the abdomen and forehead makes the pose very relaxing; the forward stretch elongates the trunk, creating space for the inner organs in the abdominal and chest cavities. The breath can diffuse into these cavities. The support for the abdomen also relaxes the lower back.

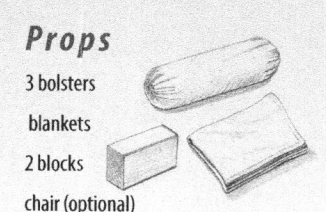

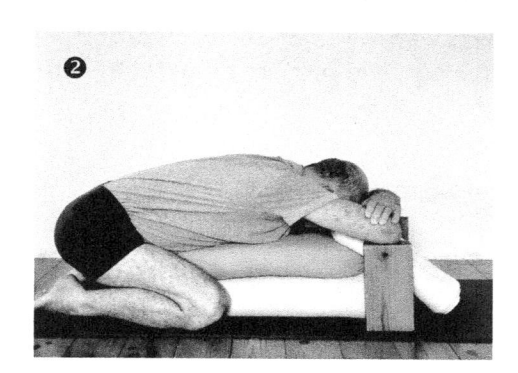

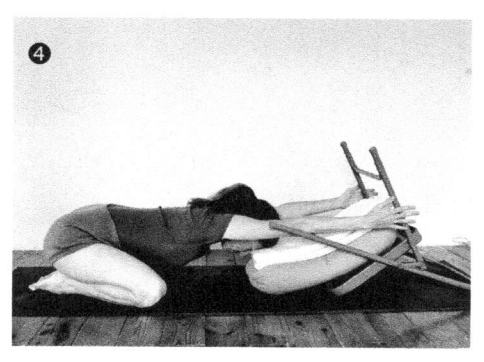

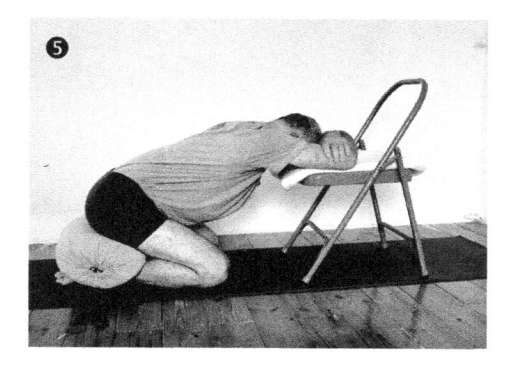

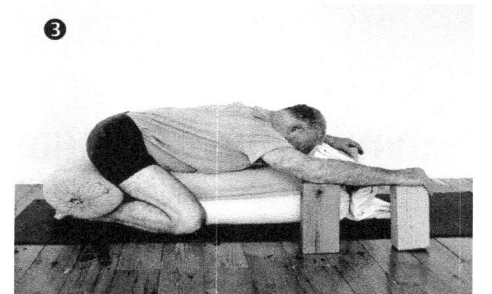

Props
3 bolsters
blankets
2 blocks
chair (optional)

For most people Adho Mukha Vīrāsana is relaxing, but with support the pose becomes restorative and very quieting. People with stiff or injured hip or knee joints, may find the unsupported pose difficult and possibly painful – in these cases bolsters' support allows them to do the pose with ease.

I. A single bolster support ❶
→ Place one bolster widthwise in front of you and when going into the pose, rest the forehead and elbows on the bolster.

II. Lengthwise support ❷
→ Place a bolster or two lengthwise in front of you. Place a folded blanket on top of the bolster for head support.

> Place the blocks in line with the bolster such that they support the entwined elbows.

> Spread the knees and adjust the support to be under the lower abdomen. The forehead support should allow for free breathing through the nose, and the blocks should provide a comfortable resting place for the elbows.

Notes:
If there is tension in the knees or hips place another bolster on the heels to support the buttocks ❸. If three bolsters are not available, place foam blocks under the lengthwise bolster, or place blankets under the buttocks.

If the arms are dropping, add more blocks to rest the palms. The upper arms should be leveled with the sides of the trunk.

III. Inverted chair ❹
→ Support the arms and head on inverted chair. Add bolster and/or blankets for head support.

IV. Chair support ❺
→ People who find it hard to bend forward can use the seat of a chair to support the forehead and arms.

Notes:
The pose can also be done with only one bolster on the heels – this helps people with stiff hip joints and/or stiff knees to do the pose with comfort (not shown).

Supta Pādāṅguṣṭhāsana I

About Supta Pādāṅguṣṭhāsana

Although Supta Pādāṅguṣṭhāsana is not usually classified as a forward extension, we chose to include it in this volume because it fits well in a sequence of forward bending. Adho Mukha Vīrāsana is a forward bend which does not stretch the hamstrings; Supta Pādāṅguṣṭhāsana is a good starting point to work on the extension of the backs of the legs, and prepare them for the other forward extensions.

Supta Pādāṅguṣṭhāsana has many other benefits. To mention just a few: it is helpful for treating lower back pain since it creates space in the sacral band. It also strengthens the bones of the legs and opens the backs of the knees.

> ⚠ **CAUTIONS**
>
> Do not practice this āsana if your hamstrings muscles are injured.

Supta Pādāṅguṣṭhāsana I

Variation 1
Bones vs. Muscles: Basic usage of belt

Effects
The belt helps to stabilize the pelvic region and open the chest. Placing the belt on the heel strengthens the bones of the legs and helps to move the femur into the hip socket. Placing the belt on the toe mounds stretches the muscles of the back of the legs.

Props
- belt
- wall
- block (optional)

a. Bones work

➡ To do the pose with the right leg lifted:

› Lie down with the feet next to a wall and have a belt next to you.

› Slightly bend the legs, move closer to the wall and place the feet against the wall.

› Roll the shoulders back, move the shoulder blades in and hold the edges of the mat ❶.

› Slowly push the legs against the wall until they are straight. Press them down attempting to touch the floor with the entire backs of the legs. This is Supta Tāḍāsana ❷.

› Now, bend the right leg and hold it at the knee. Do not shorten the right side of the trunk and do not allow the left leg to lift off the floor ❸.

› Pull the belt and slowly push the right heel against the resistance of the belt, until the leg is straight.

› Keep the leg vertical to the floor in both planes, i.e., keep the outer ankle straight above the hip joint and keep the back heel above the buttock bone.

› Leave the belt hanged on the foot and stretch the arms over the head, roll the shoulders back to the floor and open the chest.

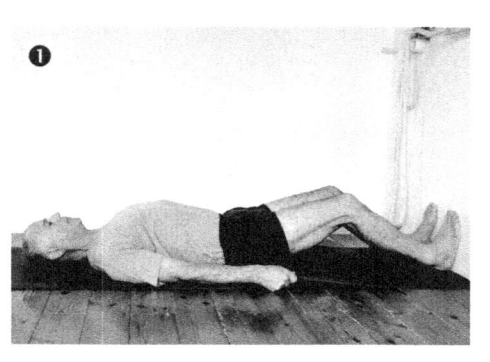

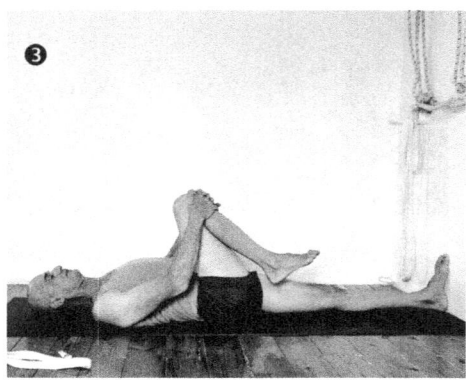

› Without lifting the shoulders, hold the belt and pull it with elbows slightly bent. As much as possible, pull the belt down toward the floor and not toward you. This places load on the bones of the leg and strengthens them; it also helps to move the femur into the pelvis.

› Move the right thigh away from the abdomen and open the entire back of the leg.

› Keep the right leg vertical; extend the inner leg up, and press the outer leg down. Open the foot and create the arch by lifting the heel and the big-toe mound ❹.

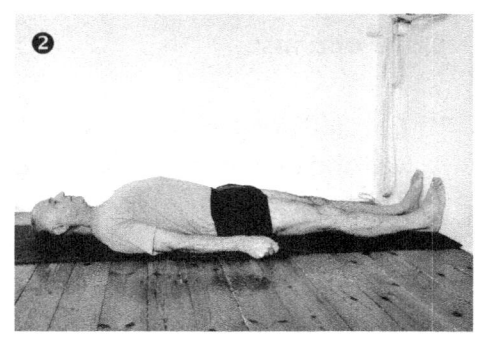

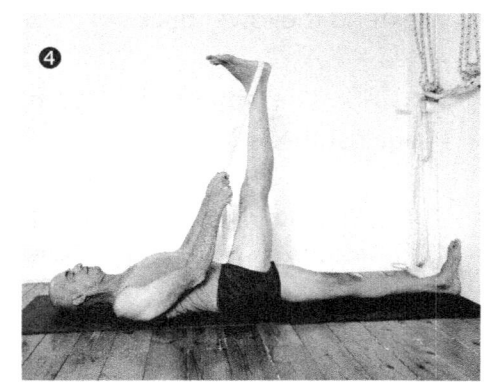

Tips

✓ Keep the abdomen soft and the breath flowing. While breathing, direct your attention to the lower abdomen and check if the breath is spreading evenly to both sides.

✓ Relax the eyes and the throat.

✓ Use both hands evenly for pulling the belt.

✓ Mentally record the sensations of the left leg when the left foot is pushing against the wall. Observe the effects on the entire body. Then, maintaining the pose, move one inch away from the wall and observe what changes take place.

Supta Pādāṅguṣṭhāsana I

Variation 1 (Cont'd)
Bones vs. Muscles:
Basic usage of belt

Other options:

→ 1. Place a block next to the wall and press the back of the left heel against it. ❺

This helps to open the back of the leg, to keep leg active and to extend the lower back.

→ 2. Use another belt to pull against the left heel.

This activates the left leg differently (and is helpful when there is no access to a wall).❻

b. Stretching the muscles ❼

→ In this variation the belt is placed on the toe mounds and the leg is drawn as close to the body as possible (without bending the knee and without shortening the right side of the trunk).

› To increase the stretch, hook the foot with a small loop, wrap the loose end of the belt around the palms and stretch the arms over the head.

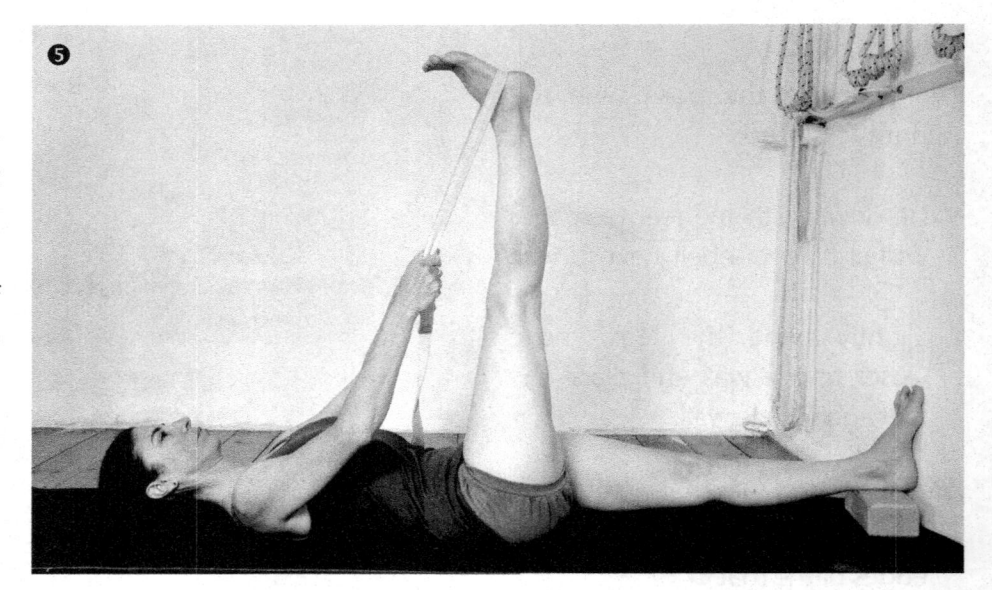

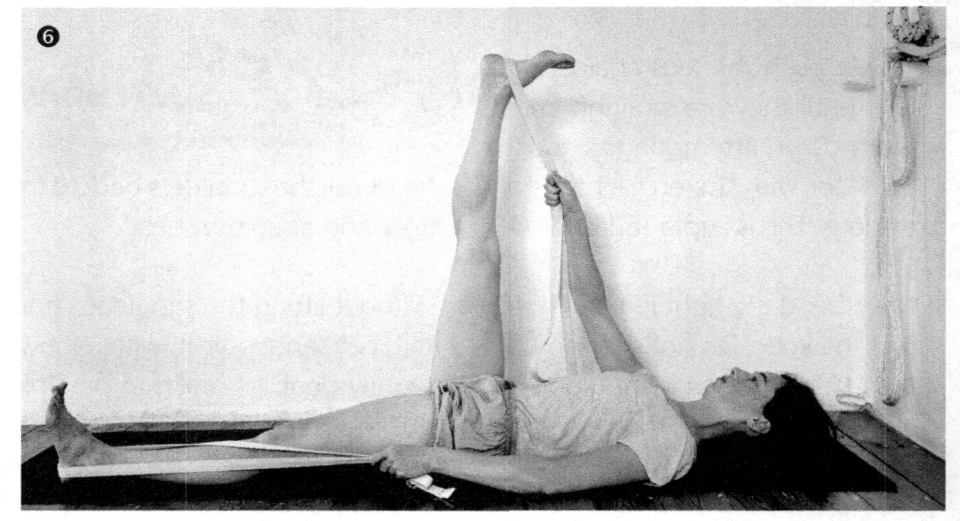

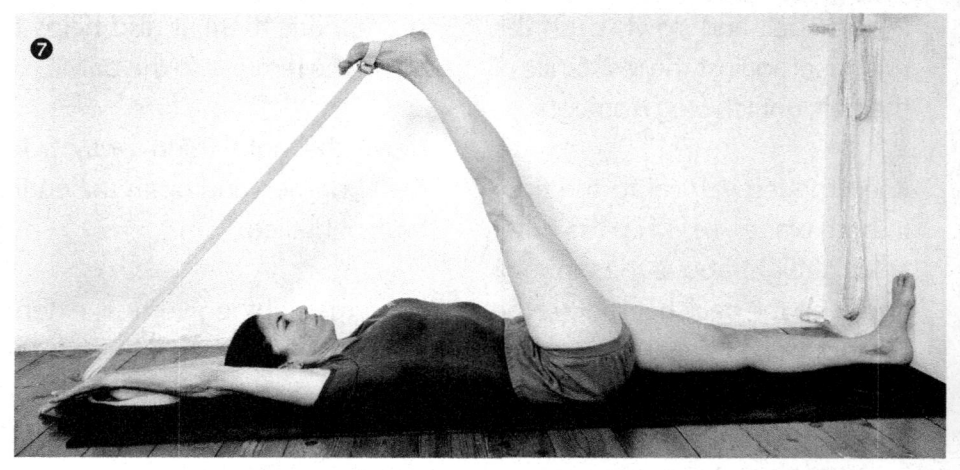

82 Props for Yoga / Chapter 3 / Supta Pādāṅguṣṭhāsana

Supta Pādāṅguṣṭhāsana I

Variation 2
Learning to keep the leg straight:
Entering from Daṇḍāsana

Effects
Entering from Daṇḍāsana helps to keep the lifted leg 'stiff as a poker' (LOY Pl 77).

Props
belt,
wall,
block (optional)

To do the pose with the right leg lifted:

→ Sit in Daṇḍāsana with your feet against the wall and place a belt on the right heel.

› Pull the belt, slightly lift the right leg off the floor and extend it against the pull of the belt ❶.

› Round the back and keep pulling the belt and resisting with the leg as you lie down on the floor ❷.

› As much as possible keep the left leg down on the floor ❸.

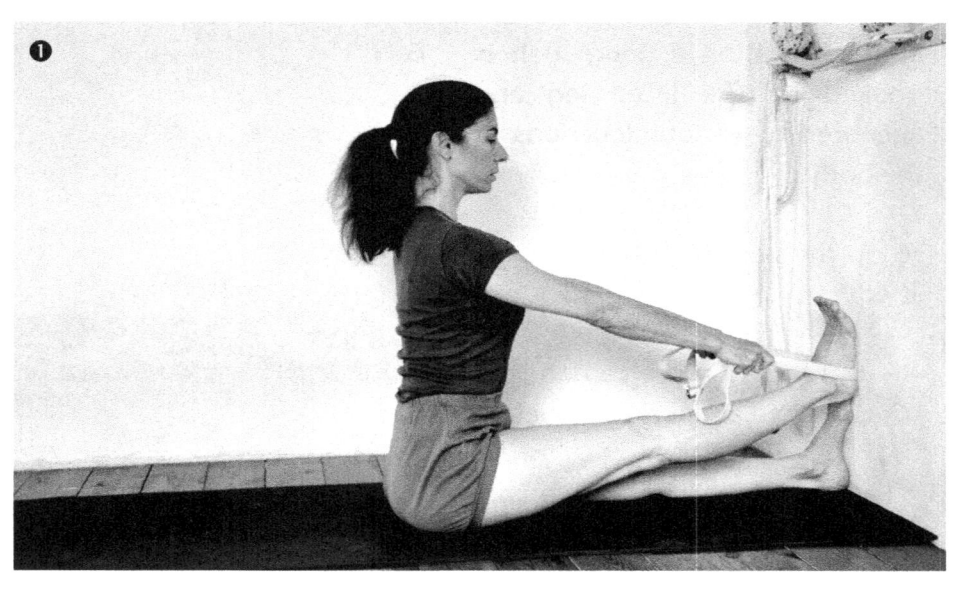

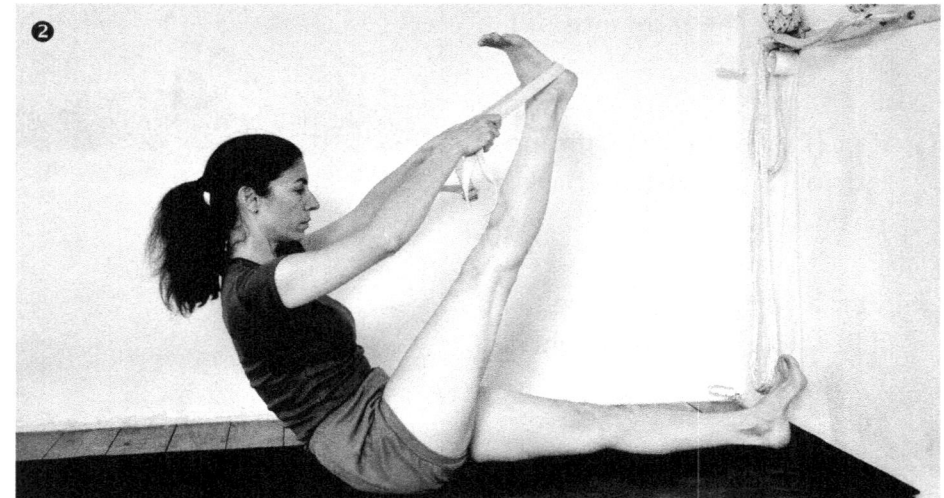

Tips

✓ Control the way you roll down to the floor; use the right leg to slow down the movement.

✓ Keep opening the back of the right knee. Extend the calf muscle to the heel.

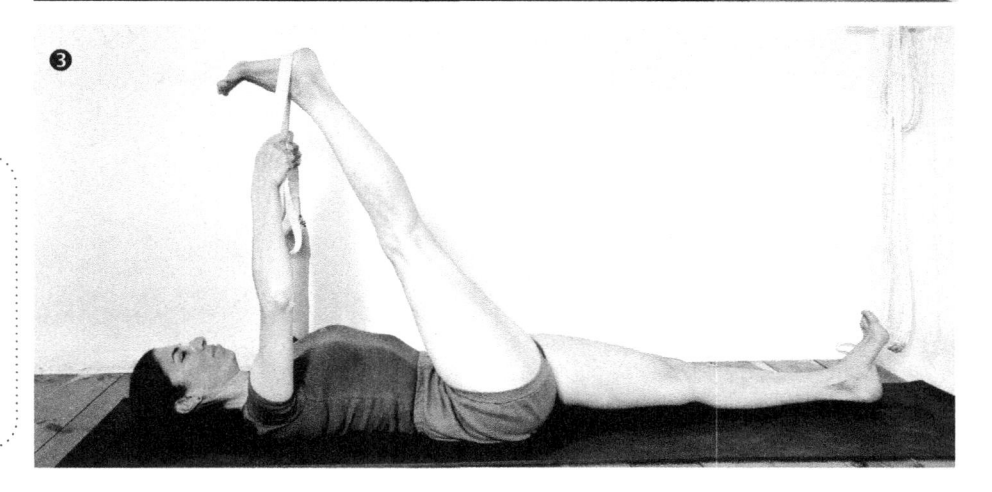

Props for Yoga / Chapter 3 / Supta Pādāṅguṣṭhāsana

Supta Pādāṅguṣṭhāsana I

Variation 3
Activating the lifted leg:
Bracing the body and the leg

Effects The pull of the belt activates the lifted leg. Compactness is created and the bones are strengthened. The arms are free and can be used to extend the torso and open the chest. The different locations of the belt on the trunk have different effects: Placing the belt on the sacrum creates compactness in the bones and joints of the leg and pelvis; the belt on the chest opens and broadens the chest and intensifies the leg stretch; finally, belt on the back of the head strengthen the neck and extends the back of the neck; this extension prepares the neck for Sarvāṅgāsana.

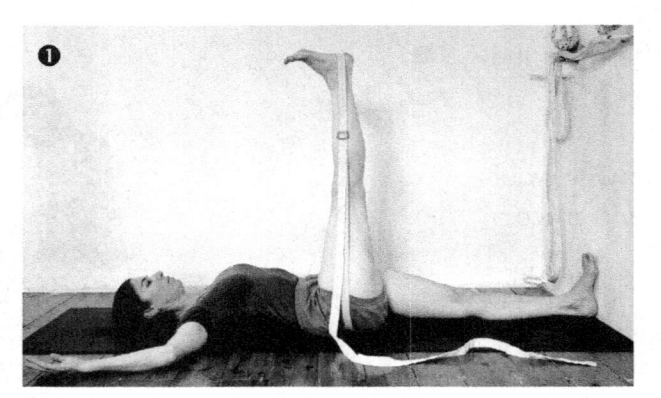

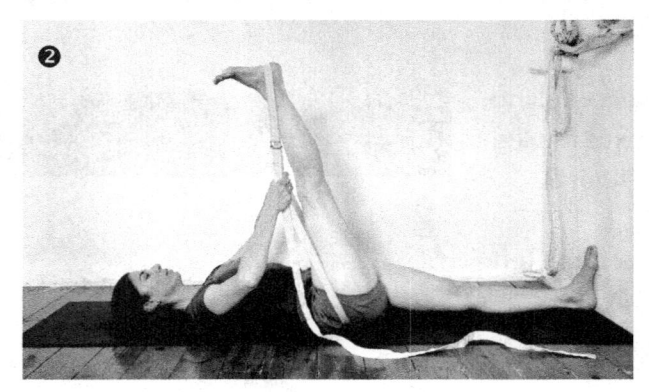

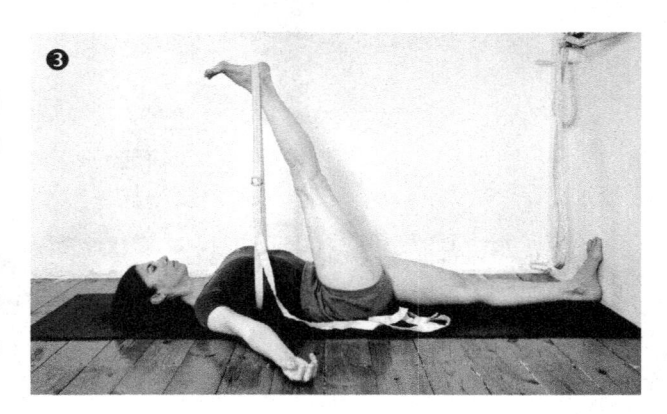

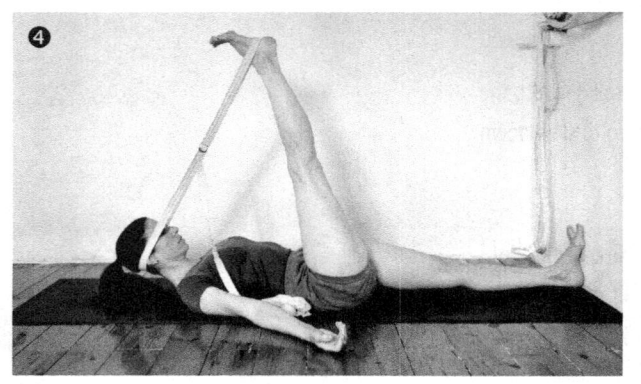

Props
long belt
wall (optional)

In this variation a (long) belt is hooked on the lifted leg and anchored to various locations in the body.

To do the pose with the right leg lifted:

⟶ Loop a long belt around the sacral band and the right heel.

> Keep the buckle accessible and, while the leg is slightly bent, tighten the belt. Then extend the leg against the resistance of the belt.

> Stretch the arms over the head and roll the shoulders back (to the floor) ❶.

> After a while catch the belt and pull it to stretch the right leg further ❷.

> Stay for 40-60 seconds and then move the belt to embrace the mid-back. You may need to adjust its length slightly ❸.

> At the final stage move the belt to the back of the head. Allow the head to lift and use its weight to stretch the belt (and the leg) ❹.

84 Props for Yoga / Chapter 3 / Supta Pādāṅguṣṭhāsana

Supta Pādāṅguṣṭhāsana I

Variation 4
Creating space in the lifted leg side: Hooking a belt from heel to groin

Effects
The pull of the horizontal belt creates space in the lower back and lower abdomen of the lifted-leg side. It teaches the strong action of the upper thigh of the lifted leg in the pose.

Props
2 belts (one of them may need to be long), wall (optional)

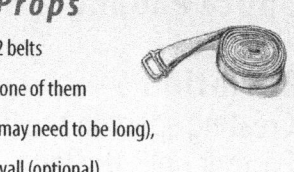

In this variation a belt is looped from the heel of the bottom leg to the groin of the lifted leg. If your legs are long, you will need a long belt.

To do the pose with the right leg lifted:

→ Start as in Variation 1 of this pose and wrap a belt around the right groin (or top leg) and onto the left heel.

> Bend the right leg and hold the knee. With the left leg slightly bent, tighten the belt. Then extend the left leg to stretch the belt such that it moves the right thigh away from you.

Note: Keep the buckle accessible to you so you can adjust the belt.

> Then place the other belt around the right heel and stretch the right leg vertically up.

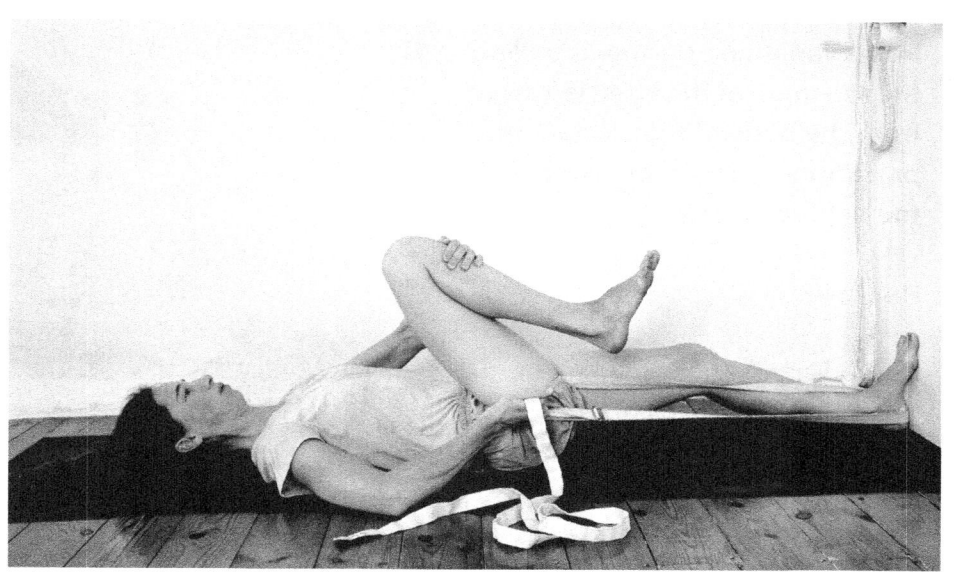

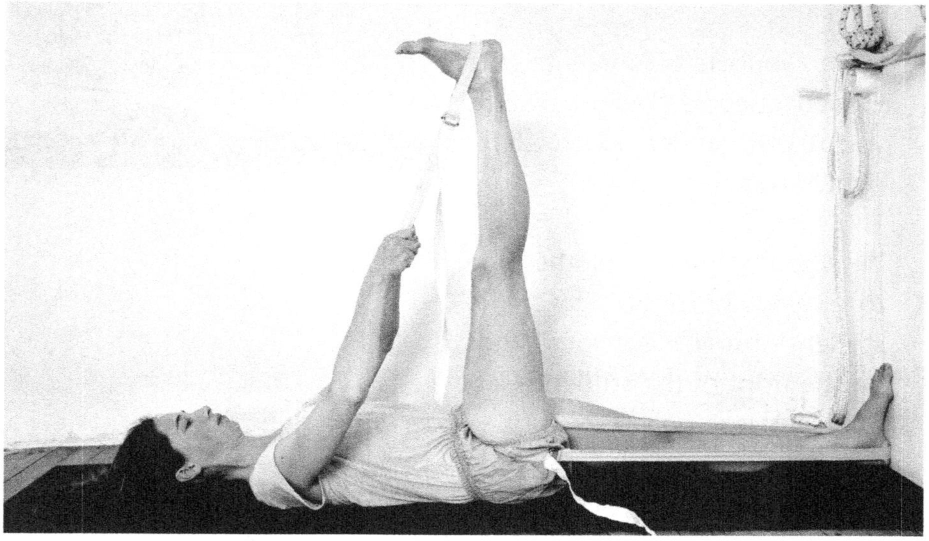

Tips

✓ Extend the left leg and use its inner heel to stretch the belt.

✓ Compare this variation with Variation 1: How is the flow of the breath in the lower abdomen?

Supta Pādāṅguṣṭhāsana I

Variation 5
Creating space in the lifted leg side: Partner pulls the leg

Effects
Similar to those of the previous variation, but the partner can provide a more sensitive and intelligent traction. The partner also presses the thigh of the bottom leg; this teaches to keep this leg rooted and to turn it from outside in.

Props
partner
rope,
belt
wall (optional)

In this variation a partner is pulling the top thigh of the lifted leg away from the body of the student (the practitioner). To do the pose with the right leg lifted:

Partner:

→ Double the rope and insert it around the student's right leg. Lower the rope to the groin.

  Note: If no rope is available, use a belt, but try to get a wide belt.

> Insert your left foot into the looped rope and stretch it towards you. Ask the student to stretch his right leg up, using a belt.

> With your left foot, pull the rope to extend the right side of the student's trunk. Place your hands on the front of the student's left thigh and lean on it ❶.

> Place your palms such that your fingers induce an inner rotation of the student's thigh ❷.

Option: Placing the rope above and below the student's knee ❸

  Effects: This option teaches how to straighten the leg and to open the back of the knee. It can aid recovery from certain knee injuries.

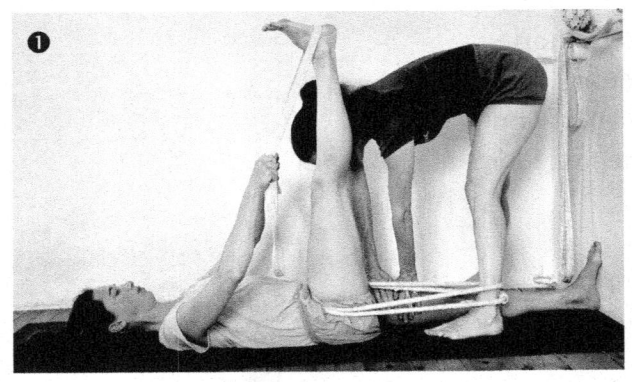

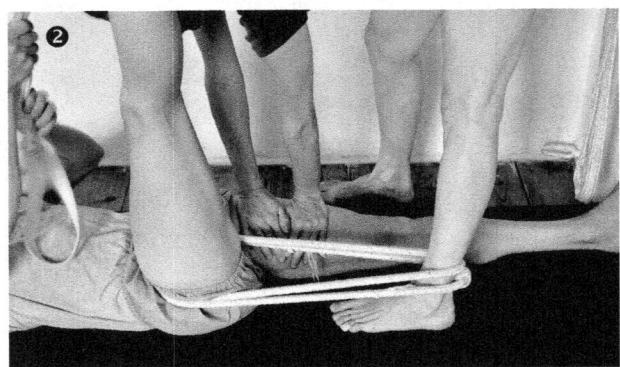

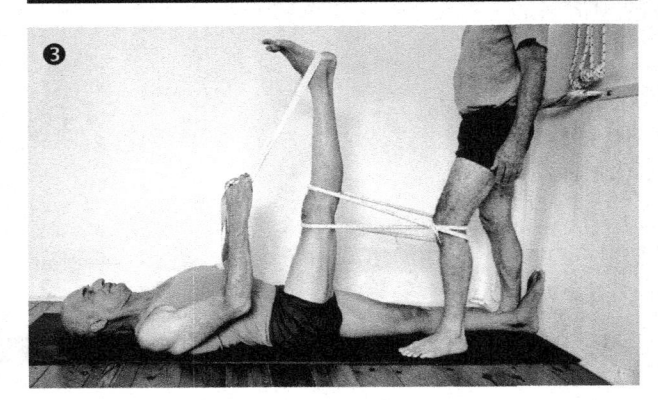

→ Place one end of the rope above the knee and the other below the knee.

> Gently pull the rope with your leg.

Tips (for the partner):

✓ When leaning on the student's left thigh apply vertical pressure to move the thigh bone down toward the floor. The direction of the fingers should move the inner thigh down toward the floor.

✓ Ask the student if you need to increase or decrease the pressure.

Supta Pādāṅguṣṭhāsana I

Variation 6
Supporting the leg at 90°:
Using a wall corner

Effects
The wall ensures precise positioning of both legs. Pressing the back of the lifted leg to the front wall and the inner thigh of the other leg to the side wall helps to align and stabilize the legs and pelvis. Supporting the lifted leg also reduces the strain of a person with limited flexibility.

Props
wall corner,
belt,
2 blocks (optional)

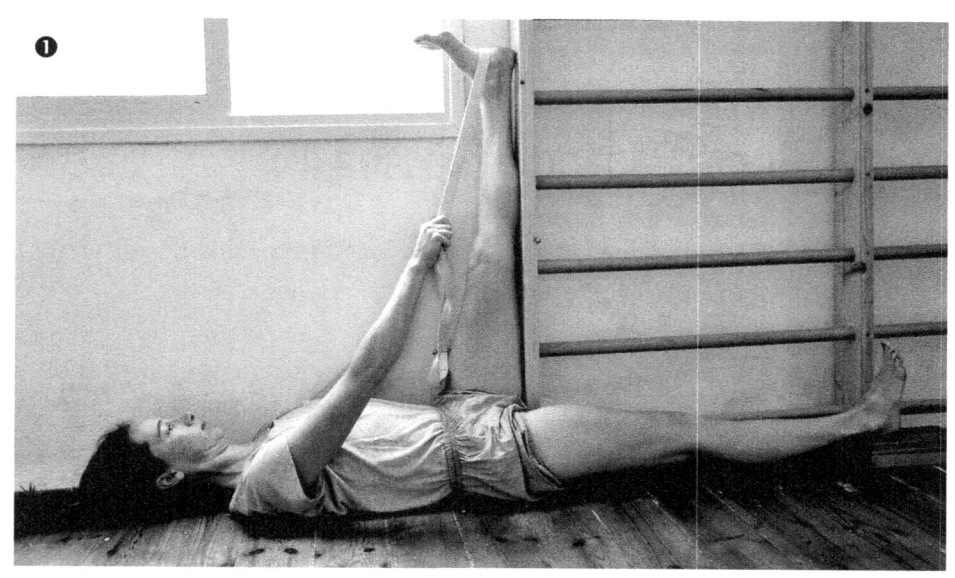

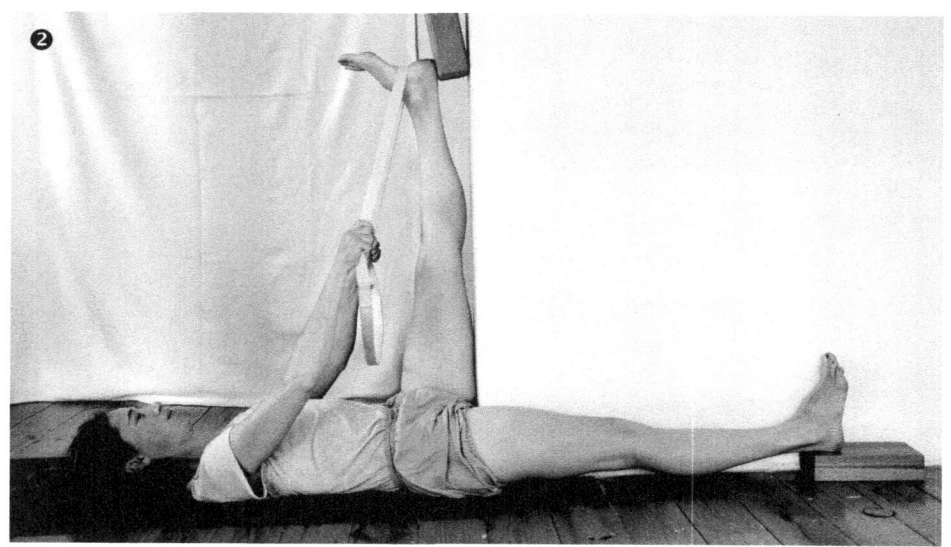

To do the pose with the right leg lifted:

→ Lie close to an external wall corner or a column. Lift the right leg and move close to the wall until the right buttock bone and the right heel touch the wall.

› Move slightly to the left to press the left inner thigh to the wall, while turning it from outside in.

› Place the left heel on a block and press the heel on the block. Use a belt to pull against the right heel ❶.

› You can also place a (rubber or foam) block in between the right heel and the wall ❷.

Supta Pādāṅguṣṭhāsana II (lateral)

About Supta Pādāṅguṣṭhāsana II

This is the third movement shown in *Light on Yoga* for this pose (LOY Pl. 77), but nowadays it is usually referred to as Supta Pādāṅguṣṭhāsana II.

This pose creates a lateral expansion of the pelvic area and the lower abdomen; it is a good preparation for Utthita Trikoṇāsana and the other lateral standing poses. It is one of the poses recommended for menstruating ladies – in a class situation they can practice this pose instead of Supta Pādāṅguṣṭhāsana I, Ūrdhva Prasārita Pādāsana and so on.

> **⚠ CAUTIONS**
>
> Do not practice this āsana if your adductor muscles are injured.

Supta Pādāṅguṣṭhāsana II

Variation 1
Stabilizing the pelvis:
Holding a belt with two hands

Effects
Holding the belt with both hands stabilizes the pose and helps to overcome the sideways rolling of the pelvis.

Props
wall
belt

We show the pose in two stages: bent leg and straight leg.

To do the pose on the right leg:

- Lie down with your feet against the wall. Bend the right leg, hold its knee with your right hand and roll it to the right side.

- Resist the tendency of the pelvis to roll to the right by tightening the right buttock and rolling the pelvis girdle from right to left.

- Put the left palm on the left thigh and stay for a while to experience the opening in the right pelvis ❶.

- Now take the belt, make a small loop and place it on the right heel. Pass the loose end of the belt under the upper back and hold the belt with both hands.

- Pull the belt and slowly stretch the right leg against the resistance of the belt.

- Keep the left leg well stretched and press the foot against the wall and the back of the leg down to the floor ❷.

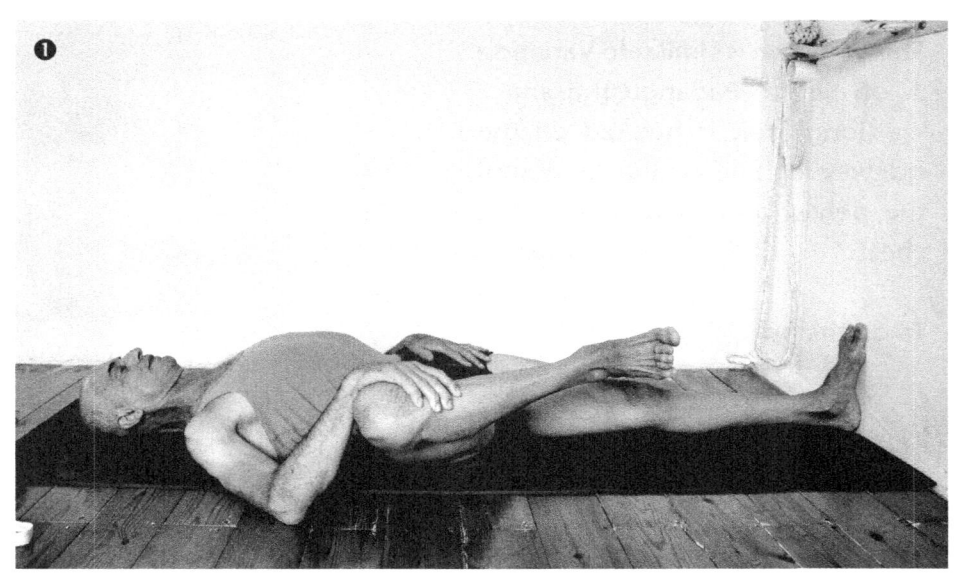

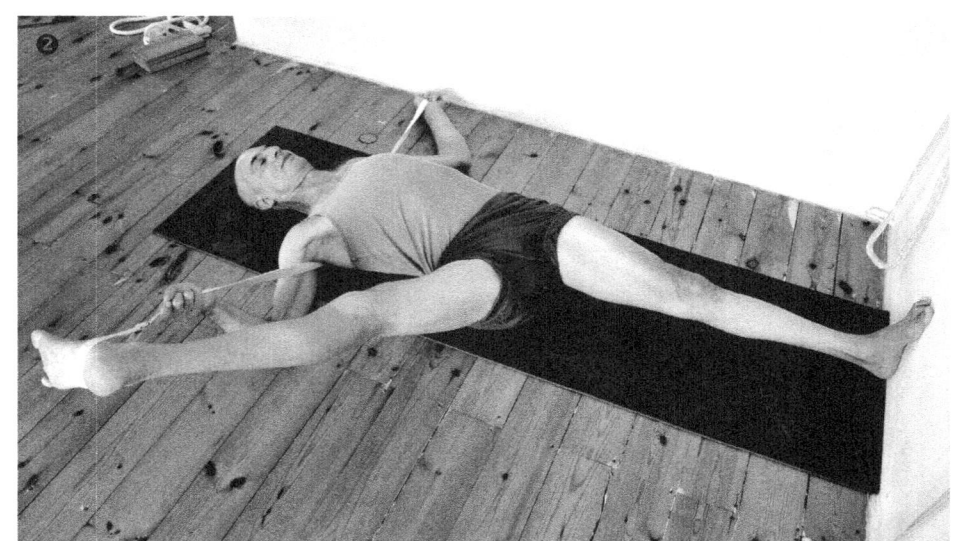

Tips

- Do not allow the right foot to turn out; keep it parallel to the floor.

- Lift the head to look at the pelvis and ensure that it is facing up, not sideways to the right.

- To increase the space in the pelvis you can move the left foot to the left and align it with the left edge of the mat (you will need to get slightly closer to the wall).

- Observe your breath in the lower abdomen region – does it spread evenly to both sides?

Props for Yoga / Chapter 3 / Supta Pādāṅguṣṭhāsana II

Supta Pādāṅguṣṭhāsana II

Variation 2
Activating the leg:
Bracing the body and the leg

Effects
The pull of the belt activates the leg that is extended sideways. Compactness is created and the bones are strengthened. The arms are free, so they can be used to extend the torso and open the chest.

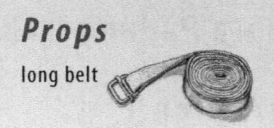

Props
long belt

This variation is similar to Variation 3 of Supta Pādāṅguṣṭhāsana I - a (long) belt is hooked on the sideway leg and anchored around the pelvis, and then around the chest.

To do the pose on the right leg:

⟶ Loop a long belt around the pelvis and the right heel. With bent knee tighten the belt such that when you straighten the leg, the belt is well stretched.

› Then move the belt to embrace the chest. You may need to adjust the length of the belt.

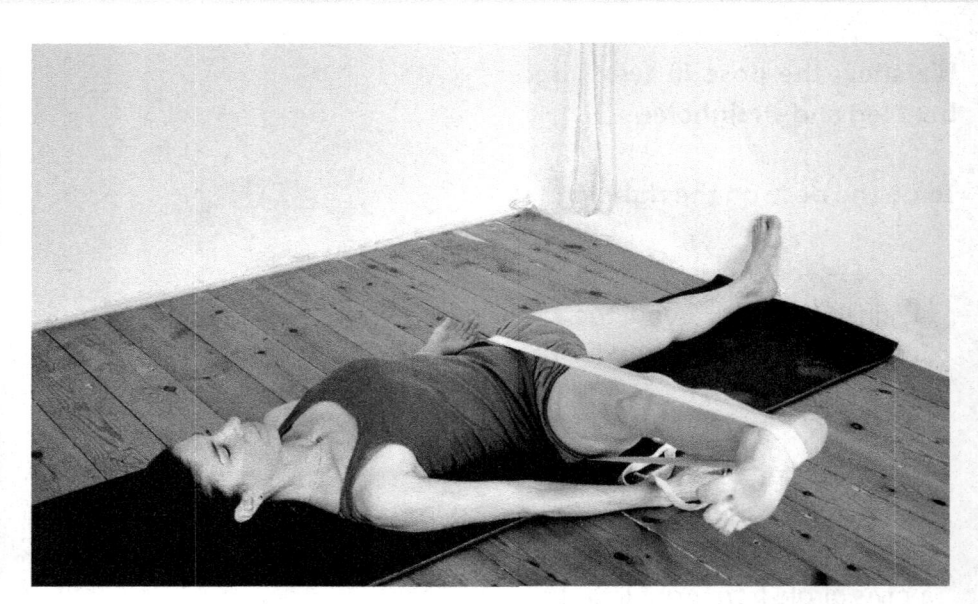

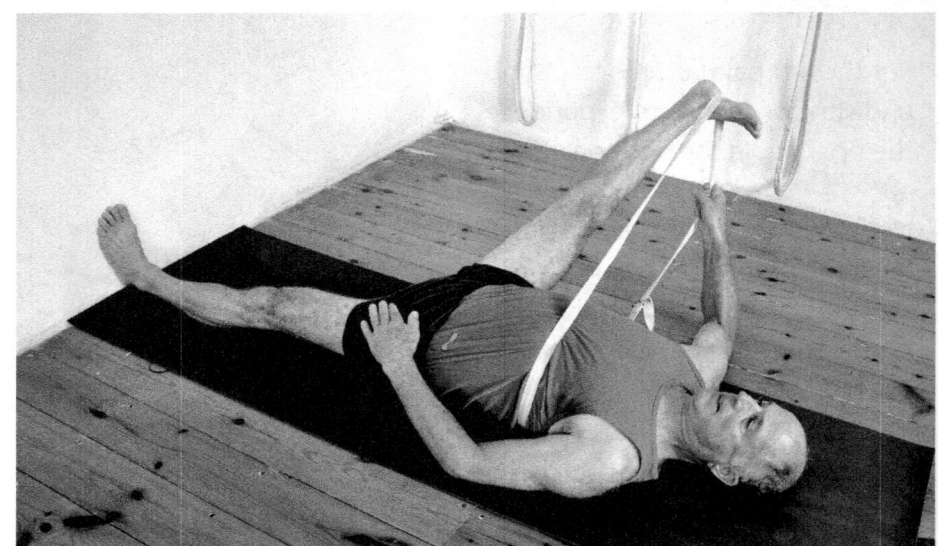

Supta Pādāṅguṣṭhāsana II

Variation 3
Creating space in the pelvis: Hooking a belt from heel to groin

Effects
The pull of the belt creates space in pelvis and teaches to maintain its evenness. A space is created for the breath in the lower abdomen.

Props
wall
2 belts
(one of them may need to be long)

This variation is similar to Variation 4 of Supta Pādāṅguṣṭhāsana I. We show here an option of using a short looped belt. To do the pose with the right leg sideways:

→ Wrap a belt from the right groin to the left heel (normally this should be a long belt).

> Bend the right leg and hold the knee. With the left leg slightly bent, tighten the belt. Then extend the left leg to stretch the belt such that it moves the right thigh away from you.

Note: Keep the buckle accessible for adjusting the belt later on.

> Fold the other belt twice to create a short and firm loop. Hook that loop on the right heel and straighten the leg up.

> Hold the short loop with the right arm straight and move the leg sideways to the right.

Note: Adjust the length of the loop or you grip as needed.

> Resist the tendency of the pelvis to roll to the right.

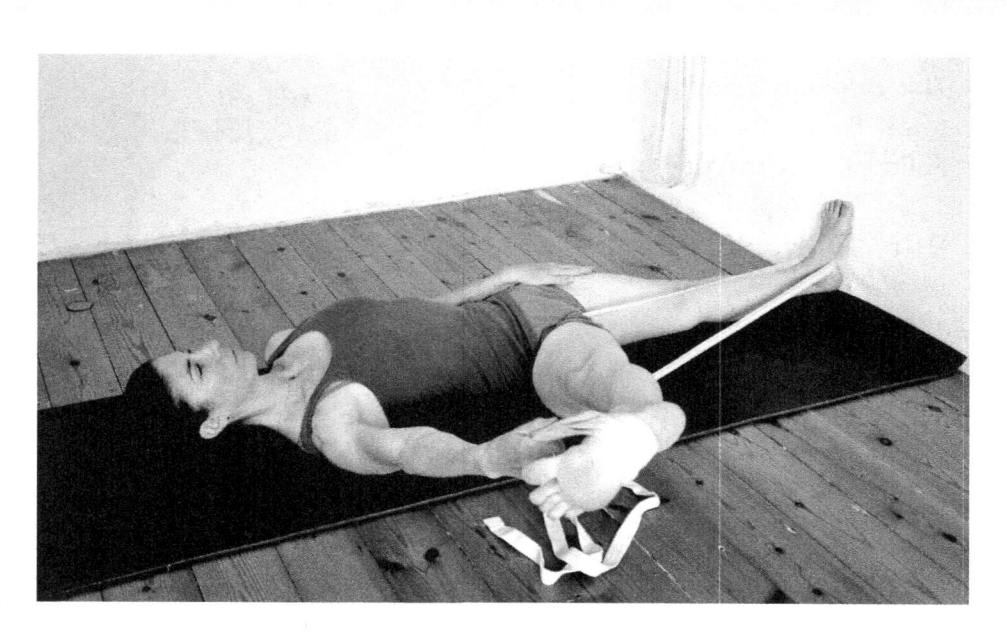

Tips

✓ When moving the leg sideways toward the floor extend the inner leg from the groin to the inner heel and move the outer leg from the outer foot toward the pelvis.

✓ Move the right leg down from the inner leg but tighten the outer leg and right buttock to resist. This prevents the pelvis from tilting to the right.

✓ Roll the pubic bone from right to left.

Supta Pādāṅguṣṭhāsana II

Variation 4
Creating space in the stretched leg side: Partner pulls the leg

Effects
This option opens the back of the leg and creates space in the knee. It can alleviate some knee injuries.

Props
partner
rope
belt
wall (optional)

This variation is similar to Variation 5 of Supta Pādāṅguṣṭhāsana I. Follow the instruction given there.

Other Options:

1. Scissors-action ❶

Partner:

→ Place your right heel against the student's top front thigh and move it towards you (to extend the right side of his trunk).

› At the same time use your left leg to gently push against the student›s calf so as to keep his leg well stretched.

› Place your right hand on the students left iliac crest to keep it grounded.

› Use the scissors-like action to open the back of the knee of the student.

> *Note:* Be sensitive in applying your force. Do not do this variation if the student has a knee problem.

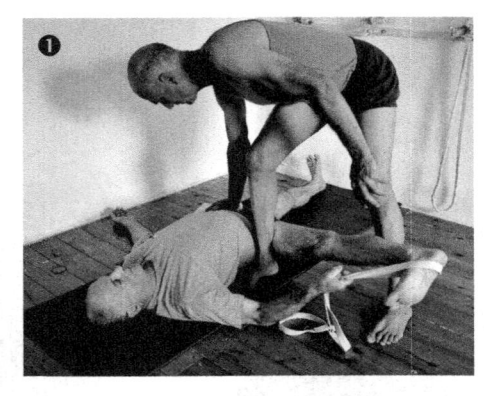

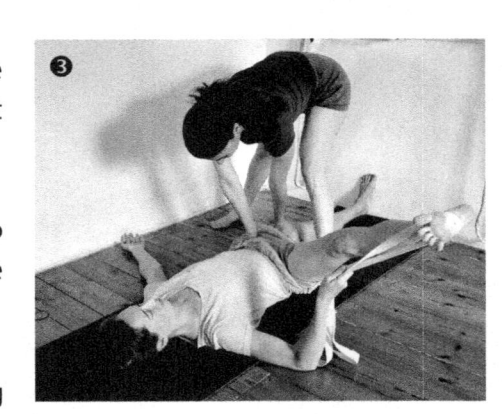

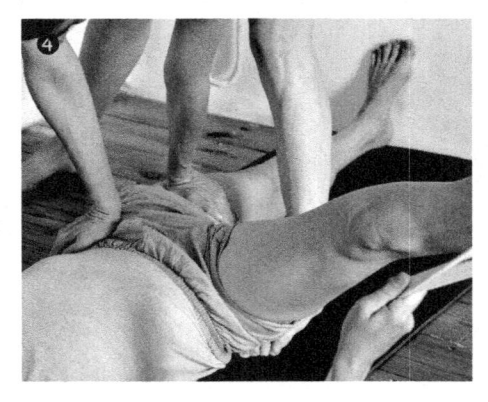

2. Foot under buttock ❷

Partner:

→ After the student has lifted her/his right leg, stand facing her/him and insert your left foot under the student's right buttock.

› With your foot and toes, extend the buttock toward you and support it ❷.

› As the student moves her/his leg to the right, lean with your right hand on the student's left iliac crest to prevent her/his pelvis from rolling to the right ❸.

› Place your left hand on the front of the student's left thigh and keep it anchored down. Place your palm such that the fingers are facing in and roll the student's thigh from outside in ❹.

> *Note:* The bony protrusion of the iliac crest is convex and sharp; curve your palm to match this shape and if the student is sensitive, do not apply strong pressure.

Supta Pādāṅguṣṭhāsana II

Variation 5
Moving the femur head into the hip joint: Side foot against wall

Effects

Straightening the leg against the resistance of the wall moves the femur bone into the socket of the hip joint – this is a very healthy action for this joint. Starting with the outer leg on the floor intensifies the sideway opening of the pelvic girdle.

Props

belt,
wall,
block (optional)

Usually in this pose we attempt to keep the pelvis stable and open the leg to the side without allowing the pelvis to roll sideways. Sometimes this can be reversed: start by moving the leg all the way to the floor and then roll the pelvis to the opposite side. This creates compactness in the pelvis, especially when placing the foot against the wall as shown here.

To do the pose with the right leg sideways:

→ Lie on a sticky mat parallel to a wall, with your right side about 75 cm (30 inches) from it (the distance should be slightly less than the length of your leg).

> Bend the right leg and place the foot on the wall. The knee should be slightly bent, the outer foot on the floor and the leg should be perpendicular to the wall ❶.

> Slowly push the wall in order to straighten the leg.

> **Note:** The sticky mat is mandatory, since it provides friction for resisting the push.

> Place the left palm on the left iliac bone. Turn the pelvis as much as possible to the left attempting to move the left buttock closer to the floor ❷.

Option: Using wall corner

→ You can do this variation such that the left foot will also push a wall. For this you have to use a wall corner as shown here ❸:

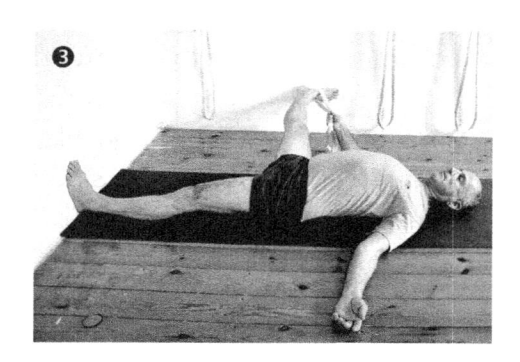

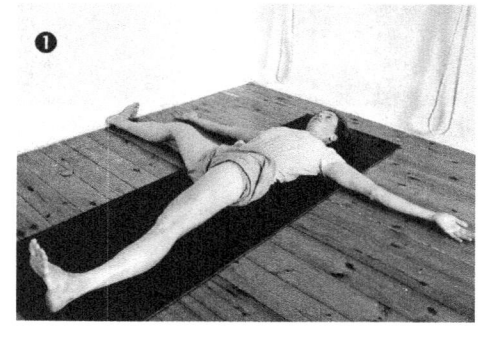

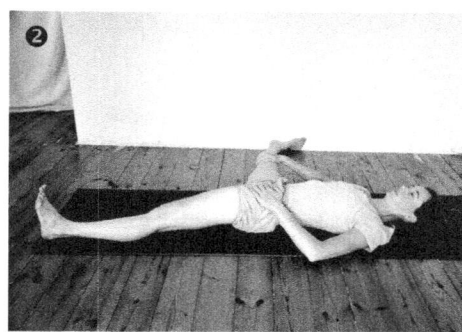

Tips

✓ Moving the femur head into the socket is most effective when the angle between the right leg and the wall is 90°; hence do not move the right foot higher than this.

✓ You can place a folded blanket, or some other support to fill the gap under the left buttock.

✓ Move the outer buttocks inward toward one another, this helps to open the front of the pelvis, keep the left side of the pelvis grounded and root the femurs into the hip sockets.

Supta Pādāṅguṣṭhāsana II

Variation 6
Moving the femur head into the hip joint: Partner pulls the buttock

Effects
The pull of the rope stabilizes the pelvis and keeps the femur bone in place. This is very soothing and allows the abdominal organs to relax and soften.

Props
partner
rope
belt

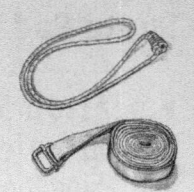

To do the pose with the right leg moving sideways:

→ Student: Lie down on the floor. Lift the right leg and hold it with a belt on the right heel.

› Partner: Sit next to the left side of the student and wrap a rope on his/her right buttock. Place your feet against the left side of the student's pelvis.

› Partner: As the student moves his/her leg to the right, pull the rope to stabilize his/her pelvis and to move the flesh of his/her buttock into the pelvis.

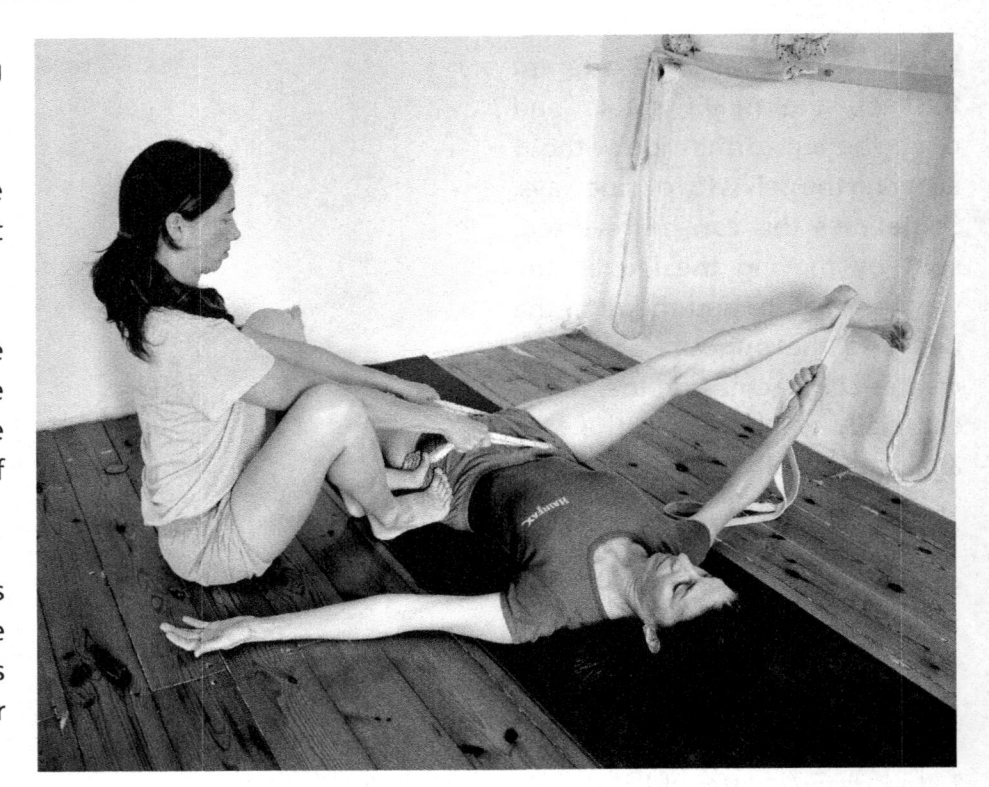

Supta Pādāṅguṣṭhāsana II

Variation 7
Restorative Supta Pādāṅguṣṭhāsana II: Supporting the outer thigh

Effects
The support enables to stay effortlessly in the pose and to enjoy the widening and relaxing effect of the pose. This variation is especially useful for women during menstruation and pregnancy (during pregnancy, use a bolster).

Props
blanket
bolster of block

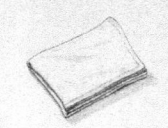

To do the pose with the right leg moving sideways:

⟶ Place a rolled blanket (or a bolster) lengthwise on your right.

› Hold the right foot using a belt and lift it up.

› Move the leg to the right side and adjust the rolled blanket to support the right upper thigh.

› Bend the right elbow and place it on the floor at shoulder-height ❶.

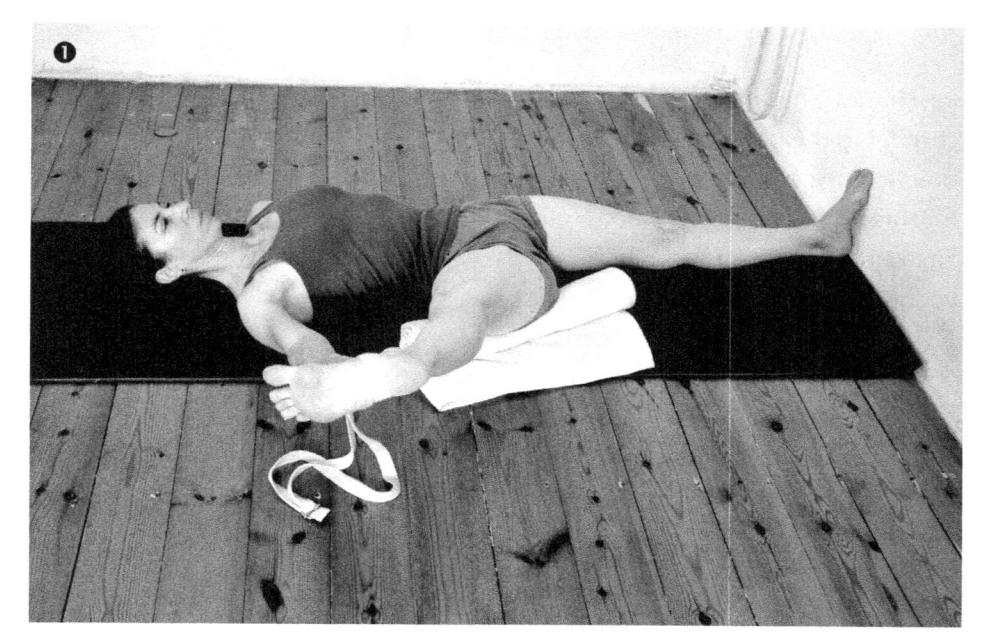

Other options: Using a hard support

⟶ You can use a wooden block ❷ or even a flat metal weight (not shown).

› Place the block or the weight so as to support the greater trochanter (the quadrilateral eminence of the top lateral femur).

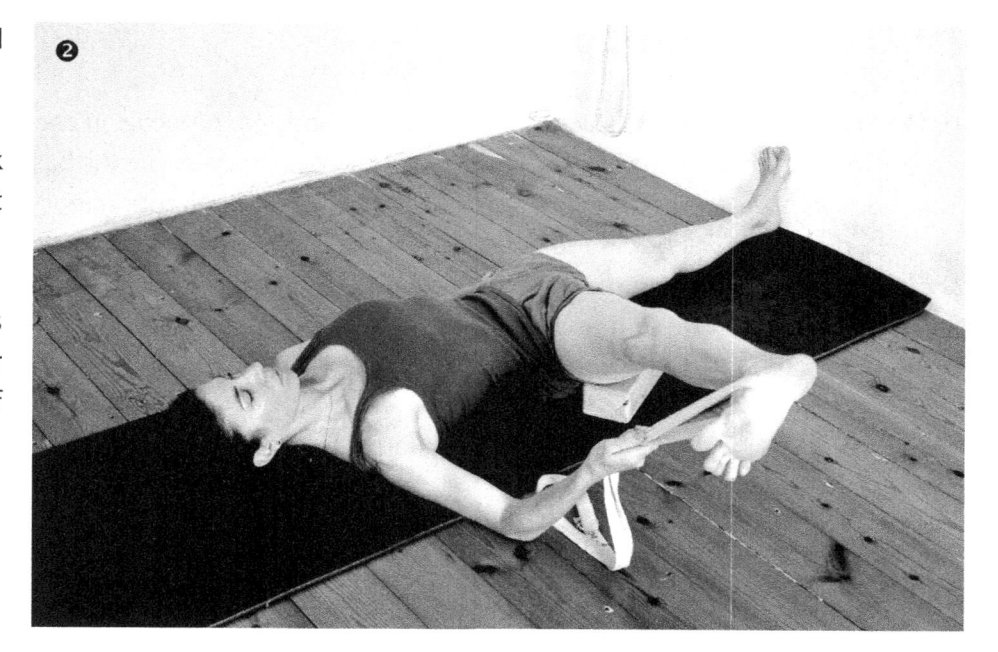

Props for Yoga / Chapter 3 / Supta Pādāṅguṣṭhāsana II 95

Paschimottānāsana
About Paschimottānāsana

Paschimottānāsana is a major forward extension. It is especially beneficial for stretching the back legs and back torso as well as for restorative and meditative practices. Hence we cover it with some length. Many of the variations shown for this pose can be easily adapted to other basic forward extensions (like Jānu Śīrṣāsana and Trianga Mukhaikapāda Paschimottānāsana). We present here variations for:

- Activating the legs
- Bending deeper into the pose by lengthening the hamstrings muscles
- Restorative prolonged stays in the pose

People with short hamstrings tend to bend from the back, which causes an unhealthy load on the back. To do the pose safely one must first learn to lengthen the hamstrings.

> **⚠ CAUTIONS**
>
> To protect the hamstrings muscles, always open the knees completely, extending them evenly on all sides. Do not allow the thighs to lift off the floor. Do not practice this āsana during or just after an asthmatic attack. Avoid this pose if you have diarrhea.

Activating the Legs

Unlike standing āsanas, in which the feet are the base of the pose, in most forward extensions, the backs of the legs – from buttocks to heels – are the base. The more you press the legs down and make them heavy, the more freedom and extension you will get in the trunk. The quadriceps (front thigh muscles) should be tight and flat on the femurs (thigh bones). One has to learn how to activate and tighten these muscles without puffing and shortening them, or pulling them away from the bones.

The following variations help to learn this action.

Paschimottānāsana

Variation 1
Activating the legs: Block between the thighs

Effects
The block activates the outer thighs; this stabilizes the hip joints and helps to extend the sides of the trunks. It also helps to roll the thighs inward and thus widen the pelvis. Pulling the belt with the arms helps to extend the spine and widen the back, thereby preventing it from bulging upward (like a "hunchback").

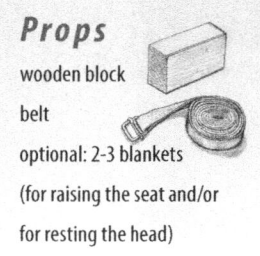

Props
wooden block
belt
optional: 2-3 blankets
(for raising the seat and/or for resting the head)

This is similar to Variation 6 of Daṇḍāsana.

> Place a folded blanket next to you for later head support (the height of the support should be adjusted according to your need).

> Sit in Daṇḍāsana. Hold the block firmly in between the thighs. Roll the thighs inward, so as to touch the block with the upper edges of the inner thighs (as in page 10).

> Bend the knees slightly. Loop a belt around the heels and hold it. Pull the belt with both hands, lift the chest, move the upper spine in, and make the back concave. Stretch your legs against the resistance of the belt and sit straight ❶.

> Inhale and lift the arms up to Ūrdhva Hasta Daṇḍāsana.

> Bend forward 45° keeping the concave shape of the back, lift the sternum; then lift the chin and look upward (this is Pādanguṣṭha Daṇḍāsana) ❷.

> Inhale and open the chest. If necessary, shorten the belt so as to keep your arms stretched.

> Exhale and move forward by bending the elbows sideways (if you reach the feet, hold them instead of the belt). Widen the elbows to broaden the chest.

> Place the naval region on the thighs, then the bottom chest and finally lower the head.

> Soften the neck as you lay your forehead gently in between the shins ❸ (or on a blanket or bolster you placed on top of them).

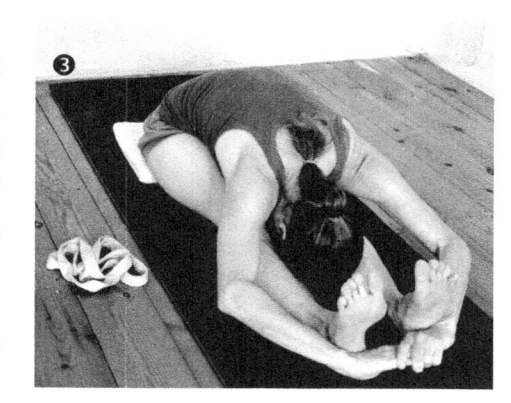

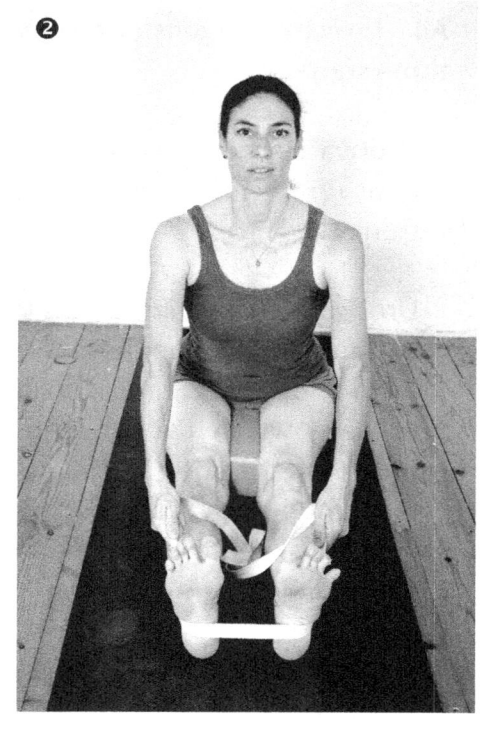

Tips

✓ Learn to activate the legs and press them down to the floor while keeping the abdomen completely passive.

✓ When an airplane lands, its rear wheels touch the ground before its front wheels; similarly, when entering Paschimottānāsana the bottom trunk should descend down before the top trunk (do not do a "crash landing").

✓ Lift the elbows to broaden the chest and to open the sides of the trunk and armpits. Do not drop the sides but move the spine down, into the back.

Note:

All forward extensions have three stages:

> **Ūrdhva Hasta** – stretching the arms up to create length in the trunk ❶.

> **Ūrdhva Mukha Dandāsana (or Pādanguṣtha Dandāsana)** – in this stage the back is made concave which creates length in the front spine. The head is facing upward, but the eyes recede to mentally observe the spine ❷.

> **Adho Mukha** – This is the final stage in which the head is brought down. The back of the trunk is long with a gentle curve ❸.

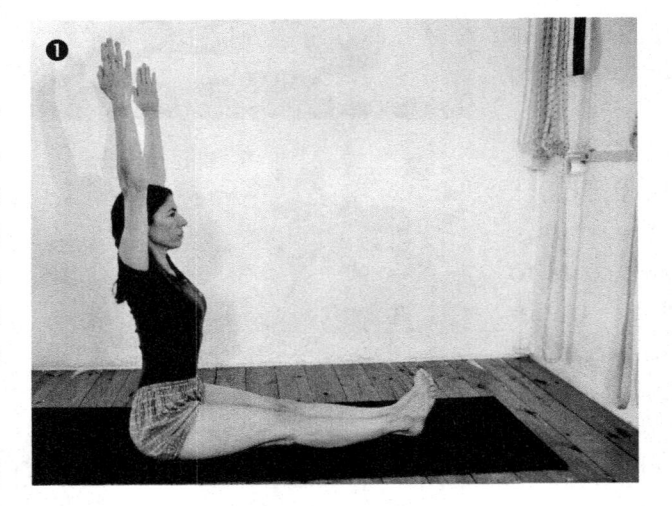

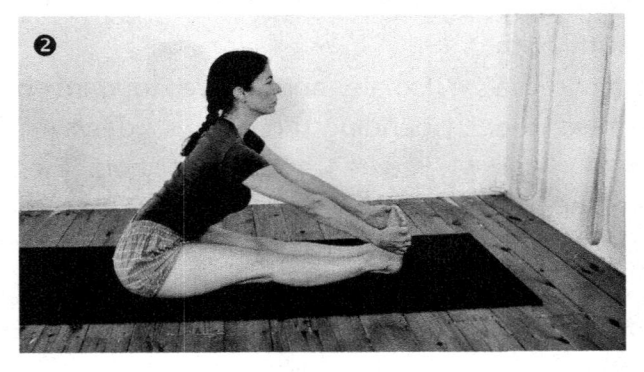

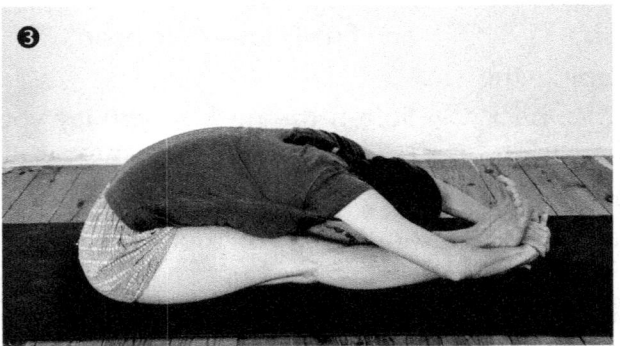

Paschimottānāsana

Variation 2
Activating the feet: Block against the soles

Effects
The flat & hard block stabilizes the feet and provides a good gripping surface for the symmetrical pull of the hands, which activates the legs further. The hip joints are stabilized and the sacrum is drawn in.

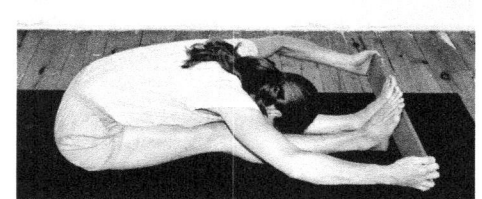

Props
block or two
blanket
(optional)

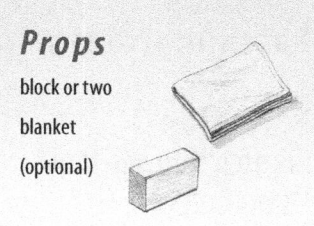

Variation 5 of Dandāsana (see page 9) is similar to this one, but here we use a block to facilitate the forward extension.

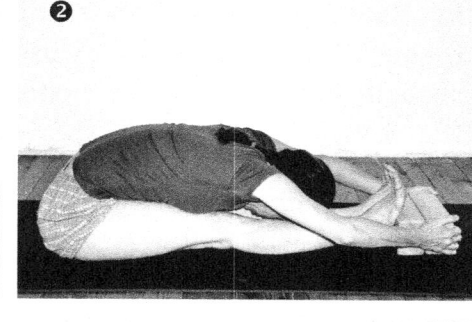

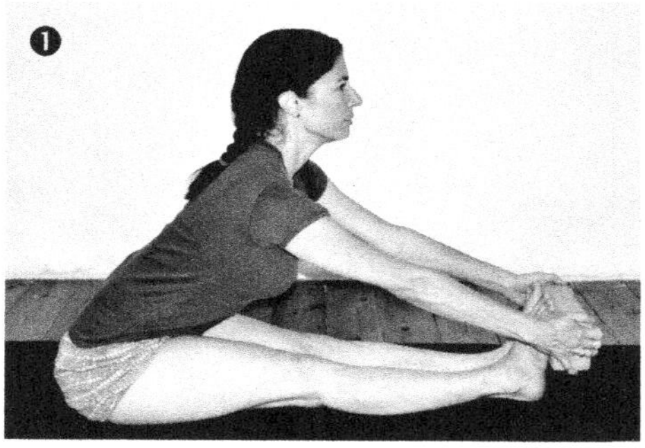

→ Sit in Dandāsana and place a block against the soles of your feet.

> Inhale, lift the arms and extend the trunk up. Exhale, bend forward from the hips, hold the sides of the block and straighten the legs; look forward and up to make the back concave ❶.

> Inhale, and with exhalation bend the elbows and extend the trunk forward over the legs.

> Rest your forehead on the shins (use a folded blanket, a bolster or even a chair, if needed).

> If possible, place another block ❷, or turn the block to its long side ❸.

Note: Instead of the block you can use a plank ❹; which induces more width in the trunk. If available, you can use a column, a wall hook, a bench ❺ or any other stable object you can grasp to increase the forward extension.

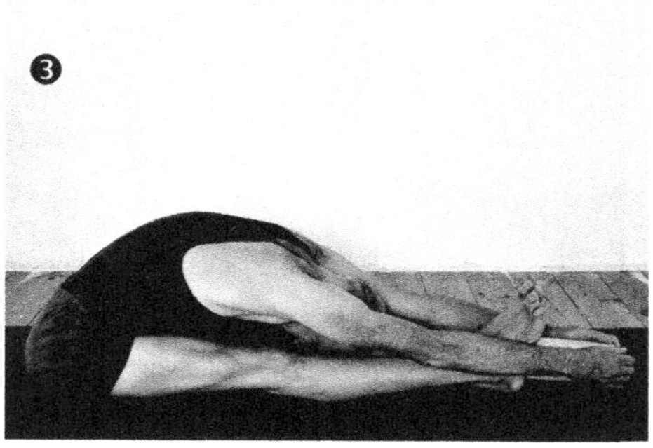

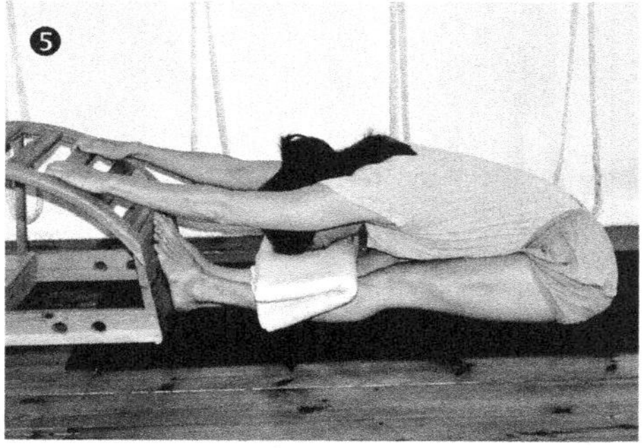

Tips

✓ Tighten the outer thigh muscles to stabilize the hip joints and broaden the pelvis girdle. This softens the abdomen.

✓ While stretching the legs, watch their top centerlines: in each leg, the centers of the front ankle, knee and thigh should be in line and facing upward.

✓ Broaden the soles of the feet and spread the toes.

Applicability
All forward bends with one or both legs stretched forward, e.g. Jānu Śīrṣāsana, Trianga Mukhaikapāda Paschimottānāsana

Paschimottānāsana

Variation 3
Compacting the legs: Using belts

Effects
The belts create compactness and sharpness in the legs and stabilize the inward rotation of the thighs. Working against the resistance of the belts activates the legs.

Props
2 belts (or more)

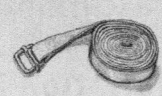

In Variation 7 of Dandāsana (page 11) we show how to use six belts to stabilize and compact the legs. This Variation shows this for Paschimottānāsana. We use here two belts; you can add belts to improve the compactness of the legs, as shown on page 11.

⟶ Sit in Dandāsana and tie one belt around the middle of the thighs, and a second belt around the middle of the shins.

› Adjust the belts such that they are tightened in opposite directions.

› Turn the thighs in, and then tighten the belts.

> *Note:* If after tightening there is discomfort at the ankle bones, place some cushioning between the ankles.

› Bend and extend forward to Paschimottānāsana.

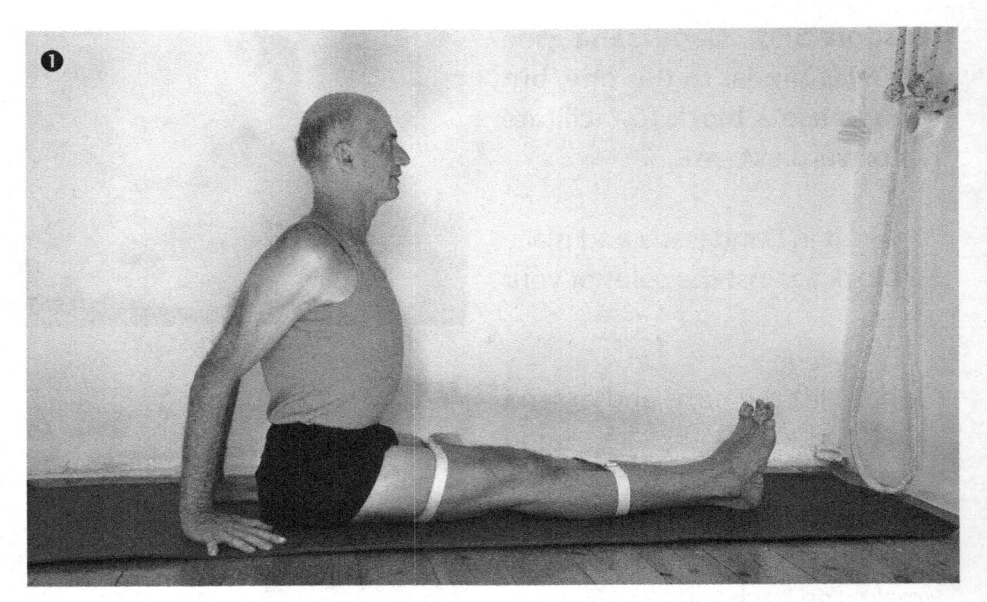

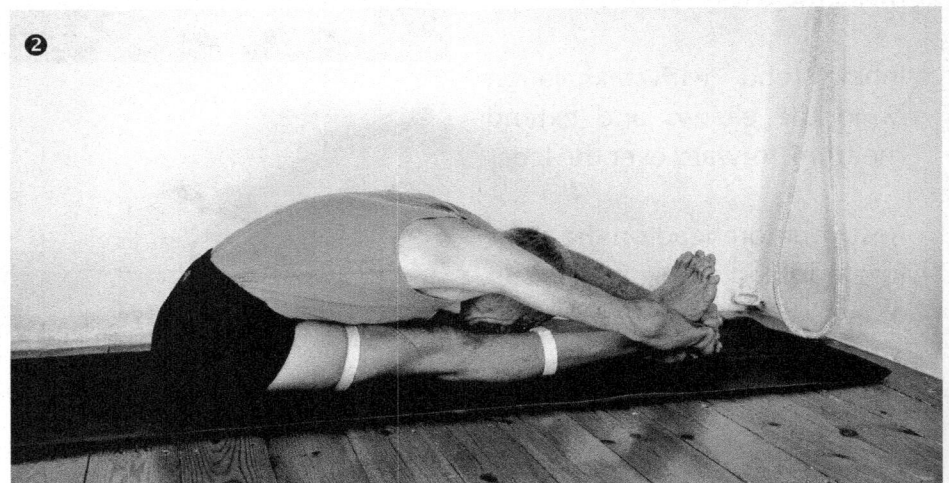

Applicability
Tying the legs with belts can be done in any pose in which the legs are joined and stretched. It can be used for Tadasana (standing near the wall), for inverted poses, and so on. You can do a cycle of Dandāsana, Urdhva Hasta Dandāsana, Paschimottānāsana, Paripurna Navasana, Ardha Navasana and so on, with the belts on the legs.

Paschimottānāsana

Variation 4
Opening the sides:
Belt around feet

Effects
Placing the belt on the feet in this way activates the feet and the legs. The palms are facing down allowing turning the arms and lifting the elbows. This opens the sides of the trunk and helps to extend them forward.

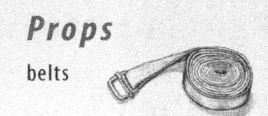

Props
belts

> Sit in Dandāsana with the legs slightly spread and wrap a belt around the middle of the feet ❶.

> Catch the far end of the belt and cross it under the closer end ❷.

> Pull the belt to bend forward. Resist with the legs. Activate and open the feet.

> Lift the elbows to the level of the shoulder blades.

> Use the pull of the belt to extend the sides of the trunk forward while descending the spine into the trunk ❸.

> When pulling with the arms do not allow the shoulders and the trapezius muscle to move closer to the neck.

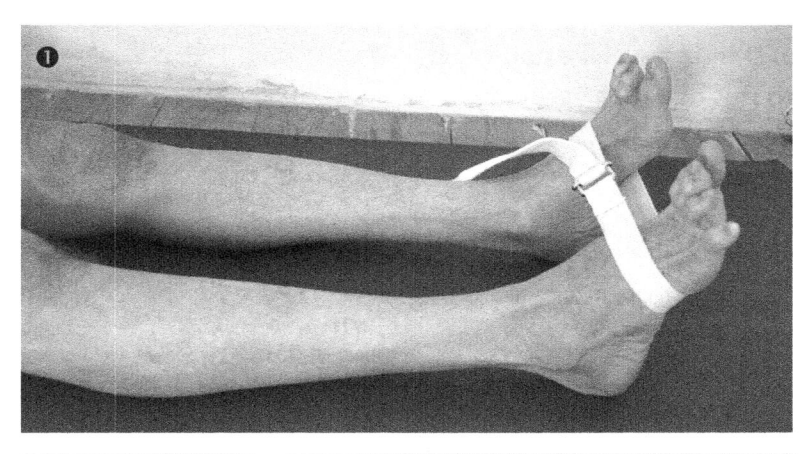

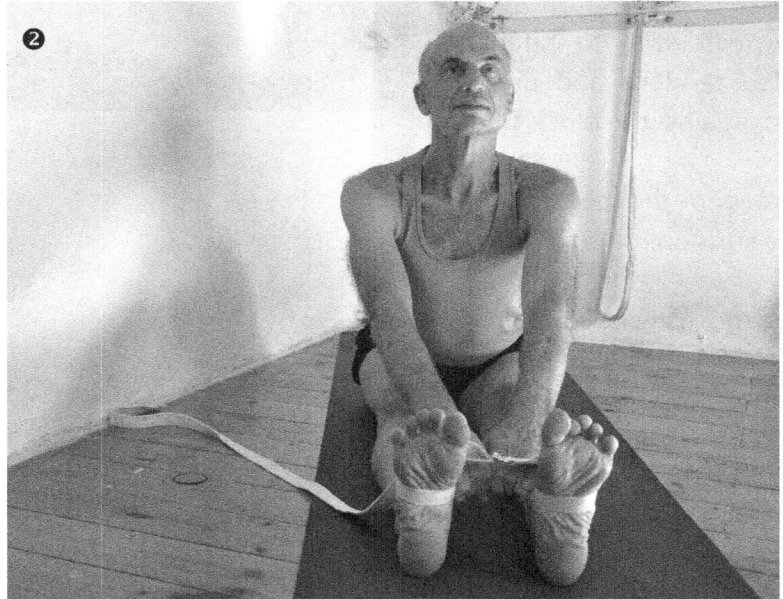

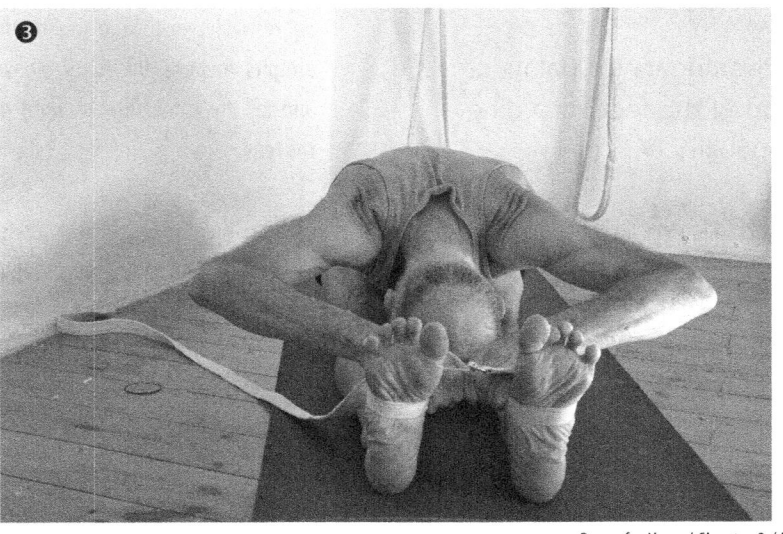

Paschimottānāsana

Variation 5
Opening the backs of the legs: Heels on block

Effects
Supporting the back heels activates and strengthens the legs. It teaches how to press the quadriceps muscles into the thigh bones, and in turn open the backs of the legs and knees. It also teaches to lengthen the Achilles' tendons.

Props
block
blanket (optional)
belt (optional)

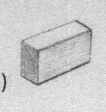

Variation 4 of Dandāsana (see page 8) is similar to this one; but here we add the forward extension.

Note: If your knees are hyper-extended, support the calf muscles as shown in Variation 4 of Dandāsana.

→ Sit in Dandāsana and place the heels on a block.

› Move the heels away to extend the Achilles' tendons and press them down against the block ❶.

› Inhale, broaden the chest and stretch the arms up.

› Exhale and go forward to catch your toes (use a belt if needed). Lift the inner arms, look up and keep the spine concave.

› Inhale, and with exhalation bend forward from the hips while keeping the trunk long.

› Interlock the fingers (or palms or wrists) around the feet according to your capability ❷.

› Push the legs down as you stretch the trunk further.

› Rest the forehead on the shins (use a folded blanket or bolster if needed).

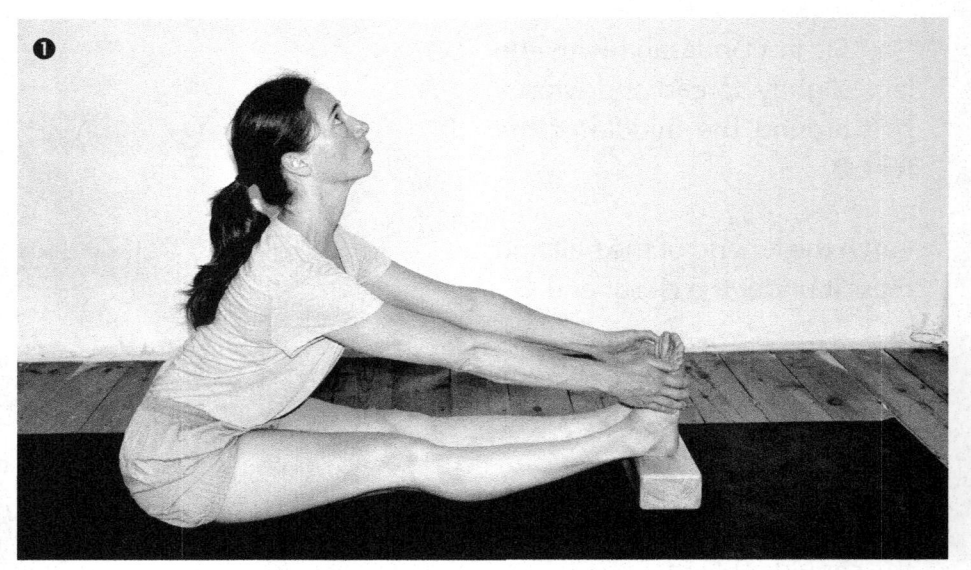

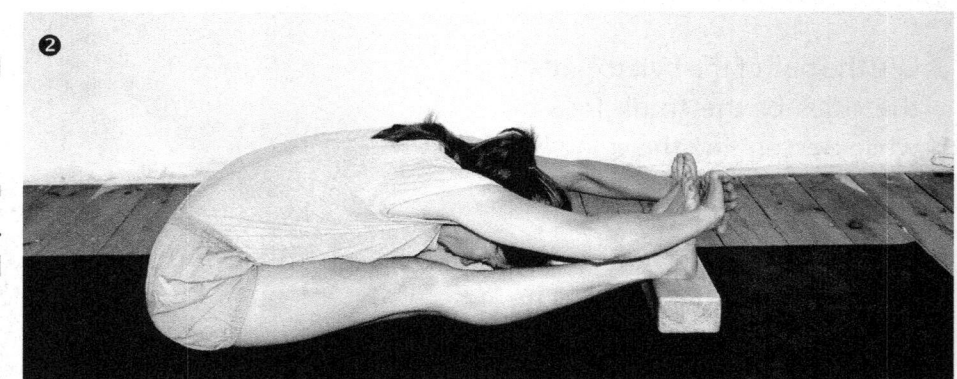

Tips
✓ Do not use the arm muscles aggressively; instead elongate the armpits towards the inner elbows and let the trunk flow forward on the legs.

✓ Flatten the front thigh muscles down so as to touch the bones while broadening the back thigh muscles. Think of the thighs being very heavy, as if weights are placed on top of them (you feel this effect by putting actual weights on the thighs).

Applicability
All forward bends with one or two legs stretched forward

Props
2 chairs

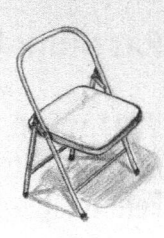

Other options:

⟶ Support both buttock bones and the heels.

› It is possible to use two blocks as shown in Variation 4 of Dandasana.

› Or to use two chairs ❶ & ❷.

Effects: Raising the body on two chairs emphasizes the four bones that you should press down (buttocks and heels). The chair that supports the heels provides anchoring points for the hands. Sitting high has a mental effect which helps to open the back of the knees further. In a therapeutic context, it also allows to hang a weight on the knees (do not do it without a guidance of a certified teacher).

Note: Avoid this variation if your knees are hyper-extended.

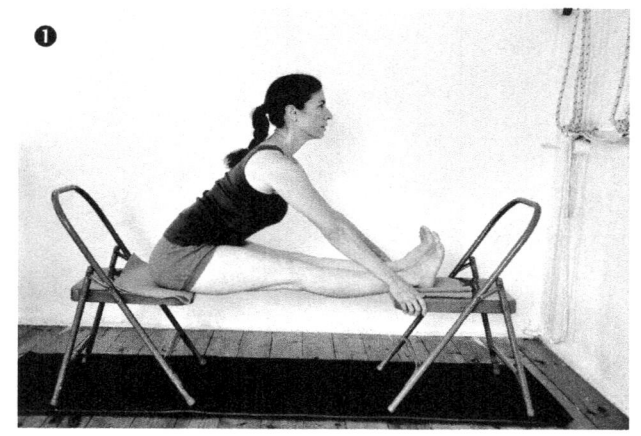

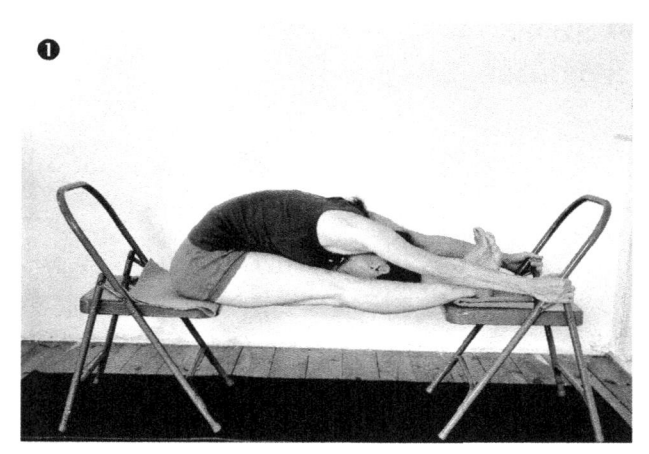

Paschimottānāsana

Variation 6
Anchoring the hands:
Feet on inverted chair

Effects
Pulling the chair against the resistance of the feet enables excellent stretching of the entire trunk forward, and teaches how to use the feet to extend the legs. The slanted seat enables one to adjust the gripping distance according to one's capability. It gives a good stretch of the arms and the trunk, while the elbows are supported on the legs of the inverted chair.

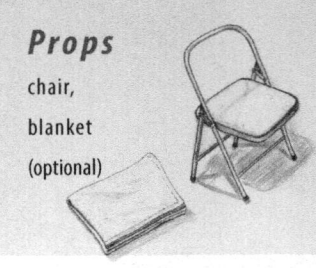

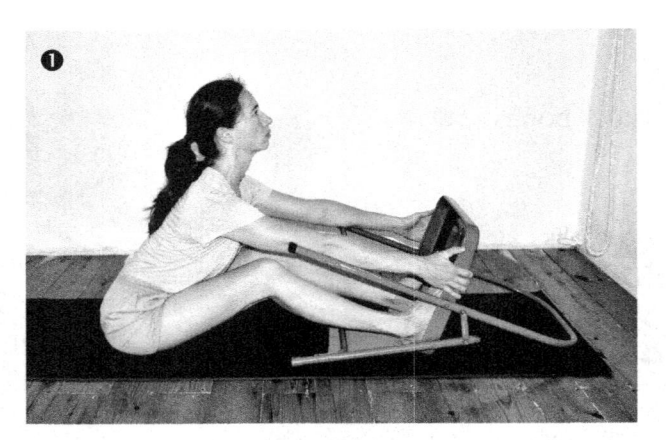

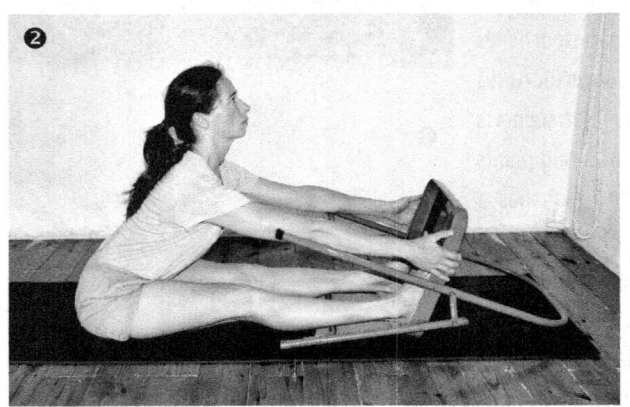

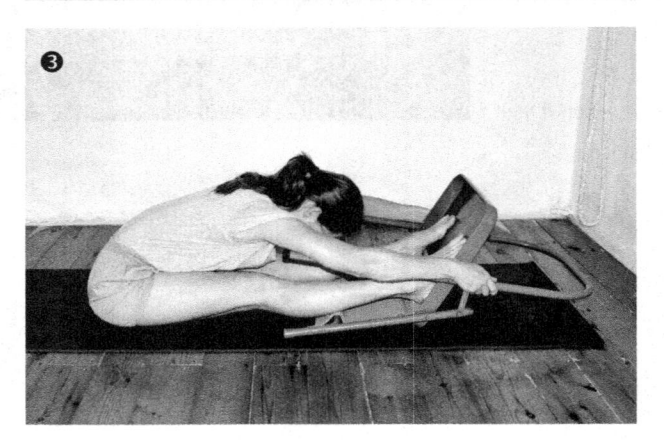

Props
chair, blanket (optional)

⟶ Turn a folded chair upside down, so that its legs are pointing toward you, back legs on the floor.

› Sit in Dandāsana with feet placed on the inverted seat (place a sticky mat piece on the seat if necessary).

› Holding the chair legs, adjust the angle of the seat to support the soles of the feet. Bend your legs and pull the chair ❶. Extend the front of the body and make the spine concave.

› With exhalation straighten the legs while keeping the back concave ❷.

› Lower the trunk on the legs in Paschimottānāsana. Place your elbows on the chair legs. Place the forehead on the chair rung or on a folded blanket ❸.

Paschimottānāsana

Variation 7
Lifting the sides:
Supporting the hips

Effects
The side support stabilizes the pose and provides resistance against which to broaden the pelvic girdle. It also lift the tailbone into the body, thus helps to extend the spine.

Props
2 rolled blanket

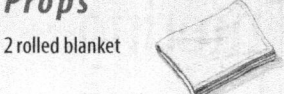

▶ Sit in Dandāsana.

> Tuck two rolled blankets diagonally along the sides of your hips such that the pelvic girdle is held compactly.

> Bend forward into Paschimottānāsana.

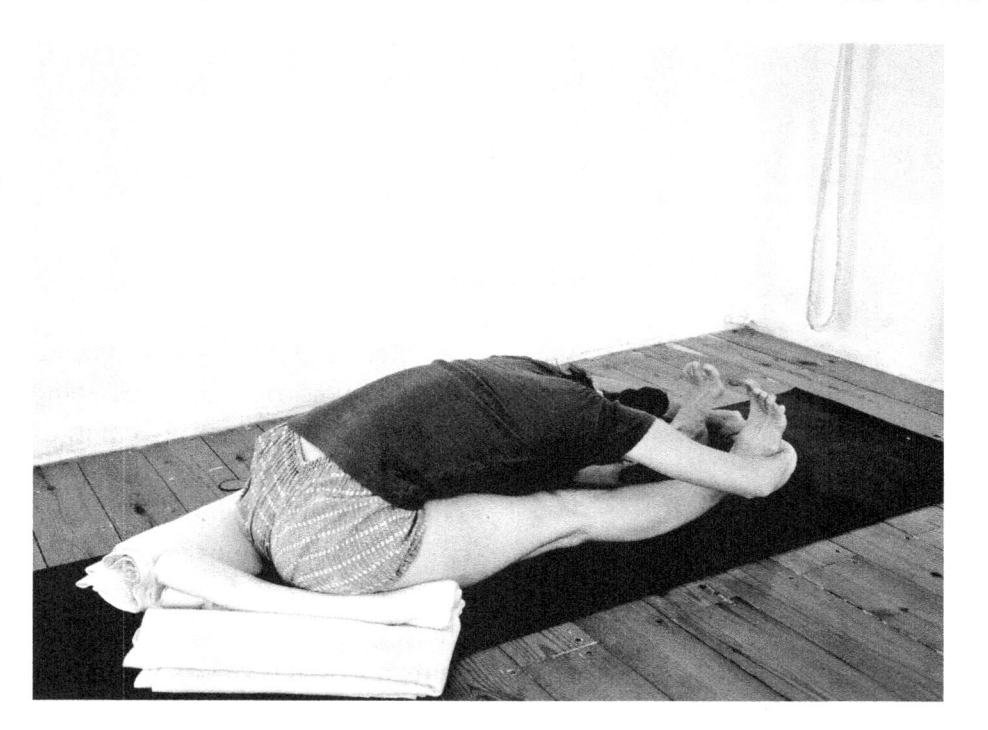

Tips
✓ Go back to Dandāsana, remove the blankets and repeat the pose. Note which muscles you needed to activate in order to re-create the compacting effect after removing the rolled blankets.

Applicability
All forward bends with one or two straight legs (one rolled blanket per straight leg).

Entering the pose with bent legs

The standard way of entering Paschimottānāsana is to keep the legs straight and firm on the floor, and move the trunk toward the legs, until the body is folded into two and the front trunk rests on the legs. If done forcefully, this can make the legs rigid, block the hamstring extension, and exert excessive pulling on the lower back. To achieve comfort in forward bends the hamstrings must be lengthened.

Entering the pose gradually with bent legs helps to lengthen the hamstrings: Sit with bent legs and lay the trunk on the thighs. Then slowly straighten the legs, keeping the trunk close to the thighs. Experience a soft and deep folding of the body into a forward bend. Patiently work to slide the heels forward (or the buttocks backward) in order to straighten the legs.

The following variations demonstrate how to enter the pose with bent legs on the floor. If padding is needed, place the heels and buttock bones on a blanket rather than sticky mat.

Paschimottānāsana

Variation 8
Sliding back into the pose: Hands grasping hooks

Effects
Sliding the buttocks back lengthen the hamstrings, a key point in the forward bends.

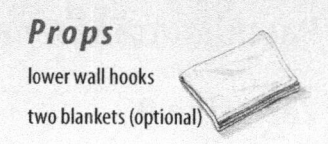

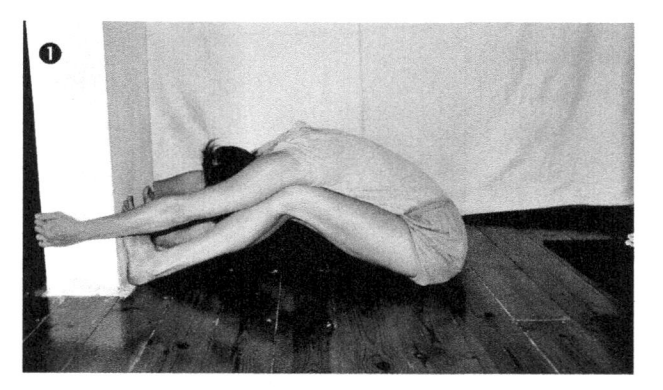

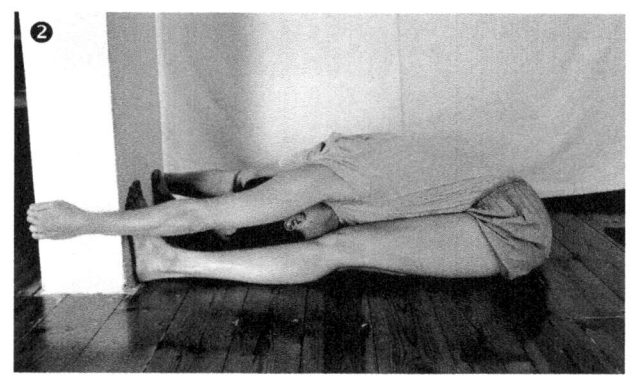

Props
lower wall hooks
two blankets (optional)

⟶ Sit on the floor or place a blanket on the floor (no sticky mat) and sit on it with your feet against the wall facing the hooks (or the column), legs bent.

› Reach forward and hold the wall hooks.

› Extend the trunk forward and lay it on the thighs. Bend the knees as much as needed to have the trunk in contact with the thighs.

› Lower the head and take a few breaths to relax in this intermediate stage ❶.

› Slowly push the wall to slide the buttocks back.

› Keep the trunk on the legs and the head down; keep sliding back until the legs are straight and the forehead rests on the shins ❷ (fold a blanket or bolster for the head rest if needed).

Notes:
When sliding the buttocks, take care not to get the buttock flesh caught under the legs, so as not to tug on the lower back.

If you do not have low wall hooks you can use any graspable heavy object like a column or a Viparita Dandāsana bench; even a closet or a piano can do the job!

Tips

✓ Work gradually. Be careful not to over-stretch the muscles and ligaments of the back of the legs and lower back.

✓ Keep your abdomen soft and breathe smoothly.

✓ When you slide back keep the forehead down and the trunk passive. Work patiently to straighten the legs; with repeated practice you will eventually be able to straighten them while keeping the trunk on the thighs and the forehead on the shins.

Paschimottānāsana

Variation 9
Rolling the pelvis forward: Belt around pelvis and heels

Effects
When sliding the heels forward the belt pushes the upper buttocks region forward this moves the trunk forward from its base. Folding deeply into the pose is done without effort, since the strength of the legs moves the trunk forward. Once the belt is well stretched it gives a framework to the body and makes the pose very stable and relaxing.

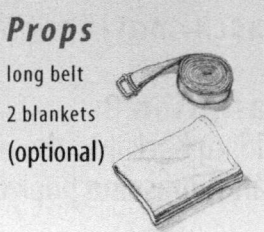

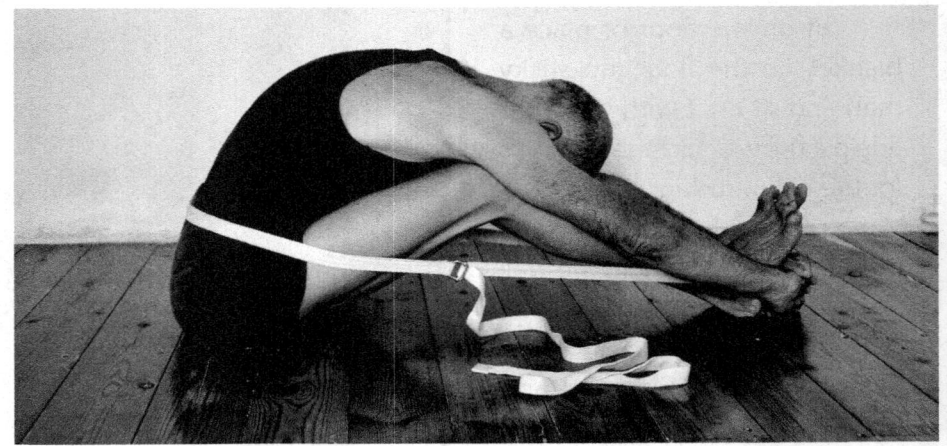

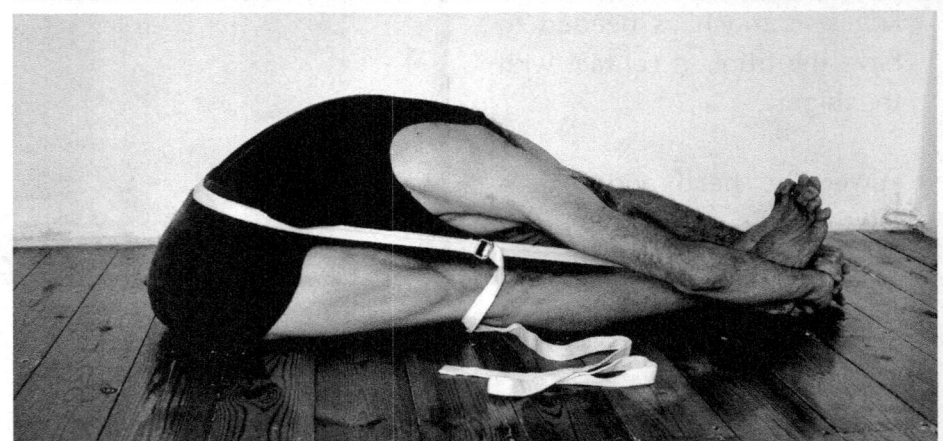

Props
long belt
2 blankets
(optional)

This is quite similar to Variation 3 of Dandāsana, but here the belt is placed slightly above the sacrum.

> Sit in Dandāsana; on the floor or on a folded blanket. Place the heels on a smooth surface, so they can slide.

> Bend the legs. Loop a long belt from the heels to the pelvis just above the sacral band.

> Tighten the belt with bent legs. Adjust as necessary to feel "braced".

> Bend forward from the upper sacral bend, catch your feet and lower the head (if needed use a folded blanket to rest the head).

> Do not allow the trunk to move away from the legs as you slide the heels forward.

> Keep the head down with forehead supported on the shins.

> Stay in the pose and slowly stretch your legs forward; if possible straighten them into Paschimottānāsana.

Tips

✓ To savor the quieting effect of the pose, rest the forehead on a folded blanket (placed on the shins).

✓ If your hamstrings are short you may not be able to straighten the legs and you may be tempted to separate the trunk from the legs – do not do that, but rather stay with your trunk on the legs and patiently check if you can slide the heels slightly forward. With time and persistence, your hamstrings will lengthen and you will be able to straighten the legs without lifting the trunk.

Paschimottānāsana

Variation 10
Rolling the pelvis forward:
Two belts around pelvis and heels

Effects
The lower belt stabilizes the pose; as you slide the heels forward, it pushes the lower back forward into the pose. The second belt helps to move the mid-back forward and down and to elongate the back muscles.

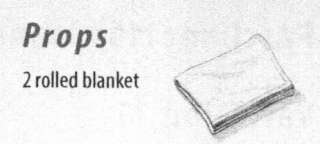

Props
2 rolled blanket

The last variation can be improved by using two long belts:

- Sit in Dandāsana and bend the legs. Loop one long belt around the heels and the pelvis, and another long belt around the heels and mid-back.

- Bend forward to Pādanguṣṭha Dandāsana. Tighten the higher belt according to the new position of the back.

- Move toward the final pose and tighten the belt such that it supports the back in the new position.

- Keep bending forward in increments, shortening the belt to support the back as you progress toward Paschimottānāsana.

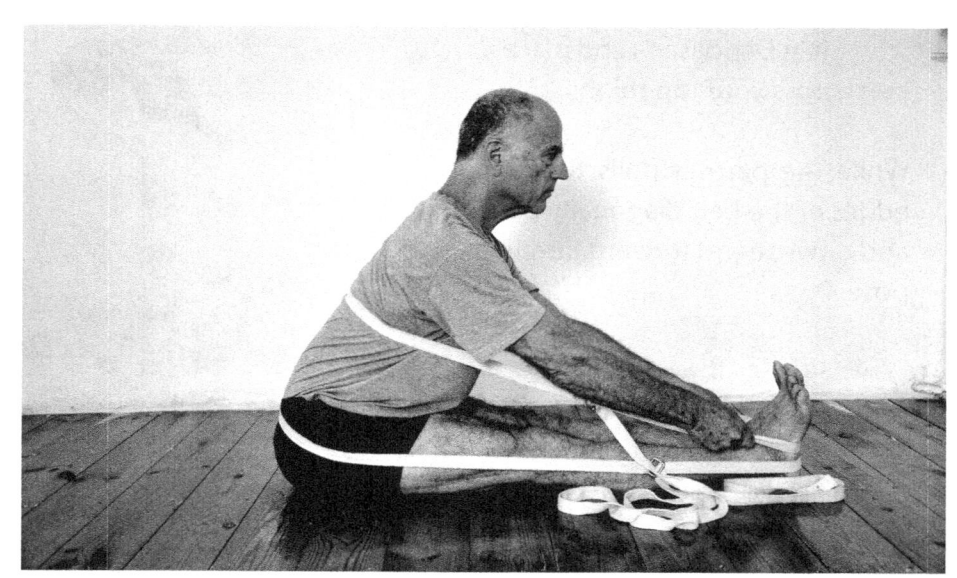

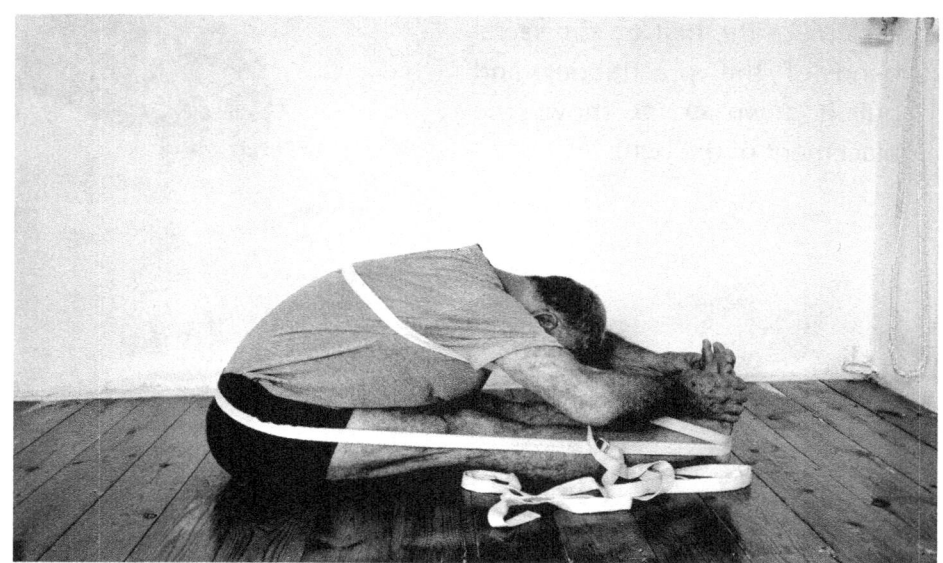

Tips
✓ Use your breathing to advance in the pose: Inhale and broaden the chest; exhale and perform a slight Uddiyana Kriyā to go deeper into the pose. Repeat this for several breath cycles until you settle in the pose.

Uddiyana Kriyā
Uddiyana Kriyā means activation of the abdominal muscles in order to suck the abdominal organs in and move them up (toward the chest). Note that this is not Bandha (which means lock), but Kriyā (which means activation).

Applicability
All the basic forward extensions.

Paschimottānāsana

Variation 11
Anchoring the base:
Partner pulls back and down

Effects
The pull clarifies the directions involved in the pose; the groins should be soft and stable and descend down. The buttock bones should not lift. The lower back should remain round and quiet. From this base the trunk can be extended forward without disturbing the quietness of the pose.

Props
partner
belt

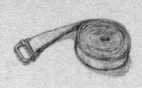

→ Sit in Dandāsana and place a belt across your top thighs.

> While the partner pulls the two edges of the belt diagonally back and down, bend forward into the pose ❶.

> *Note:* If you have a low wall hook you can use it for the belt anchoring and do this variation on your own.

> Another option for the partner is to place the belt on the sacral band of the practitioner and pull it down ❷ (❸ shows the placement of the belt).

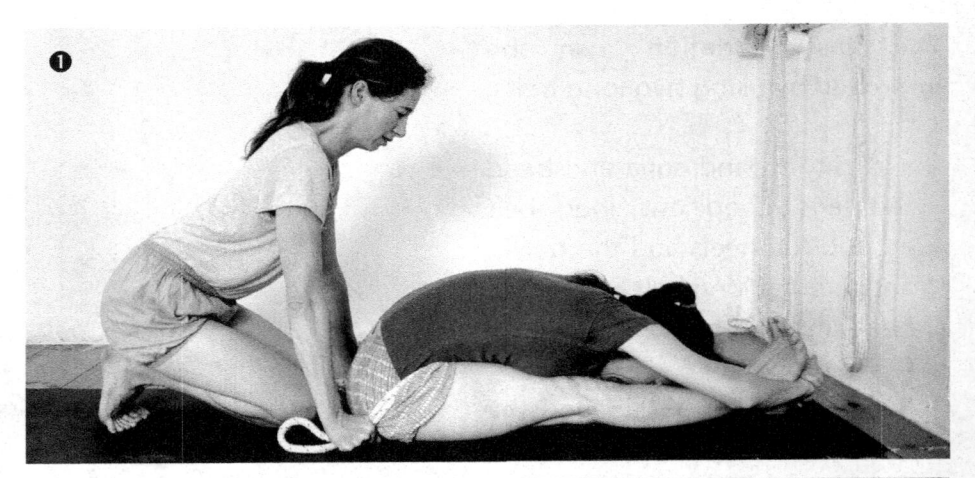

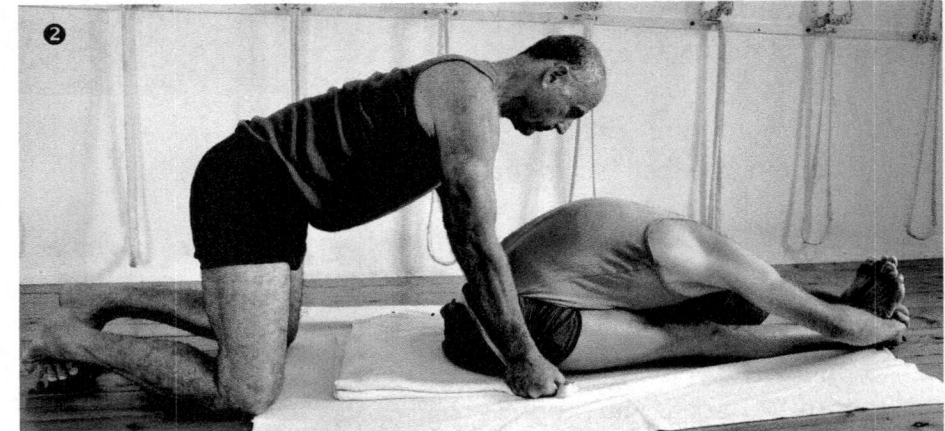

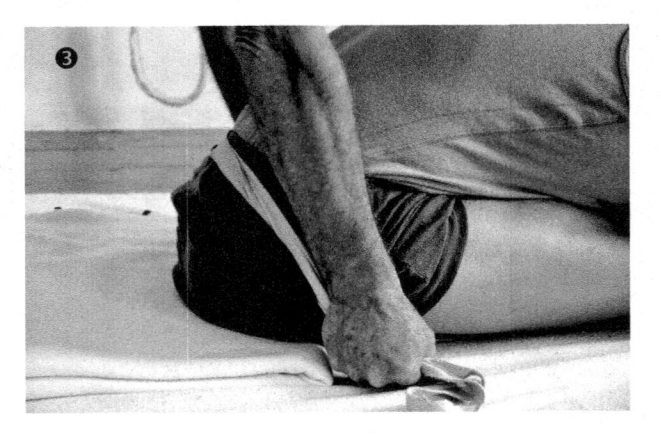

Tips
✓ Sense the quietness that the pull induces; then ask the partner to release the pull and learn to generate a similar sensation on your own.

Paschimottānāsana

Variation 12
Bending deeper into the pose:
Belt around thighs and back

Effects
The belt helps to fold deeper into the pose and to stay in it effortlessly.
Extended, relaxed stay in the pose lengthens the hamstring muscles.

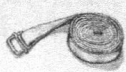

The contact of the belt allows you to sense the shape of the back.

Props
belt

Note: This is an advanced variation for people who can bend easily into the pose.

→ Sit in Dandāsana; bend slightly forward and bend the legs. Then tighten a belt around the thighs and the back. Keep the buckle on your side.

> Slowly stretch the legs with concave upper back (to Pādanguṣṭha Daṇḍāsana).

> Bend forward into Paschimottānāsana, tightening the belt as you move forward and down.

Note: An alternative to this variation is to place heavy weights on the back (or have a partner do Mayurāsana on your back, like in the famous Pl. 162 of LOY).

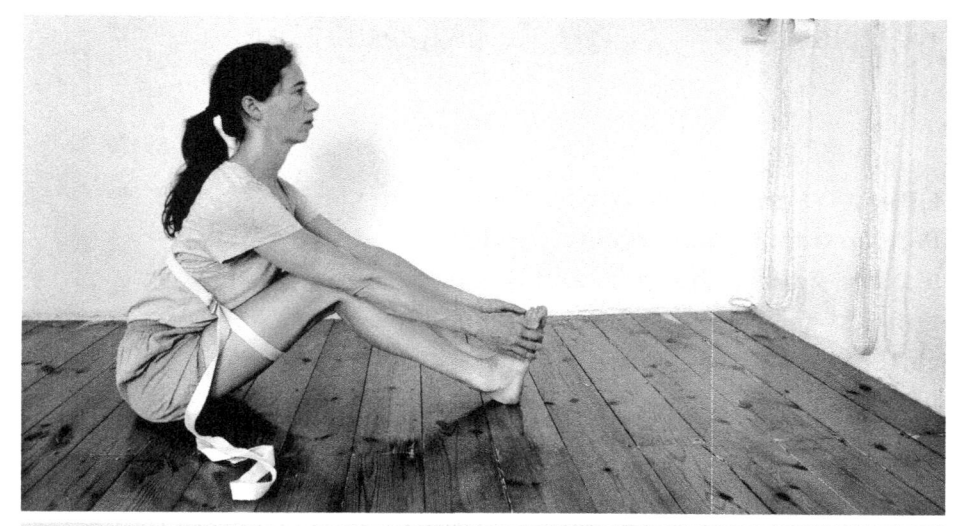

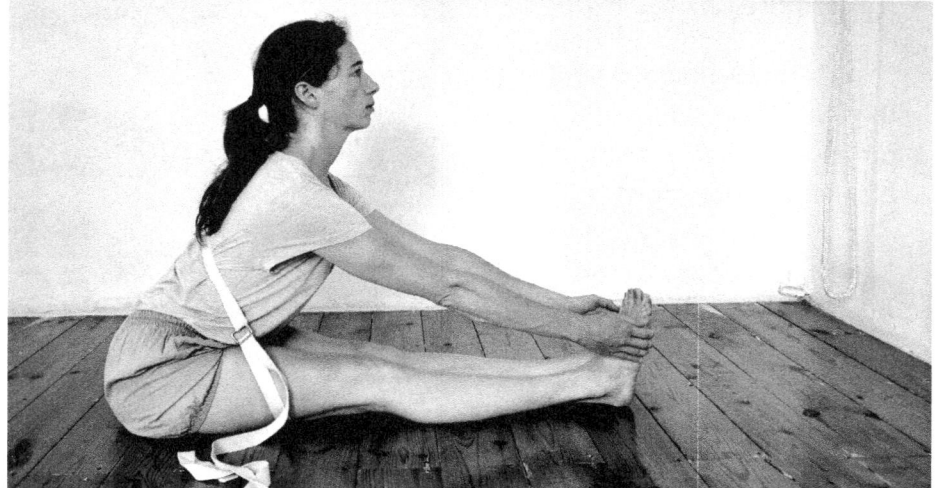

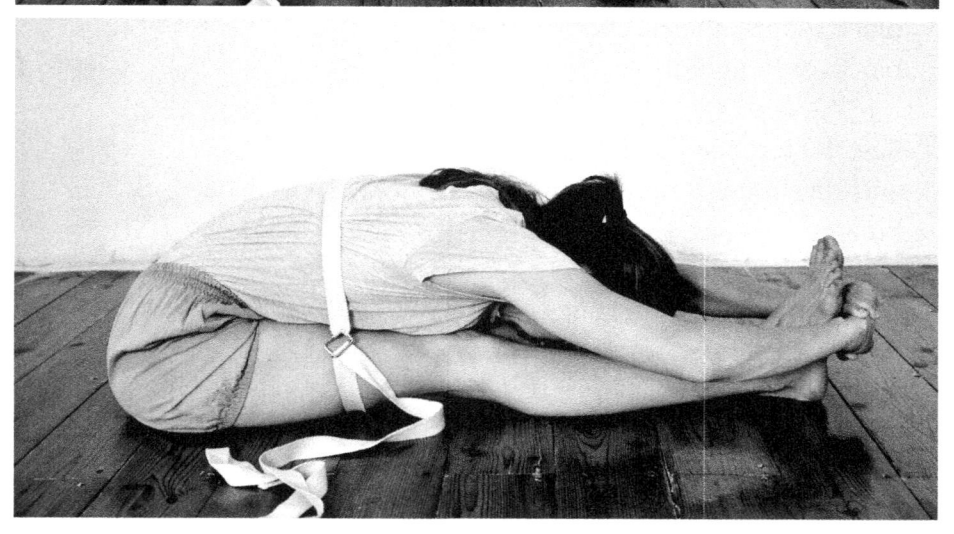

Restorative Paschimottānāsana

Variation 13
Opening the sides of the body: Supporting the elbows with blocks

Effects
The blocks support the elbows and help lifting the upper arms and shoulders. When done this way, the pull of the arms opens and stretches the sides of the body and widens the back.

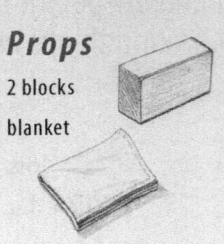

Props
2 blocks
blanket

Lifting the elbows in Paschimottānāsana opens and lifts the sides of the trunk and the armpits; this helps to move the vertebrae into the body and to flatten the back. The blocks help this action and provide supports for the elbows for extended stays in the āsana.

→ Sit in Dandāsana and place the two blocks symmetrically, one on each side of the legs. Place a blanket on your shins.

› Bend the elbows, widen and lift them as you move forward to Paschimottānāsana.

› Hold the feet and place each elbow on the corresponding block. Adjust the position of the blocks as required.

› Rest the forehead on the blankets and stay in the pose with smooth breathe.

Note: An inverted chair can also be used to support the elbows; this was shown in Variation 5 above.

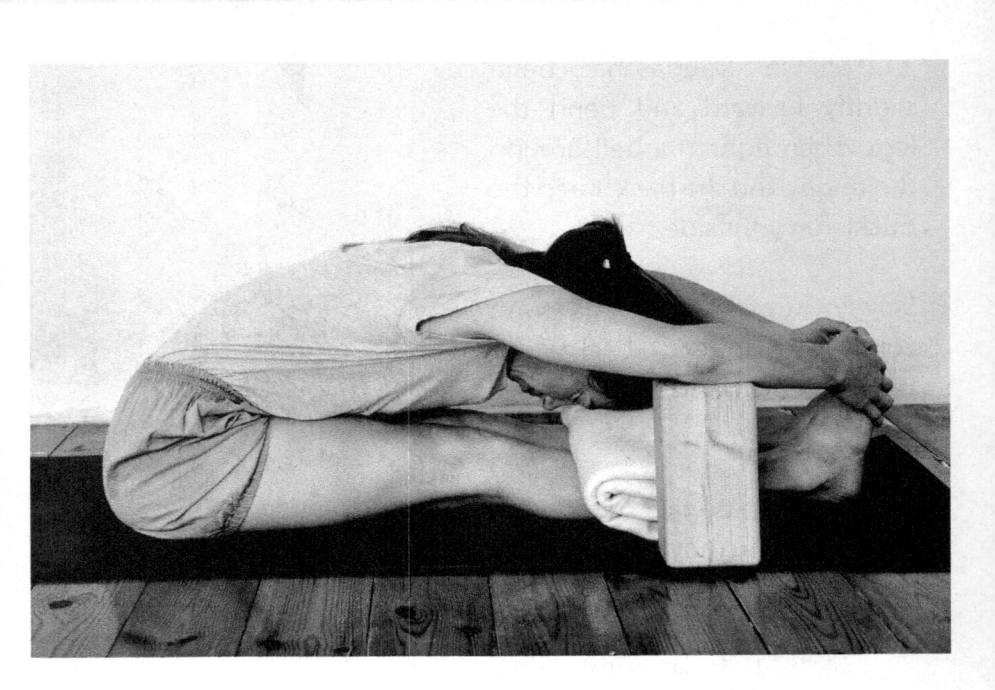

Tips
✓ Extend the sides of the trunk to the middle of the armpits, lower the armpits down. Widen the elbows by extending the inner arms from the center of the armpits to the inner elbows.

✓ To re-create the effect without the blocks, rotate the elbows upward as your chest goes down. Make sure the elbows and the shoulder blades are at the same level.

Restorative Paschimottānāsana Variation 14
Relaxing the head: Forehead on chair

Effects
The head support relaxes and cools the brain. Using a chair gives a high support which creates space in the trunk and allows for smooth breathing. The chair also provides many options for the hand grip, thus enabling a range of experiences, from active stretching to passive resting.

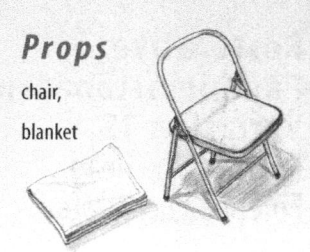

Props
chair, blanket

> Sit in Dandāsana in front of the chair and place your feet against the back rung. Prepare a folded blanket on the seat to support the head.

> *Note:* if the back rung is too high, place a wooden block on the floor in front of it and press the feet against it. If there is no back rung, you can replace it by tightening a belt across the back legs of the chairs.

> Hold the sides of the seat and pull to extend the trunk forward.

> Exhale and bend forward. Move the hands to grip the backrest of the chair.

> Lower the trunk and rest the forehead on the seat ❶.

> *Note:* If needed, a bolster or a block may be used for head support.

> To go further in the pose, grip the back edge of the seat with your hands.

> To go still further, grip the back legs of the chair and stretch forward, inserting your head and trunk below the seat. Rest your forehead on the front rung ❷.

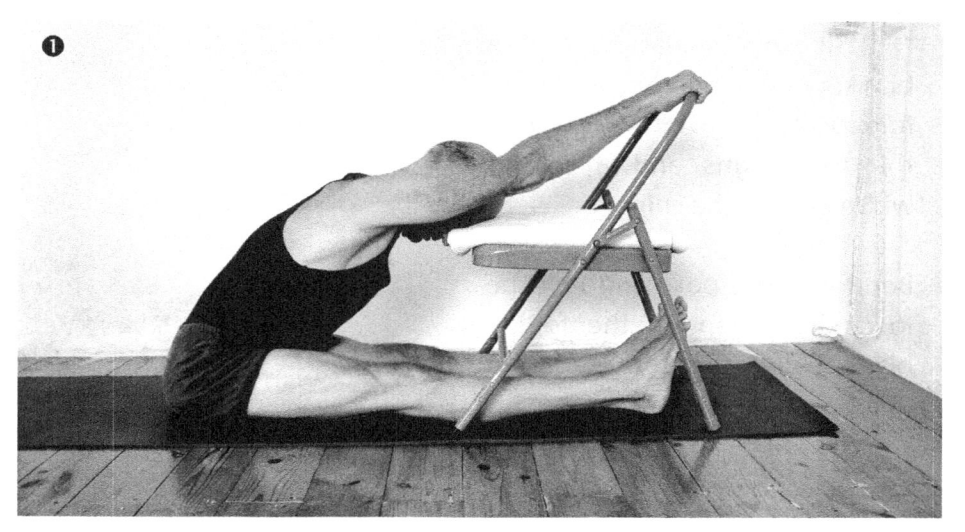

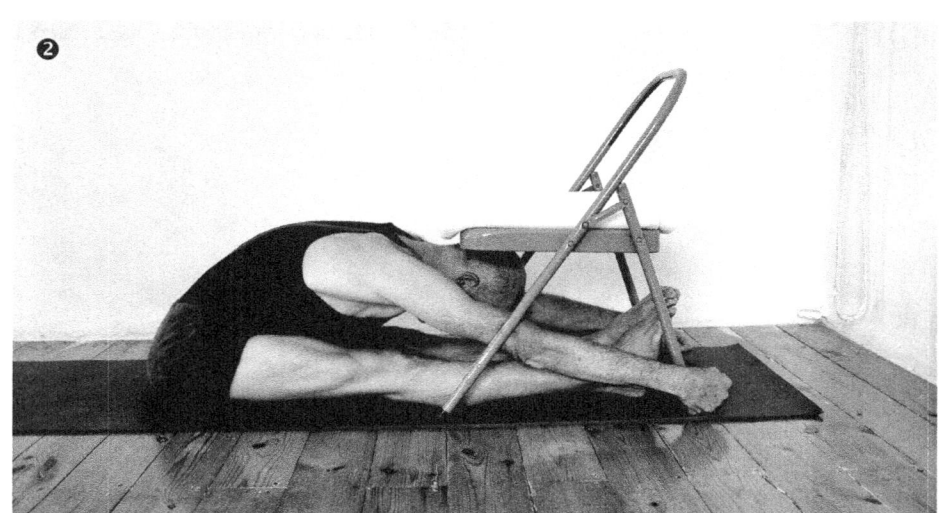

Tips
Try different hand positions and see the effects on your stretching.

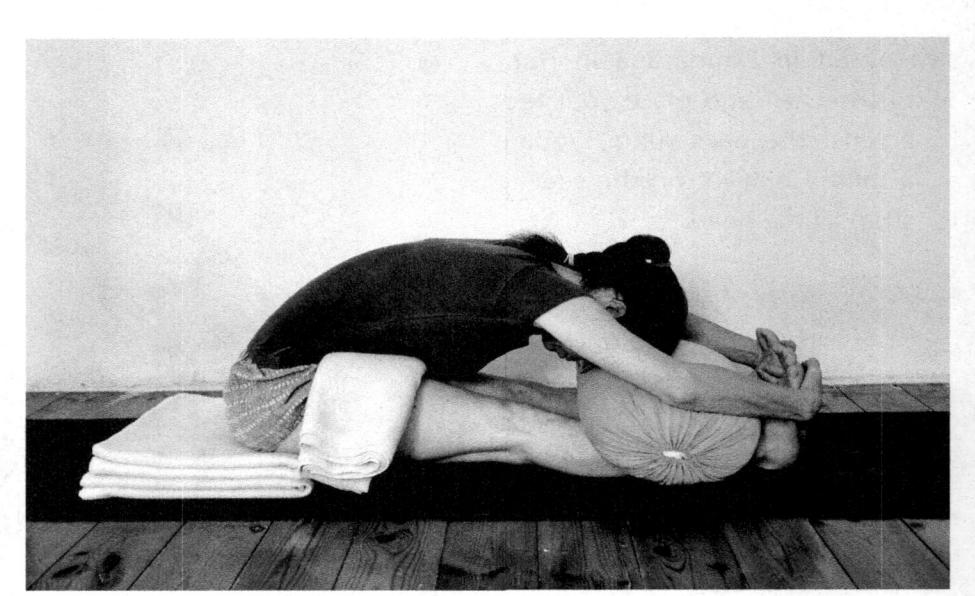

Restorative Paschimottānāsana Variation 15
Relaxing the head: Forehead on bolster

Effects
the bolster provides very soft support and hence induces relaxation and placidity. The blanket, supporting the abdomen and lower back, increases the soothing effect of the pose.

Props
bolster
2-3 blankets

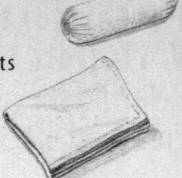

→ Sit in Dandāsana on a blanket or two and place a three-folded blanket widthwise across the top thighs and a bolster widthwise on the shins.

› Bend into the pose and rest the lower abdomen on the folded blanket and the forehead and elbows on the bolster.

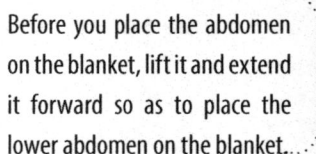

Tips
✓ Before you place the abdomen on the blanket, lift it and extend it forward so as to place the lower abdomen on the blanket.

Restorative Paschimottānāsana Variation 16
Using gravity: Sitting on a chair

Effects
The gravitational pull helps the back muscles to extend gradually.

Props
chair
wall
belt (optional)
bolster or folded blanket

⟹ Place a chair on a sticky mat in front of the wall. Place a sticky mat on the seat and sit on the front edge in Daṇḍāsana, feet against the wall.

› Place a bolster on the top shins.

› Bend forward, hold the feet, make the back concave and look forward to the wall. If you do not reach your feet, use a belt to hook the feet ❶.

> *Note:* Note: If you happen to have upper wall hooks, you can use them to extend the trunk as shown in ❷. This is especially beneficial for people suffering from back pain due to compression of the vertebrae.

› Bend further forward and rest the forehead on the support ❸.

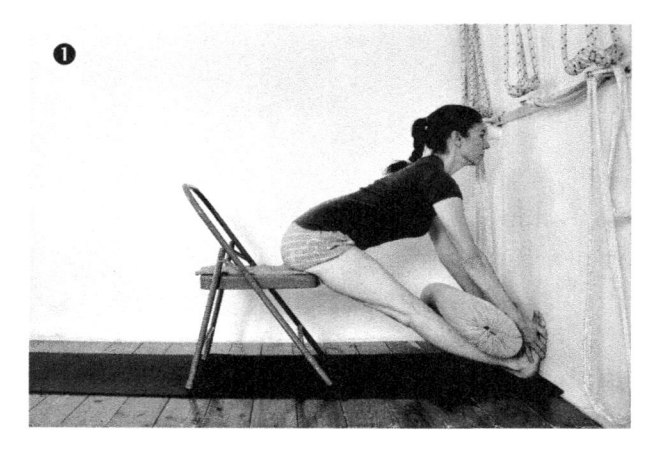

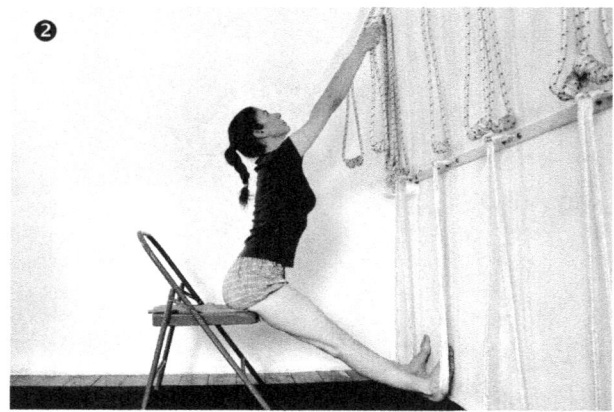

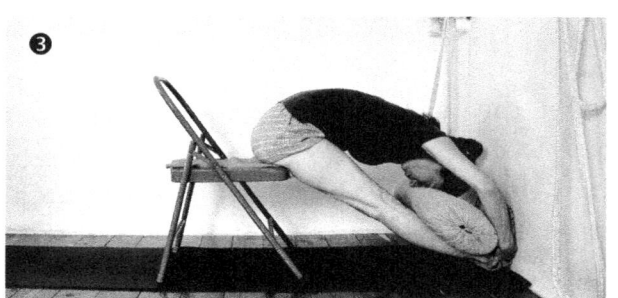

Tips
✓ Keep the groins and the abdomen soft as the trunk is lowered to the legs.

Props for Yoga / Chapter 3 / Restorative Paschimottānāsana 115

Using Wall Ropes

Note: The following three variations are advanced and require good flexibility and coordination.

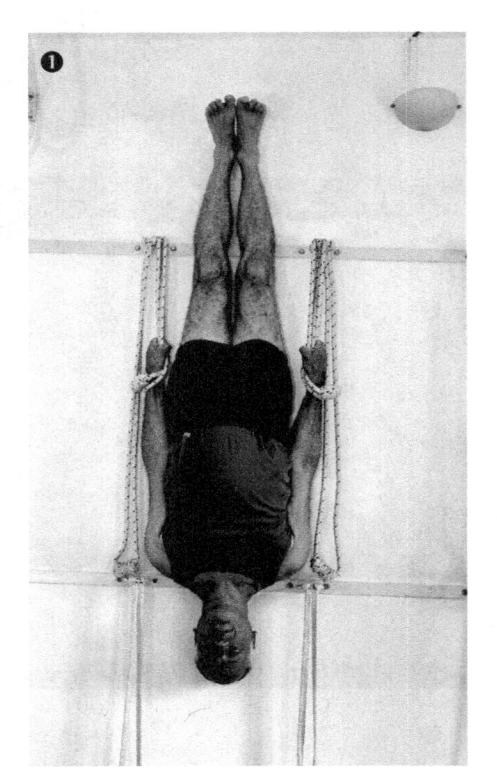

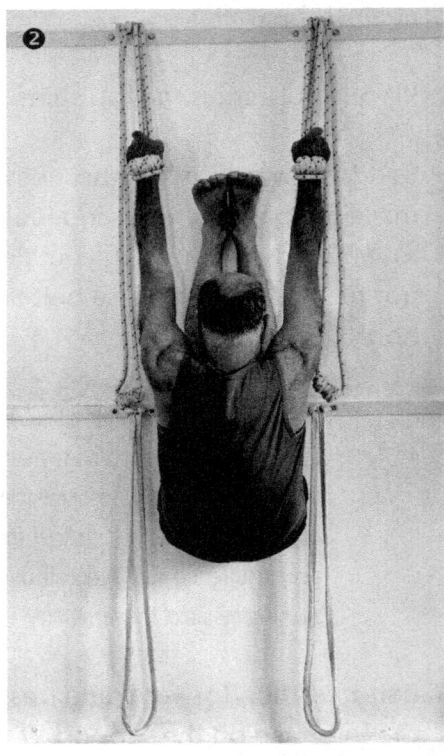

Ūrdhva Mukha Paschimottānāsana Variation 1
Ūrdhva Mukha Paschimottānāsana I
Using wall ropes

Effects
The weight of the body helps to fold into the pose; this variation improves the flexibility of the back and the stretches the backs of the legs almost effortlessly.

Props
wall ropes, partner (optional)

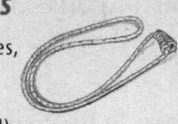

This variation is a good preparation for Paschimottānāsana, as gravity helps to fold the body.

The standard top wall ropes should be folded into two for this variation.

⟶ Catch the ropes and climb on the wall.

> Option: climb up until the whole body is inverted in hanging Adho Mukha Vṛkṣāsana ❶.

> Then slide the buttocks down to fold into Ūrdhva Mukha Paschimottānāsana I (LOY Pl. 168)❷.

> A helper sitting on a mat can help you fold into the pose while reducing the load on your arms. This is very useful as it releases load from the hands, and helps to bend deeper into the pose ❸.

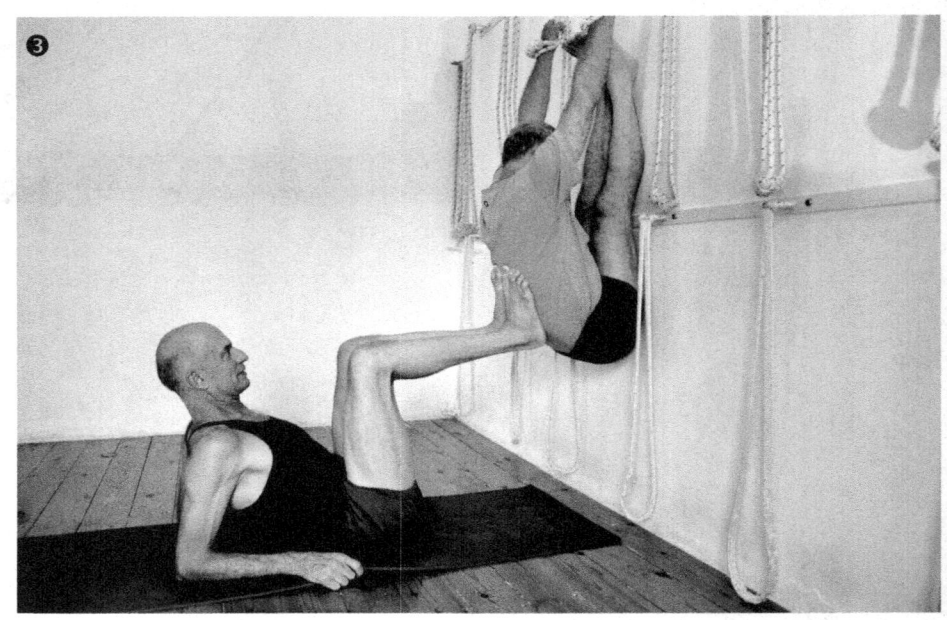

116 Props for Yoga / Chapter 3 / Restorative Paschimottānāsana

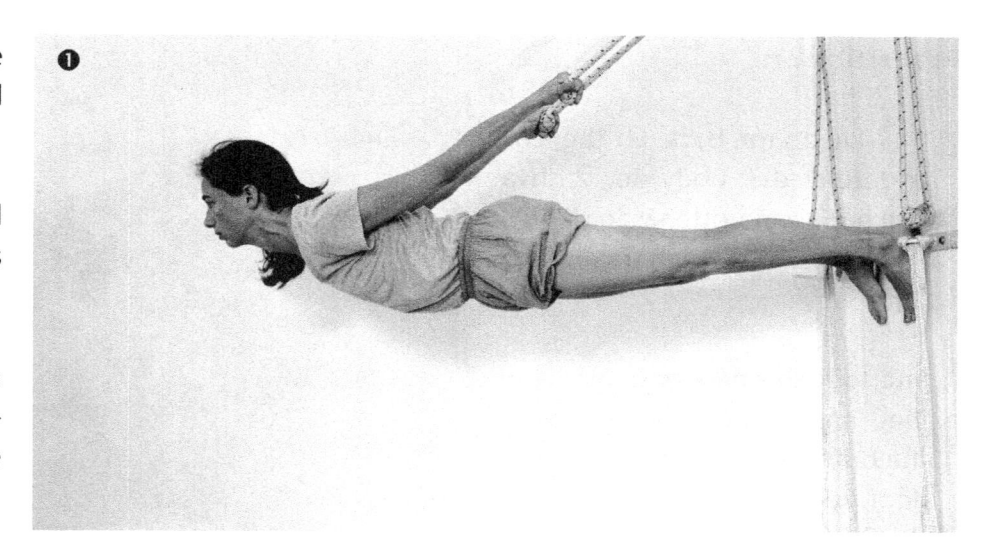

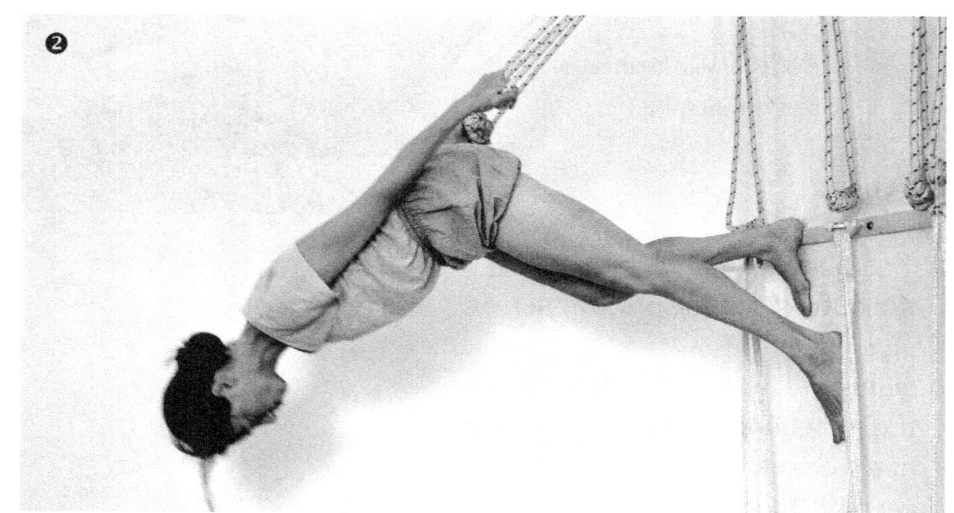

Ūrdhva Mukha Paschimottānāsana Variation 2
Ūrdhva Mukha Paschimottānāsana II
Using wall ropes

Effects
The gravitational pull helps to fold the body. The challenge of entering the pose in this way develops coordination and confidence.

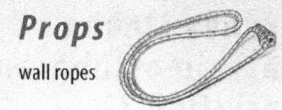

Props
wall ropes

> Stand with your back to the wall and catch the upper wall ropes.

> Climb with your feet pressed against the wall until the body is parallel to the floor ❶.

> Now, simultaneously, step down on the wall and fold the body – coordinate the stepping with the folding ❷.

> Roll the buttocks down and fold into Ūrdhva Mukha Paschimottānāsana II (LOY Pl. 170) ❸.

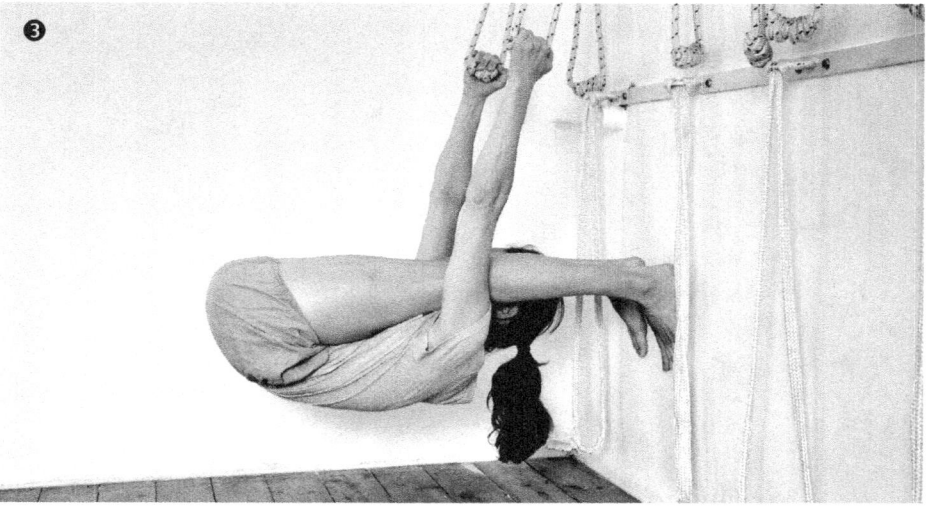

Ūrdhva Mukha Paschimottānāsana Variation 3
Ūrdhva Mukha Paschimottānāsana II
Helper presses down

Effects
Extends and tones the back muscles and hamstrings. The external weight induced by the helper allows you to fold deeper into the pose, keeping the groins and the abdomen very soft.

Props
blanket
belt (optional)
partner

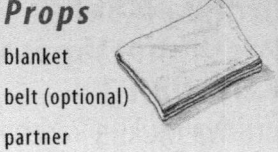

Practitioner:

⟶ Lie on the back, lift the legs and fold the body to Ūrdhva Mukha Paschimottānāsana II (LOY Pl. 170); keep the legs straight and tight.

› Interlock the fingers behind the feet and simultaneously lower the buttocks and feet toward the floor, keeping the legs parallel to the floor.

Note: If your hands do not reach your feet, use a belt.

Partner:

⟶ Place a folded blanket on the buttocks of the practitioner.

› Simultaneously and gently push the practitioner's buttocks and heels or ankles toward the floor, keeping the legs parallel to the floor.

Note: choose a partner of your same gender.

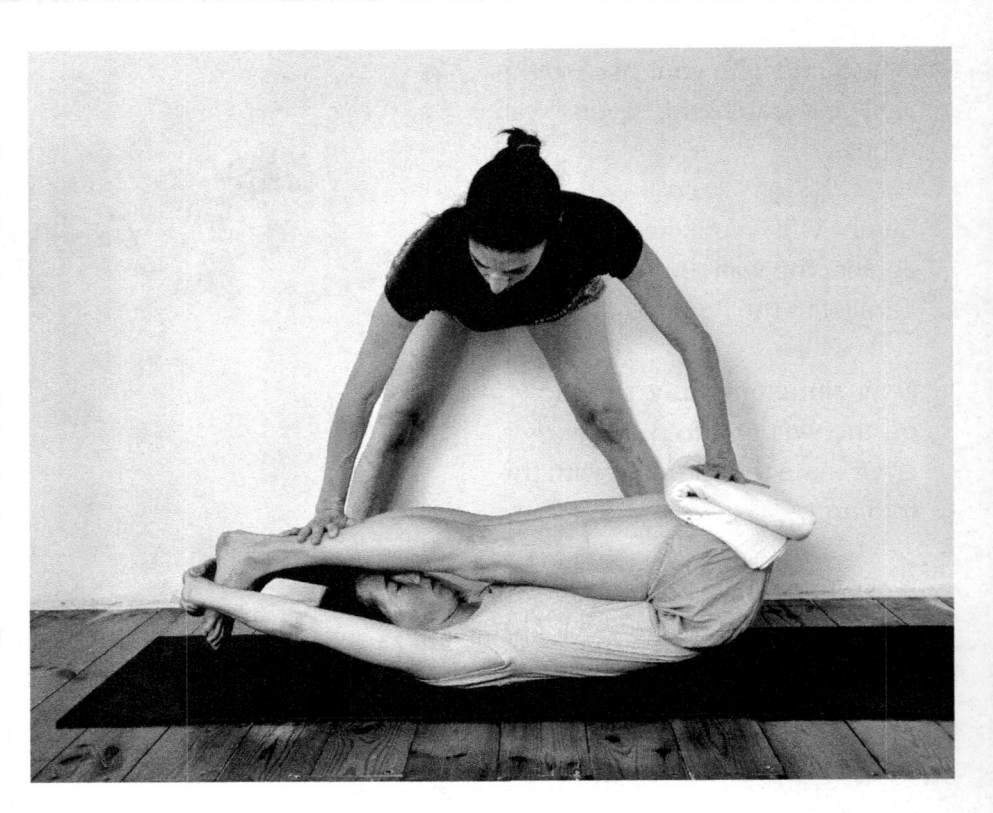

Tips

✓ Open the backs of the knees and stretch the legs well as the partner pushes you down.

✓ As much as possible keep the back on the floor (do not go toward Halāsana).

Jānu Śīrṣāsana
About Jānu Śīrṣāsana

Jānu Śīrṣāsana is a non-symmetrical pose, which requires simultaneous action in several axes. Bending one leg and rolling the thigh out, tends to pull the corresponding side of the trunk back and make it more convex. Nevertheless, we still inspire to keep the back as symmetrical as the back of Paschimottānāsana. This is challenging and requires practice. The following variations help to learn these actions.

> ⚠ **CAUTIONS**
>
> To protect the hamstrings muscles, always open the knee of the outstretched leg completely, extending it evenly on all sides. Do not allow the thigh of that leg to lift off the floor.
>
> If you have a knee injury or suffer from knee pain avoid doing this pose or ask advice from a knowledgeable teacher.
>
> If your hamstrings are over extended and feel sore, work softly in order to prevent injury.

Jānu Śīrṣāsana

Variation 1
Turning sideways:
Using a belt

Effects
The belt provides leverage for the turning action.

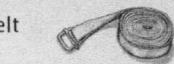

Props
belt

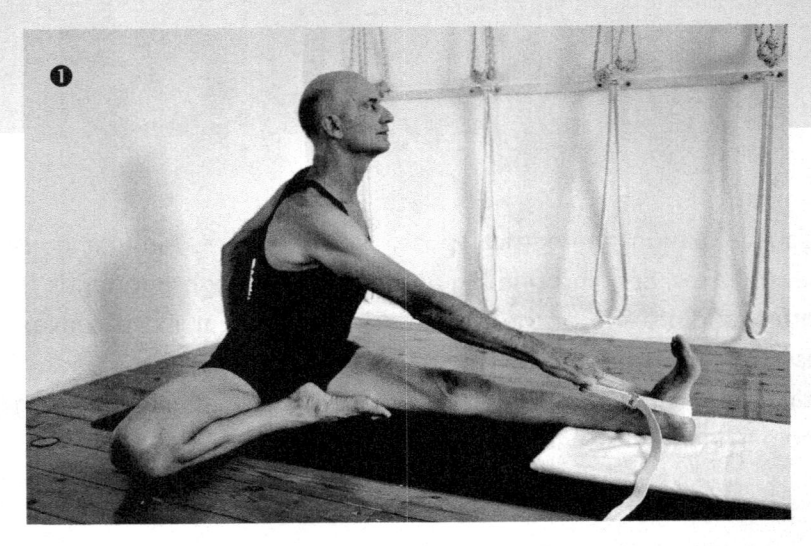

This is a preparatory stage in which one learns to turn the body sideways until it faces the straight leg.

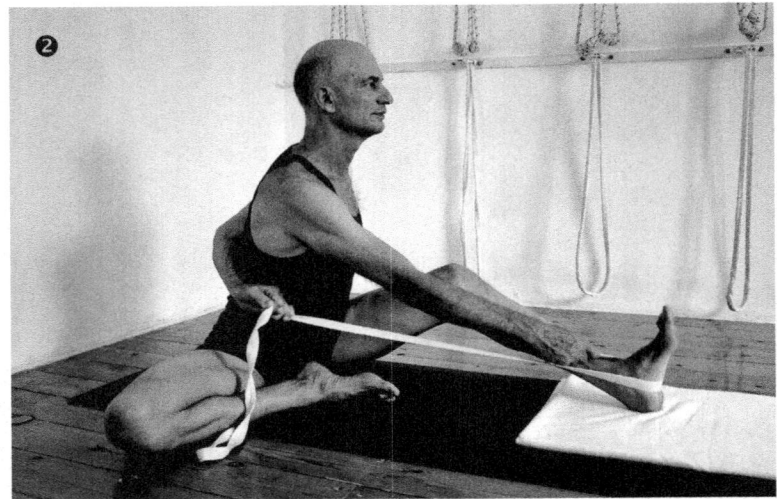

To do the pose with the right leg bent:

⟶ Sit in Dandāsana and bend the right leg to the right side.

› Place a belt on the left foot and catch it with your right hand.

› Place the left hand on the floor and use the hands to turn the trunk from right to left ❶.

› Now make a small loop and take the long loose end of the belt around the right side of the trunk to your back.

› Bend slightly the left knee, move the left arm behind the back and catch the belt with your left hand. Catch it as far and deep as you can behind the back ❷.

› As you straighten the left leg, roll the left shoulder back and turn the trunk from right to left ❸.

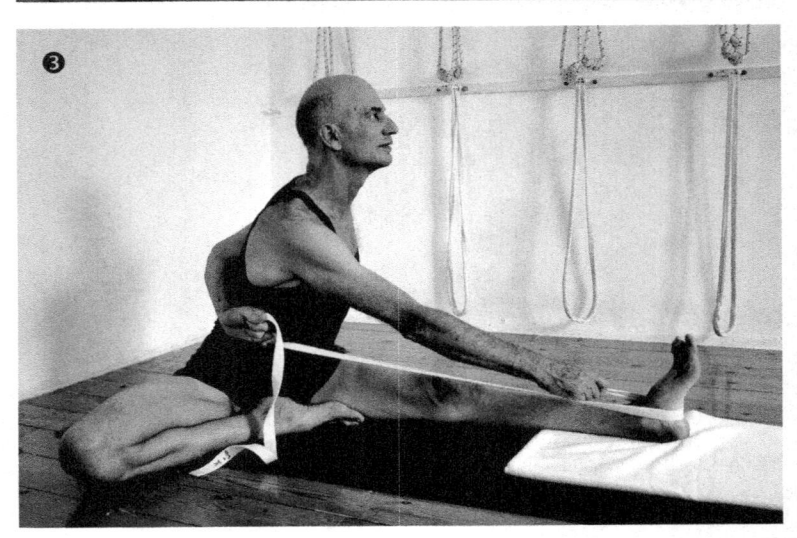

Applicability
Ardha Padma Paschimottānāsana,
Triaṅga Mukhaikapāda Paschimottānāsana,
Marīchyāsana

120 Props for Yoga / Chapter 3 / Jānu Śīrṣāsana

Jānu Śīrṣāsana

Variation 2
Rolling the bent leg out:
Using bolster against the heel

Effects
Placing the heel against the bolster teaches to move the knee back to form an obtuse angle between the thighs.

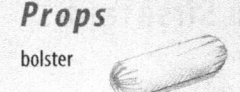

Props
bolster

Turning sideways as shown in Variation 1 above is challenging when the bent leg is rolled out and moved back. *Light on Yoga* says: "The angle between the two legs should be obtuse." (Para. 3 of the Technique for this pose). This means that the right thigh should be moved more the 90° sideways and the right heel should be place next to the right groin.

This preparatory stage teaches to place the bent leg at the correct angle.

To do the pose with the right leg bent:

➤ Place a bolster across the mat and sit in Dandāsana on its right edge.

➤ Bend the right leg by folding it from the inner knee. Move the knee back and place the heel against the right side of the bolster, next to the right groin ❶.

> **Note:** If the knee cannot be kept on the floor rest it on a folded blanket.

➤ Using your hands, rotate the waist and chest until your entire trunk faces the left leg.

➤ Inhale, open the chest, and with exhalation bend forward into the pose ❷.

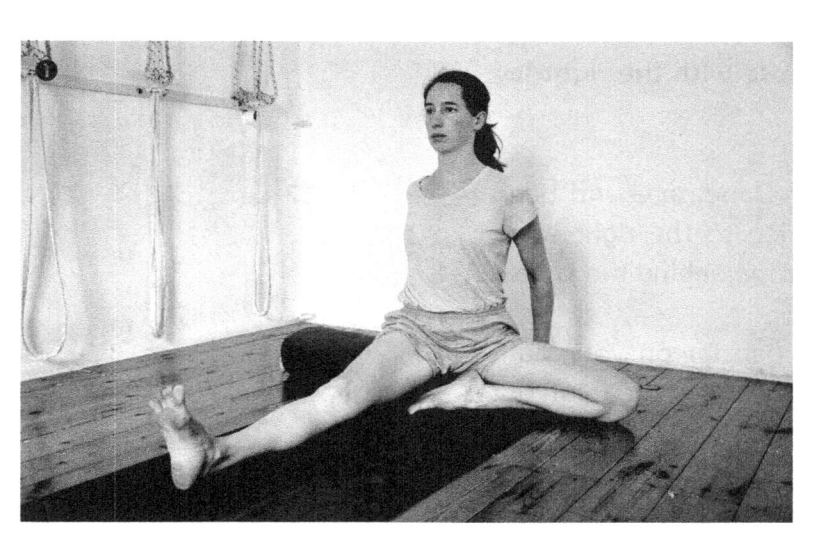

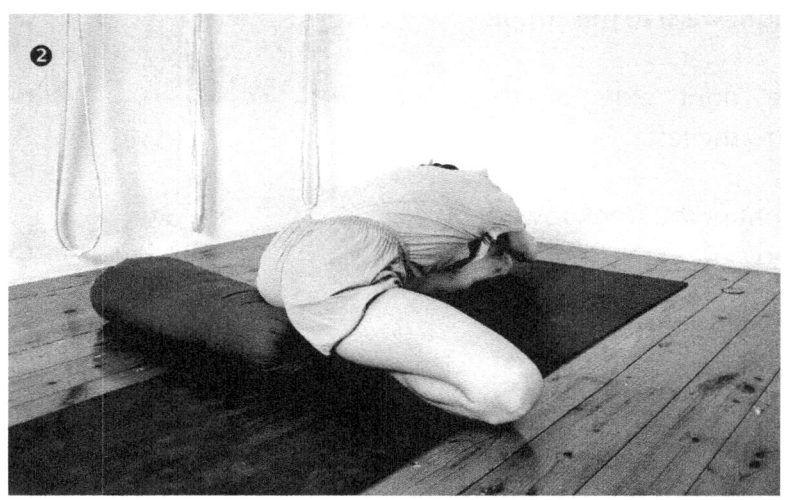

Notes:
If needed, place a folded blanket or another bolster under your forehead.

To turn more to the left, try to place the right cheek on the head support.

Props for Yoga / Chapter 3 / Jānu Śīrṣāsana 121

Jānu Śīrṣāsana

Variation 3
Rolling the bent leg out:
Partner pulls the thigh back

Effects
Rolling the thigh back with one end of the rope helps to create the bi-directional stretch of this pose (the thigh rolls back while the trunk moves forward). At the same time, the other end of the belt extends the inner thigh.

Props
partner
rope
(or belt)

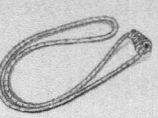

To do the pose with the right leg bent:

⟶ Sit in Daṇḍāsana and bend the right leg to the right while placing a rope behind the knee.

> Have the partner on your right pull the rope to roll the thigh out and back.

> Extend the right side of the trunk, from the right waist to the armpit.

> Move the right side of the abdomen to the left.

> Roll the front of the trunk toward the left leg and extend forward into the pose.

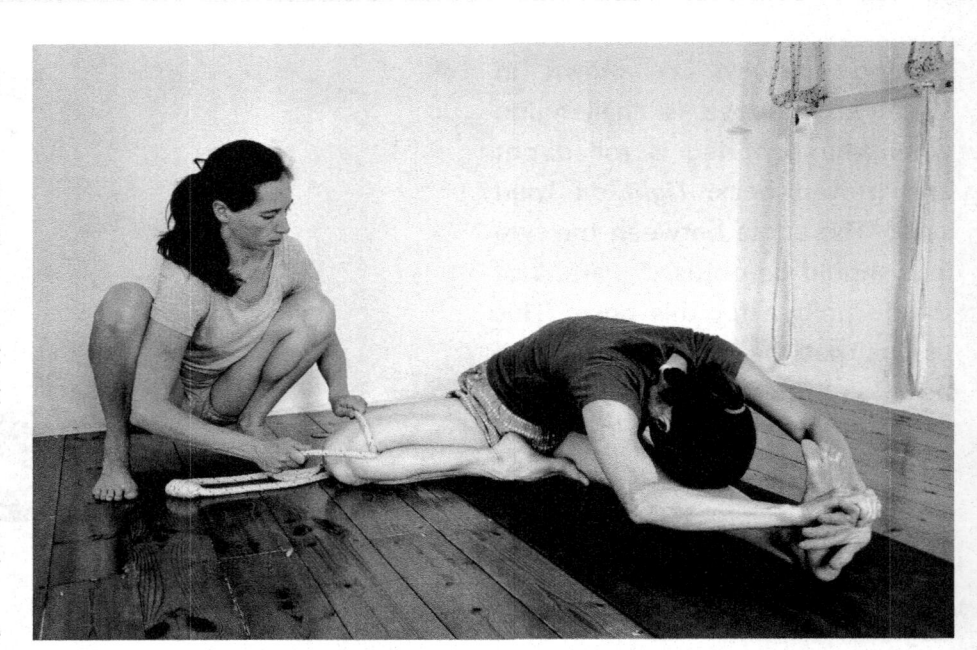

Tips
✓ When helping, separate the two ends of the rope and use one of them to extend the inner knee out, and the other to roll the thigh back (see photo).

Jānu Śīrṣāsana

Variation 4
Keeping the bent knee backward: Knee against wall

Effects
Placing the knee against the wall helps to keep the knee from sliding forward; it also helps to extend the thigh.

Props
wall
blanket or bolster (optional)

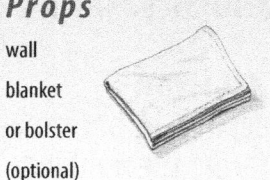

This variation achieves the same purpose as the previous one, without a partner.

To do the pose with the right leg bent:

⟶ Sit with your right side facing the wall at about 50 cm (20 inches) away from it.

› Bend the right leg and move to the right until the right knee is placed against the wall.

› Move yourself slightly forward. The wall prevents the knee from moving; hence, as you shift forward, the angle between the thighs increases.

› Keep extending the right thigh so as to press the knee against the wall while bending forward into the pose.

> *Note:*
> if the pressure of the wall on the knee feels uncomfortable, place a piece of sticky mat in between knee and wall.

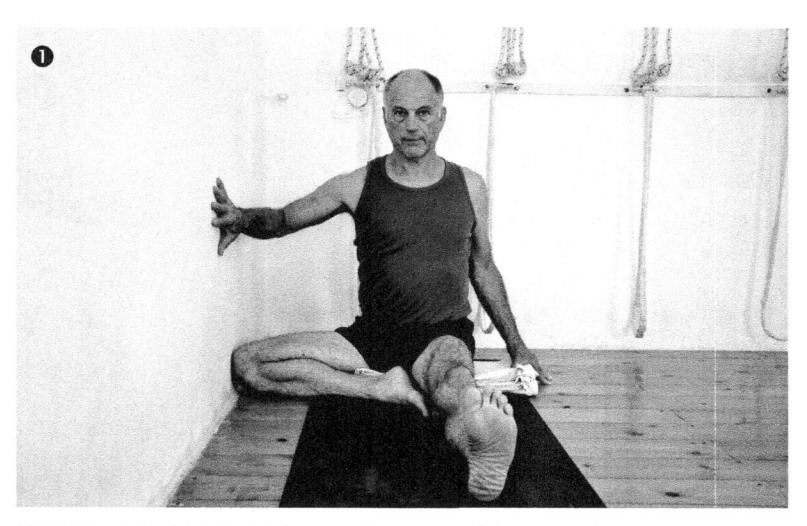

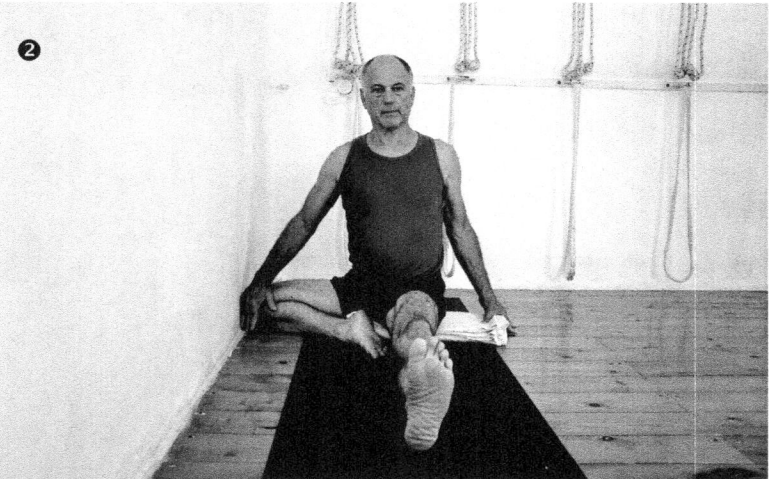

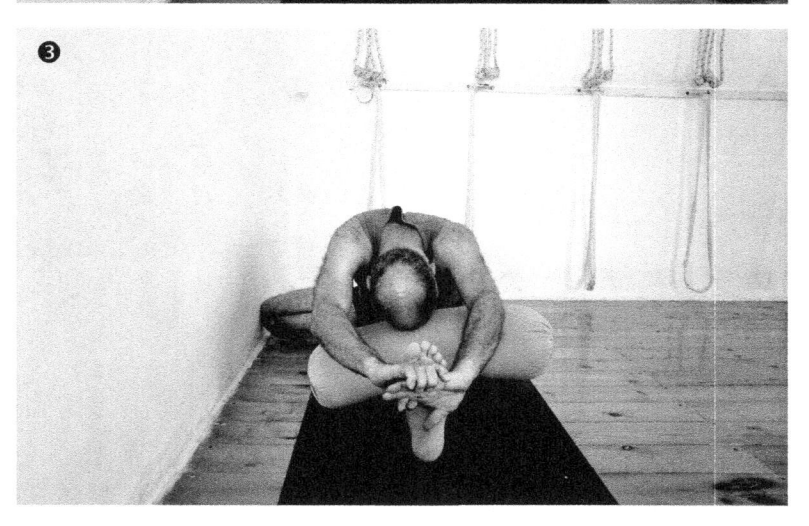

Jānu Śīrṣāsana

Variation 5
Keeping the bent knee backward:
Bracing the right leg

Effects
The belt bracing the leg keeps the femur head inside the hip joint. When grasping the foot it helps to turn the trunk sideways. These actions sharpen the awareness to the bent knee and help roll it out and back.

Props
belt

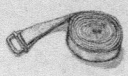

To do the pose with the right leg bent:

⟶ Sit in Daṇḍāsana and bend the right knee sideways.

❯ Insert a looped belt over the head and tighten it around the pelvis and bent knee.

❯ Move the left shoulder and arm back and catch the belt with the left hand. Use it to turn the trunk to the left ❶.

❯ Keep stretching the belt with the bent knee as you go to Jānu Śīrṣāsana ❷.

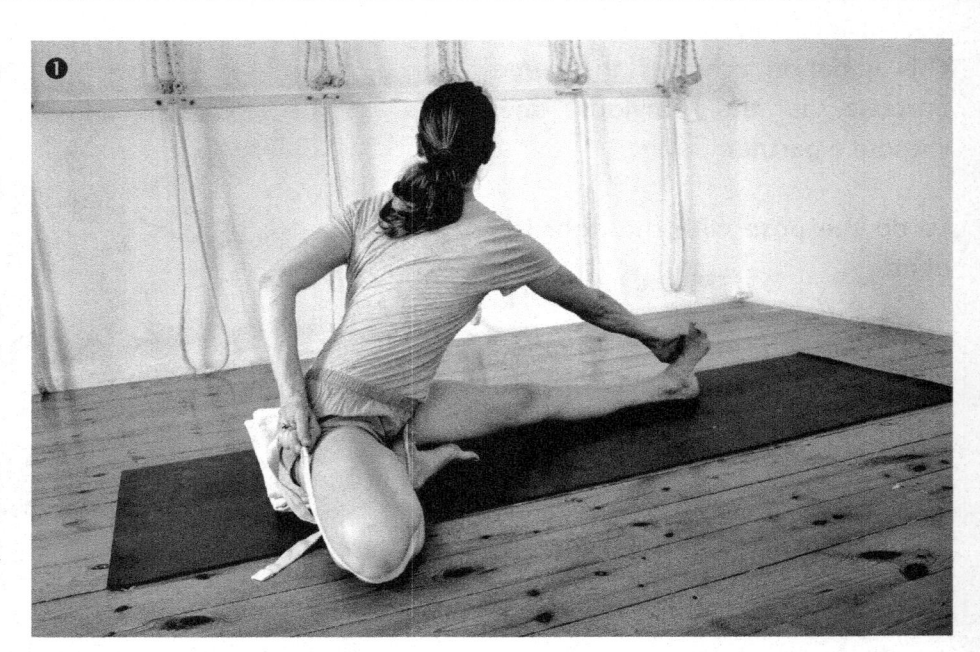

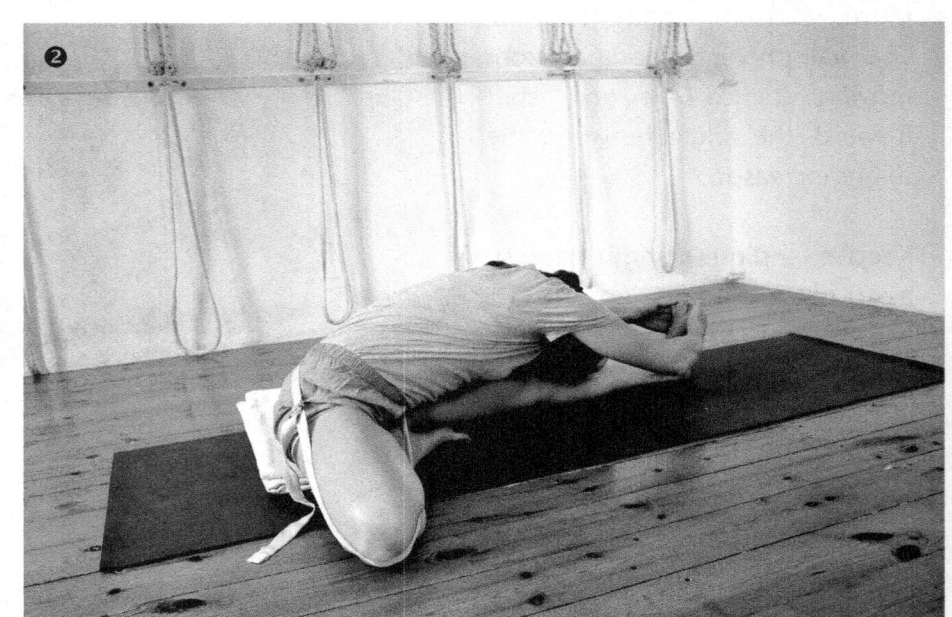

Jānu Śīrṣāsana

Variation 6
A different way to enter the pose: Sliding the knee back

Effects
This way of entering the pose helps to keep the back in a symmetrical shape even after moving the knee back. This helps to keep the abdomen quiet.

Props
blanket

The previous variations help to move the knee back and keep it there, but at the same time the back may be tilted toward the bent knee side. So, after moving the right knee back we have to struggle in order to lower and flatten the right side of the back.

This variation takes an opposite approach: first enter the pose with the knee taken only about 60° sideways; then, while keeping a "Paschimottānāsana back" (see the section About Jānu Śīrṣāsana above) slide the knee backward to form 90° or even a wider angle.

To do the pose with the right leg bent:

⟶ Spread a blanket (do not use sticky mat) and sit on it in Daṇḍāsana.

› Bend the right leg; move the knee about 60° to the right.

› Turn from right to left and bend forward keeping both sides of the waist moving evenly forward ❶.

› Lower the trunk down and stay a while.

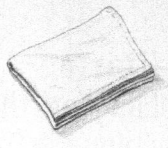

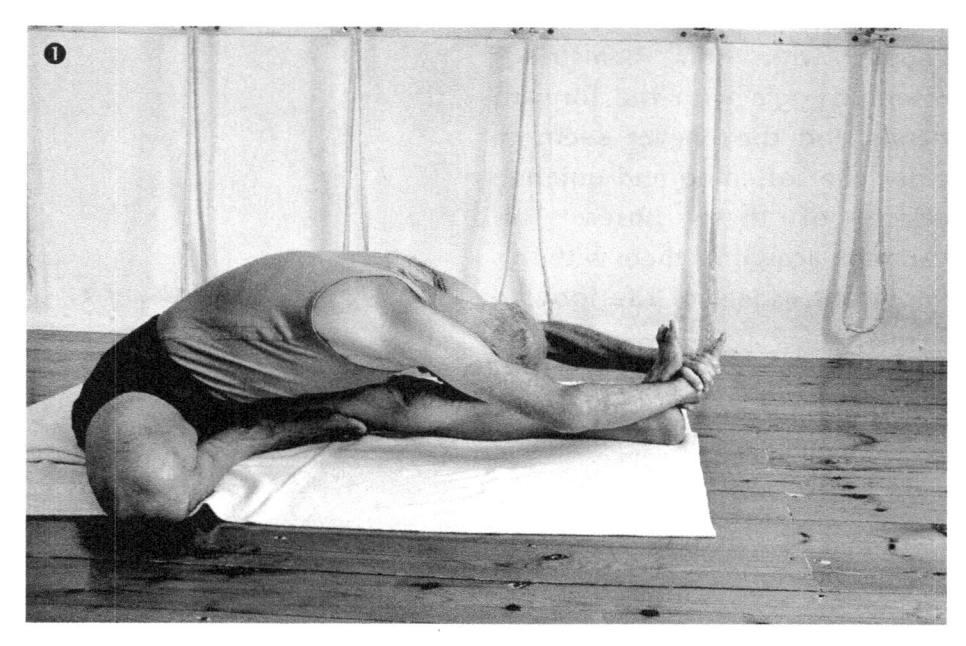

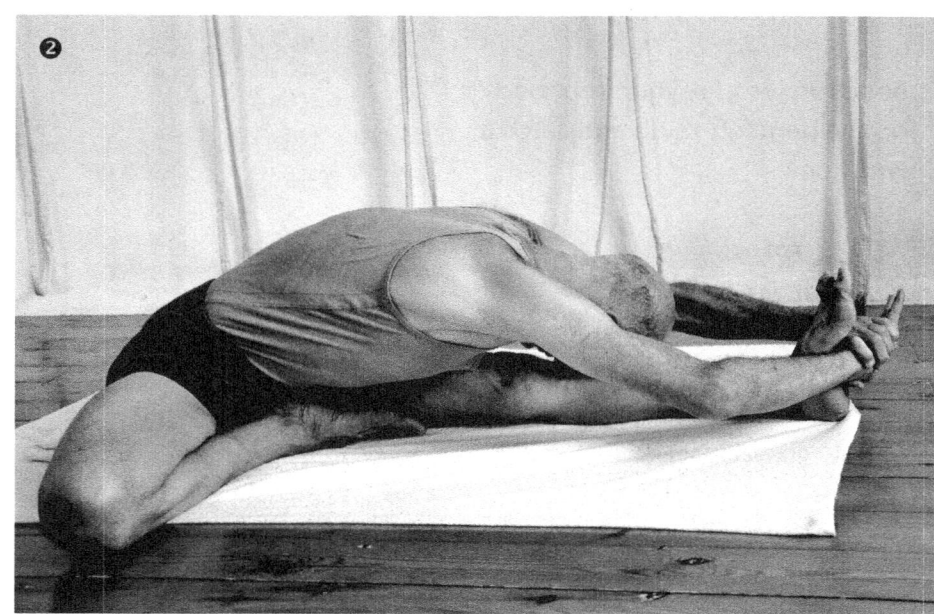

› Then, without allowing the right side of the back to become convex or move sideways, slide the right knee backward to form an obtuse angle between the thighs ❷.

Jānu Śīrṣāsana

Variation 7
Folding into the pose: Start by bending the Dandāsana leg

Effects
Keeping the front body in contact with the straight leg clarifies how the back side of the body needs to be stretched in the final pose.

Props
blanket, low wall hook

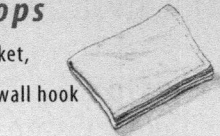

People with stiff hamstrings often struggle with the forward bends and they never seem to enjoy the softening and quieting effects of these poses. This variation acquaints them with this important aspect of the forward bends.

To do the pose with the right leg bent:

→ Sit in Dandāsana on a blanket (not on a sticky mat) and bend the right leg to the right.

› Slightly bend the left leg at the knee.

› Bend forward, lay your front body on the bent left thigh and catch a wall hook.

> **Notes:**
> If you do not reach the hook, use a belt.
> You can use a column (as shown here) or any other stable and graspable object.

› Grip the hook firmly and gradually straighten the left leg by pushing against the wall and sliding back. Keep going without letting the trunk lose touch with the thigh.

> **Note:**
> If you cannot straighten the leg, keep it bent and work slowly on sliding back.

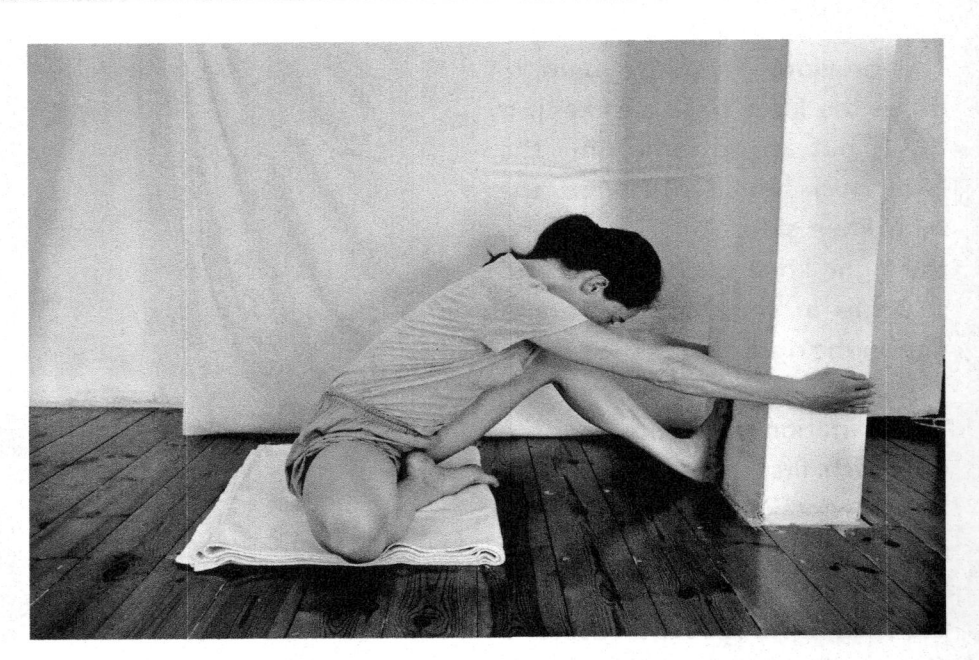

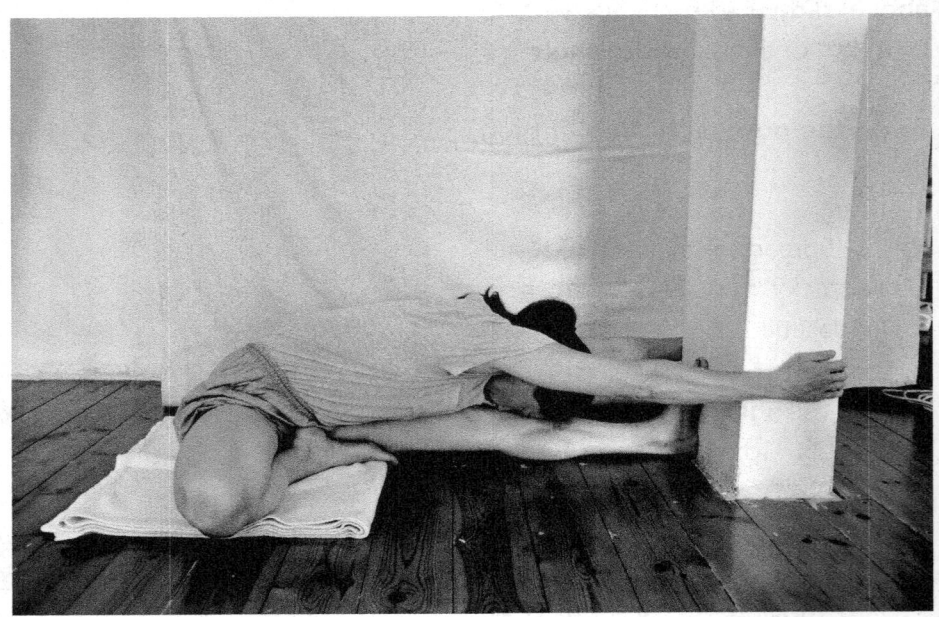

› Rest your forehead on the left shin (add a blanket if needed).

Tips
✓ Keep the abdomen close to the spine as you stretch forward. This will help you extend the lower back and breathe more easily.

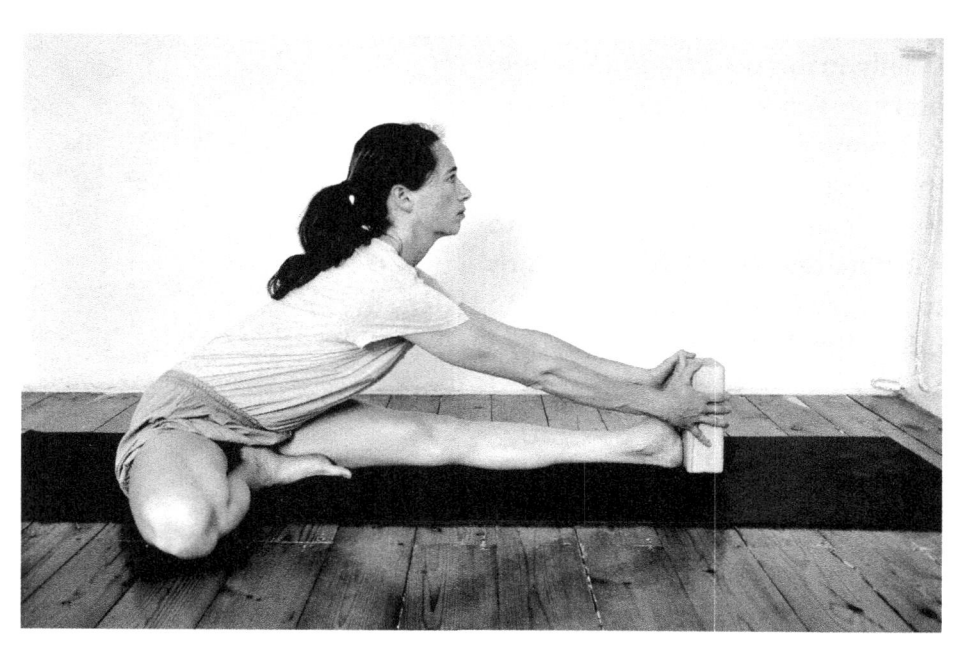

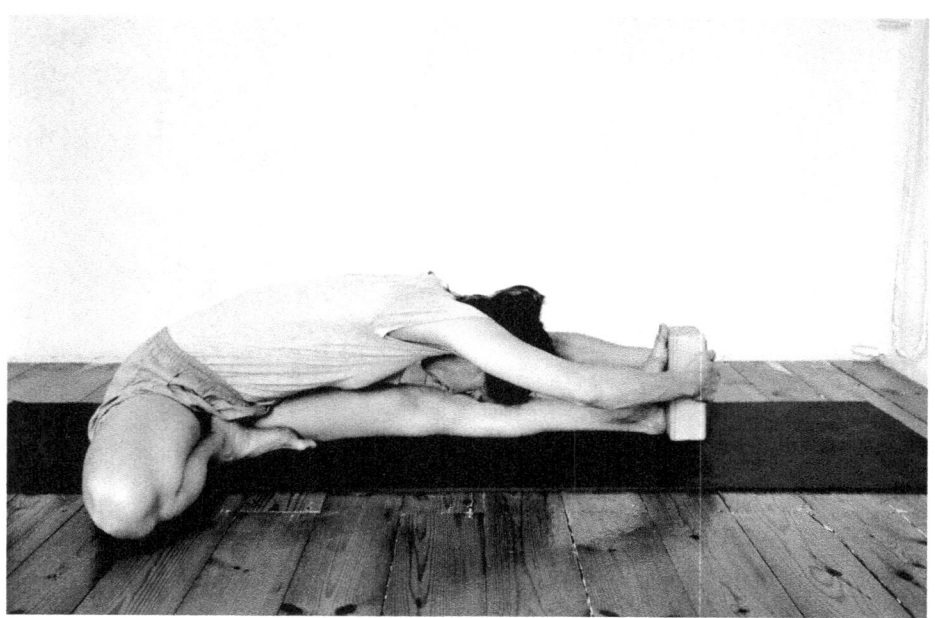

Jānu Śīrṣāsana

Variation 8
Activating the straight leg:
Foot against a block

Effects
Pulling the block helps to activate the Dandāsana leg. The block also provides a better anchoring place for the hands and helps to sensitize the foot.

Props
block

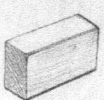

This Variation is similar to Variation 2 of Paschimottānāsana.

To do the pose with the right leg bent:

→ Sit in Dandāsana with a block in front of the feet. Bend the right leg.

› Catch the block with your hands and pull it toward you. Resist the pull of the arms by tightening the left leg.

› Make the back concave and look up.

› Pull the block to extend the trunk forward and go into the pose.

Jānu Śīrṣāsana

Variation 9
Aligning the trunk:
Rolled blanket on top thigh

Effects
The pointed shape of the rolled blanket lifts the left waist and helps to roll the abdomen to the left — a challenging action for most people. The blanket also supports the abdomen and helps to relax it.

Props
blanket

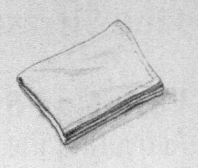

Ideally, in this pose the back should be even and symmetric, similar to Paschimottānāsana. When doing the pose with the right leg bent, the left side of the trunk tends to shorten, and the right side tends to bulge. This variation helps to bring the back to a more even shape.

To do the pose with the right leg bent:

⟶ Sit in Daṇḍāsana.

› Roll a 4-folded blanket around one of its corners to form a conic roll ❶.

› Bend the right leg and place the rolled blanket on your lap. Tuck the narrow end into the left groin from the left side, with the wide end hanging out to the left.

› Turn the waist from right to left; then bend forward, allowing the roll to support the left side of the lower abdomen.

› Catch the left foot, move the abdomen to the left and flatten the right side of the back.

› Rest the forehead on the left shin (or folded blanket) and stay in the pose ❷.

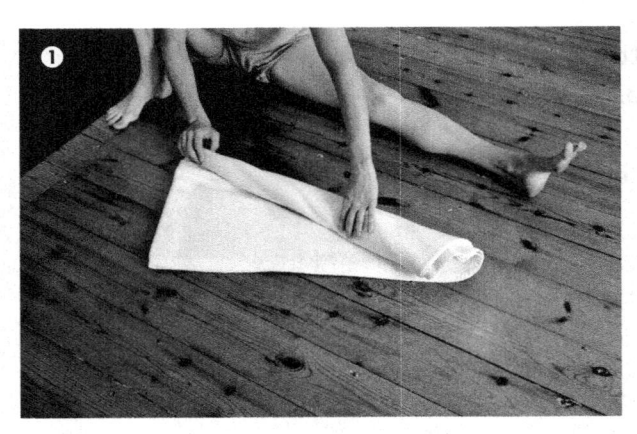

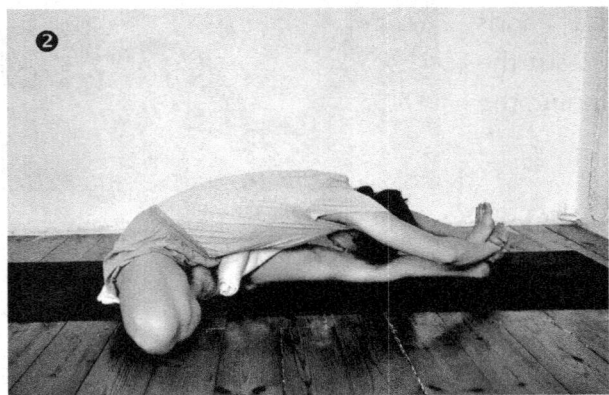

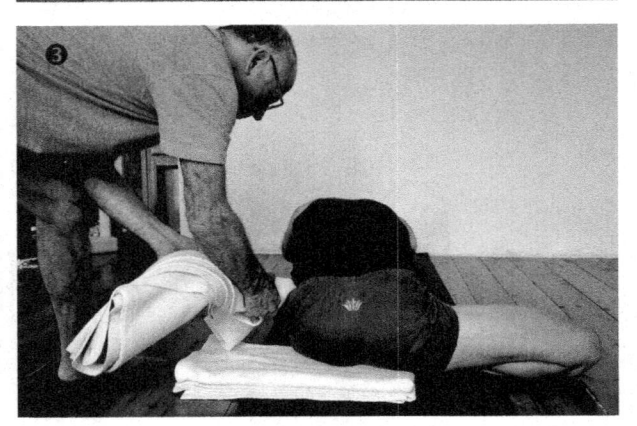

› If a partner is around he or she can pull the blanket from the left side in order to help turning the abdomen from right to left ❸.

Tips
✓ Experiment with the blanket to find the most suitable roll thickness. It is possible to use the blanket's corner even without rolling it. Find out what works best for you.

128 Props for Yoga / Chapter 3 / Jānu Śīrṣāsana

Upaviṣṭha Koṇāsana

In Chapter 2, we presented variations for Upaviṣṭha Koṇāsana as a sitting pose (or Utthita Upaviṣṭha Koṇāsana). Here we present variations for the pose as a forward bend (or Adho Mukha Upaviṣṭha Koṇāsana).

Upaviṣṭha Koṇāsana

Variation 1
Stabilizing the base:
Supporting the lower abdomen

Effects
The support for the lower abdomen helps to maintain the rounded shape of the lower back and induces quietness in the pose.

Props
blanket

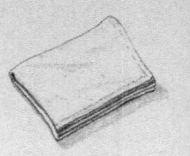

The forward movement of the trunk in this pose tends to roll the thighs forward. This creates pressure on the lower back and abdomen and makes the pose aggressive. In a relaxed pose the sacral band should remain convex and the lower abdomen should remain soft and in close proximity to the anterior (front) spine. This variation teaches this action.

→ Sit in Upaviṣṭha Koṇāsana.

› Prepare an 8-folded blanket and hold it on the floor against your pubic bone ❶.

> *Note:* You may even try to replace the blanket with a harder support like a block.

› Bend forward, resting the lower abdomen on the support.

› Rest your forehead on the floor (or on a folded blanket).

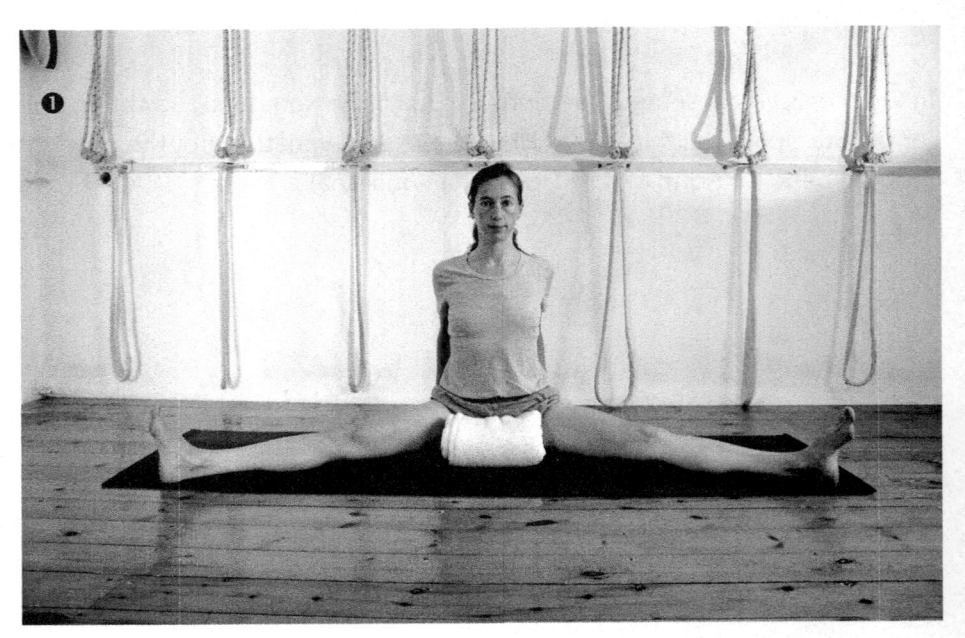

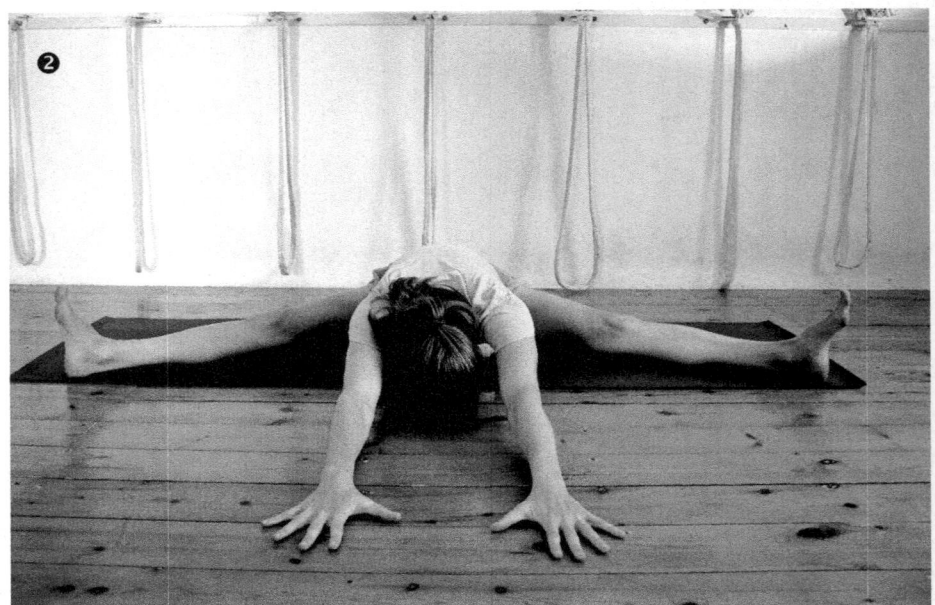

Tips
✓ Keep your abdomen soft and long.

✓ Record the sensations you have in the lower trunk with the support and then repeat the pose without the folded blanket.

Upaviṣṭha Koṇāsana

Variation 2
Restorative bending forward:
Supporting the trunk

Effects
Upaviṣṭha Koṇāsana is a very relaxing pose because of the widening of the legs and pelvis. This relaxing effect can be deepened by a longer, supported stay in the pose.

Props
1 or 2 bolsters, blanket

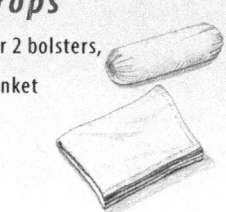

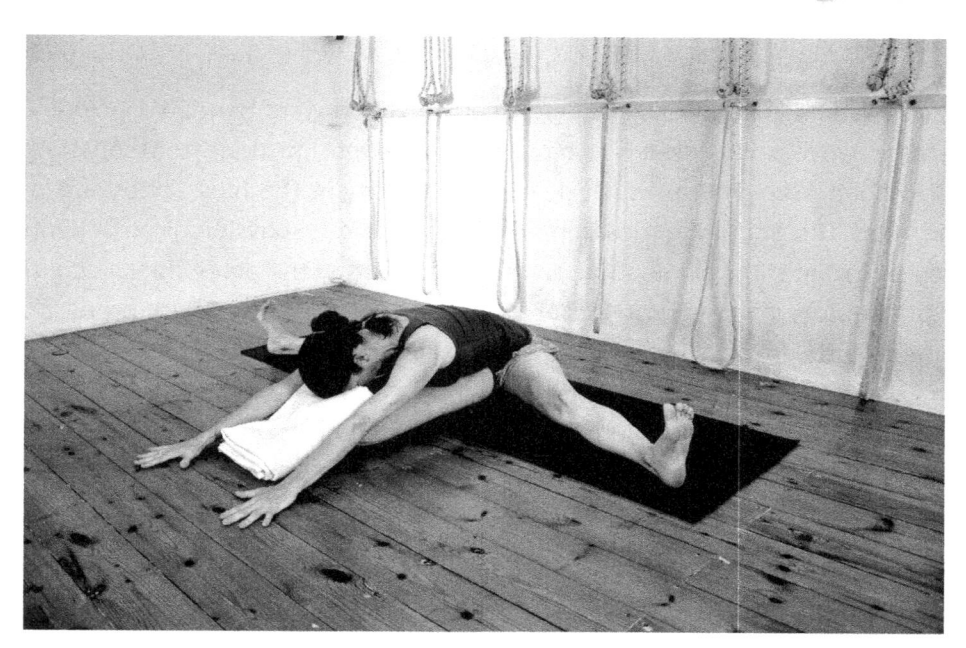

⟶ Sit in Upaviṣṭha Koṇāsana.

> Place a bolster lengthwise in between the legs. Place a folded blanket on the bolster for head support.

> Extend the trunk forward and rest the abdomen and chest on the bolster.

Note: If the support of one bolster is too low for you, place another bolster on the top of the first one.

Mālāsana
About Mālāsana

Mālāsana (LOY Pl. 321 & 322) is quite an advanced forward bend. We include it here for two reasons: First it is a unique forward extension, done from squatting rather than from sitting, which develops flexibility in the hips, knees, ankles and feet. The squatting position also offers unique physiological benefits regarding digestion, elimination, and the relaxation of the pelvic floor. Second, its preparatory stage (shown in LOY Pl. 317) is easy to perform; with props it is suitable and beneficial for most students, including beginners.

In the modern world people rarely squat, so the ankles and knees lose their flexibility; constipation and poor digestion are also common. Many westerners find it hard to squat with the heels on the floor; the shins cannot move forward sufficiently and hence the body tends to roll backward. The following variations help to improve the flexibility and to prepare for the final pose.

> **⚠ CAUTIONS**
>
> Do not practice this āsana if your ankles are injured. Avoid this pose if you are menstruating (since it tends to contract the lower abdomen).

Mālāsana

Variation 1
Preparation: Using chair

Effects
Sitting high on a chair makes it easy to fold the body forward. The front and back rungs of the chair provide stable gripping points for the hands, which are used to intensify the stretch.

Props

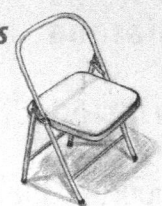

chair

➢ Sit on a chair with your buttock bones close to the front edge of the seat.

➢ Widen the feet and knees.

➢ Extend the trunk forward and then slowly lower it in between the thighs. Relax the back muscles as gravity pulls you down.

➢ Place the hands at a comfortable distance on the floor and stay in this position for a minute or two ❶.

➢ Now, lower yourself, catch the front rung of the chair and pull to increase the forward bending. Stay for a while.

➢ If you wish to bend further, hold the back rung of the chair and pull the trunk further down ❷. Stay for a while and then release the grip and come up slowly.

> *Note:*
> This variation is also a preparation for Kurmāsana (LOY Pl. 363 & 364).

➢ Another option is to turn around and to place the backs of the knees on the backrest of the chair and to lean over the knees ❸.

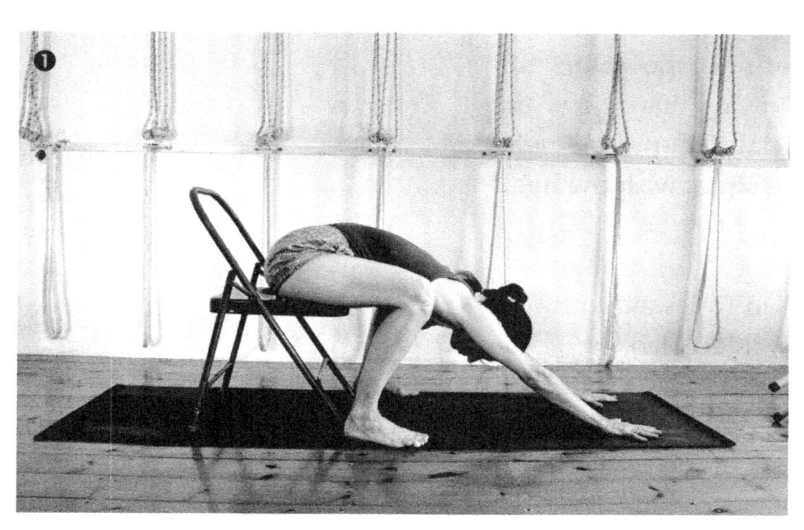

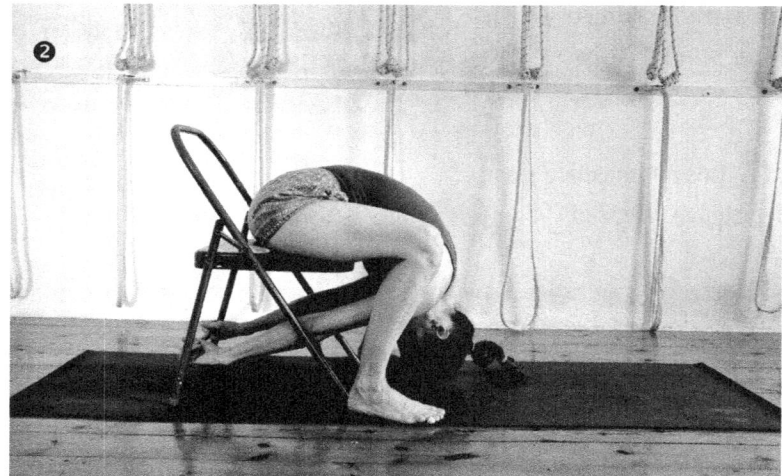

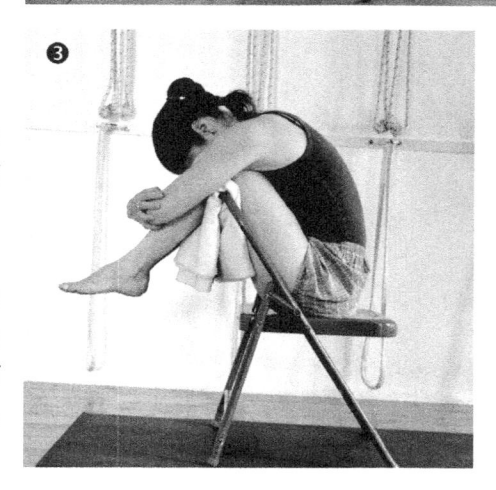

Tips

✓ Do not rush into the final stages of the pose. Allow your back muscles time to relax into the forward bending and experience the quietness it induces.

Mālāsana

Variation 2
Preparation: Supporting the heels

Effects
The support under the heels allows even stiff people to squat with comfort.

Props
blanket

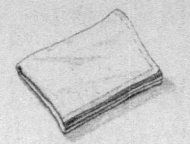

The preparations shown in this and the following variations are very beneficial for people who find it hard to squat with the heels on the floor.

⟶ Stand in Tādāsana with your heels on a folded blanket.

> Keep the legs joined and bend them to a squatting position.

> Extend the arms forward ❶ or hug the knees and stay in the pose.

Note: This intermediate stage is depicted in Pl. 317 of LOY.

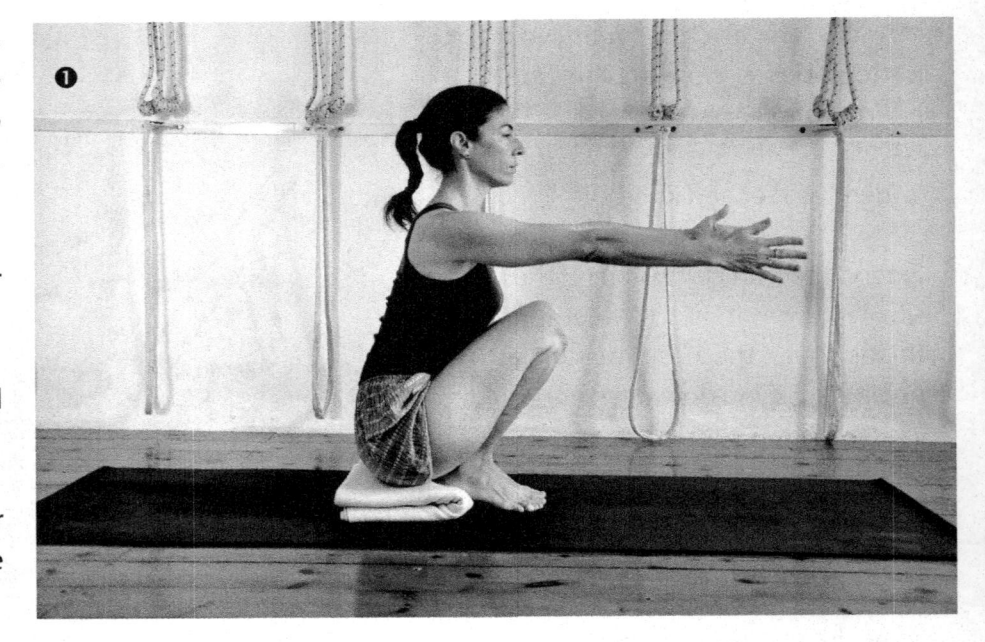

Mālāsana

Variation 3
Preparation:
Sitting on a bolster

Effects
The bolster prevents the rolling backwards, thus one is able to squat with comfort and stay in the pose longer.

Props
bolster
blanket (optional)

⟶ Place a bolster on the floor and stand in front of it.

> Squat to lower the buttocks until you sit on the bolster. If needed use a folded blanket to raise the support.

> Extend the arms forward or hug the knees and stay in the pose.

> If possible move the arms backward and catch the back of the ankles. This is Mālāsana II (LOY Pl. 322).

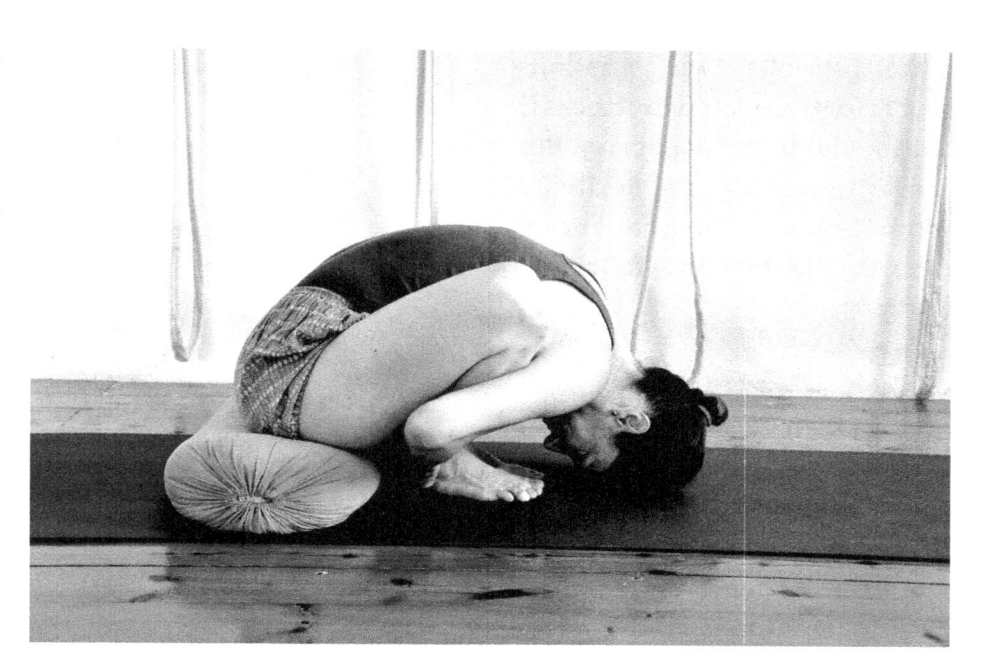

Mālāsana

Variation 4
Preparation:
Sacrum against the wall

Effects
The wall pushes the sacrum forward and helps to move the shins and the trunk forward. This enables to develop ankle flexibility gradually.

Props
wall

In the previous two variations support for the heels or buttocks is used to enable the squatting. But in order to improve the flexibility and to become independent of supports, practice the following variations.

→ Squat with the back against the wall, feet together, knees slightly apart, heels on the floor.

› Press the sacrum into the wall, lift the back up and away from the wall, extend the arms forward and look forward. Stay for a minute or two.

› Then wrap the arms around the bent legs and move the outer armpits to touch the shins.

› Extend your body forward and bring the head down.

› Push the shin bones with your upper arms in order to bend the trunk further down.

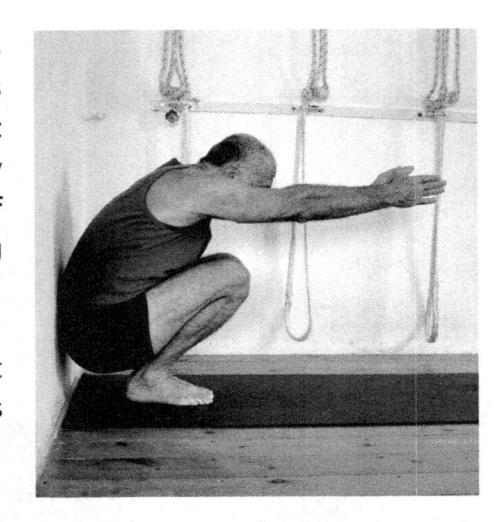

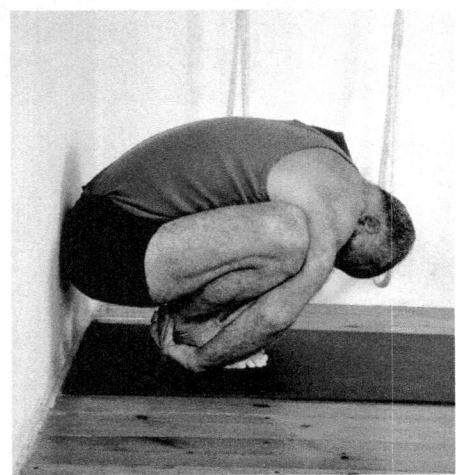

Tips

✓ If you find it difficult to keep the heels on the floor as you move forward - spread the feet slightly. You can also grab the heels and place the thumbs underneath to provide support, as shown.

✓ Using the wall, learn to lower both the pelvis AND the head at the same time. You can use a blanket or bolster to support the head.

✓ To advance in the pose, rise and move slightly away from the wall. Squat again and do the pose with your sacrum barely touching the wall.

Mālāsana

Variation 5
Flexing the ankles: Holding a wall anchor

Effects
Anchoring the hands reduces the effort of the legs and helps develop flexibility in the ankles gradually. This variation is especially effective for people who cannot squat with the heels on the floor and tend to roll back when trying to lower the heels.

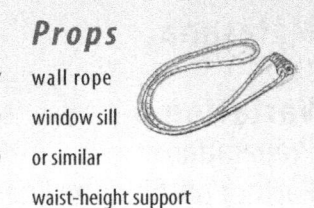

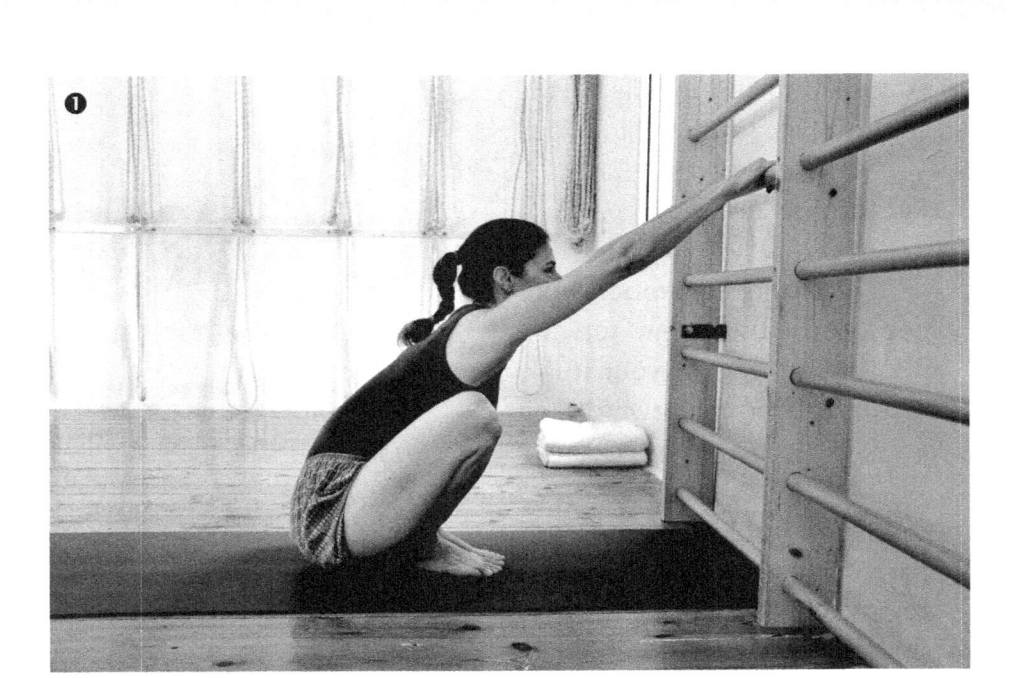

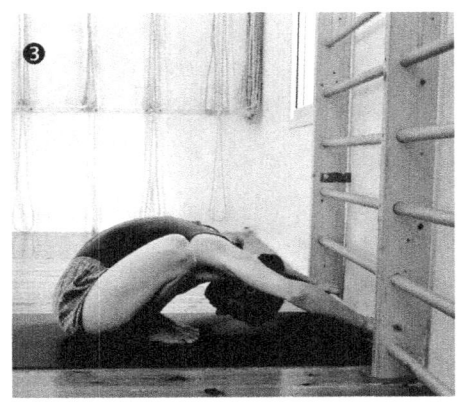

Props
wall rope
window sill
or similar
waist-height support

▶ Squat in front of a wall hook, a window sill (or any other waist-level anchor), feet together, knees apart, and heels on the floor.

▶ Hold the anchor with straight arms.

▶ Move the sacrum in, and lower the buttocks toward the floor while stretching the trunk forward and up ❶.

✓ *Tip* If you have a column or a ladder (as in ❷ and ❸), gradually catch at lower heights until finally you are ready for the final pose of Mālāsana I (LOY Pl. 321) ❹.

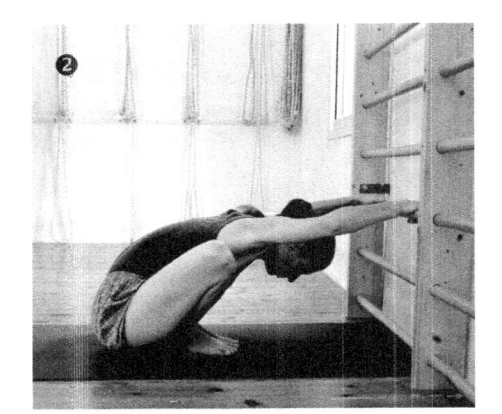

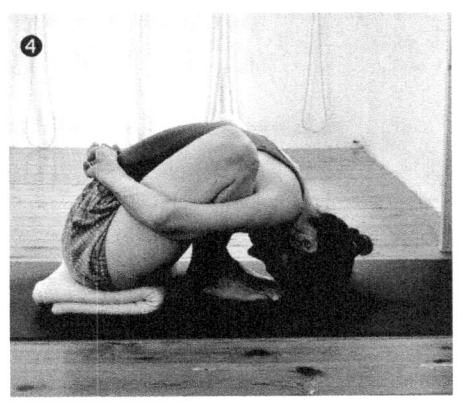

Tips

✓ Soften your armpits and let your body weight stretch the arms and the back muscles as you lower yourself towards the floor.

✓ If you tend to roll backward, support the buttocks as shown in ❹.

✓ In the final pose, the arms are clasped around the legs and back, creating a *Mālā* or garland ❹.

Mālāsana

Variation 6
Preparation:
Partner pushing the knees

Effects
Stabilizing the knees releases the groins and helps to develop flexibility in the hips, knees and ankles.

Props
partner
blanket (optional)

⟶ Stand in the middle of the room with a partner behind you.

› Start to squat down.

› Ask the partner to support your knees and push them forward and down as you lift your trunk, extend the arms forward and look forward ❶.

› Now extend the trunk and arms forward, while the partner gently presses on your sacral band and upper back ❷.

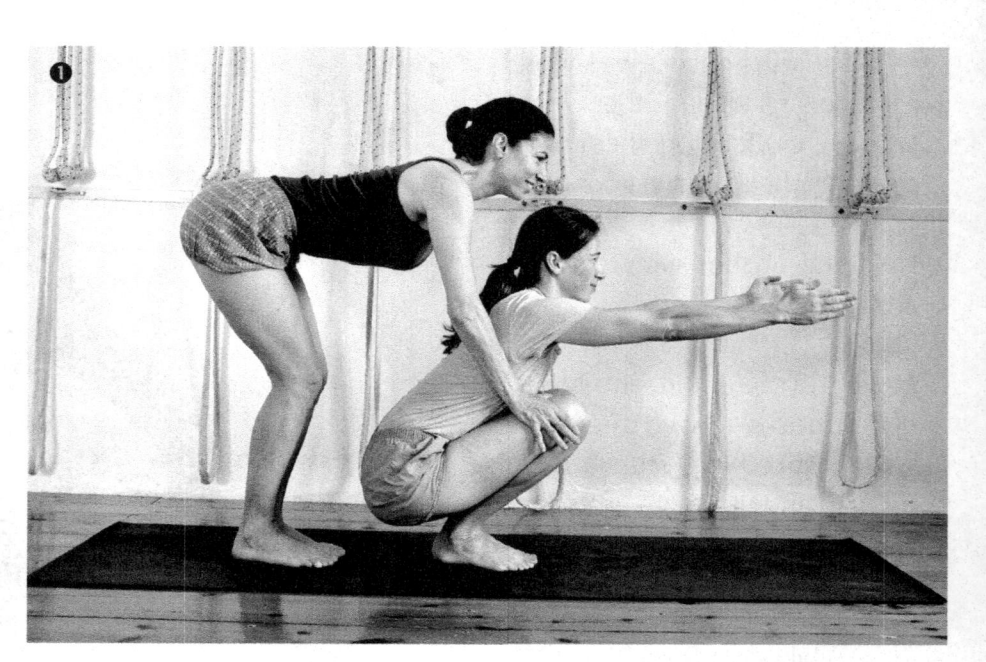

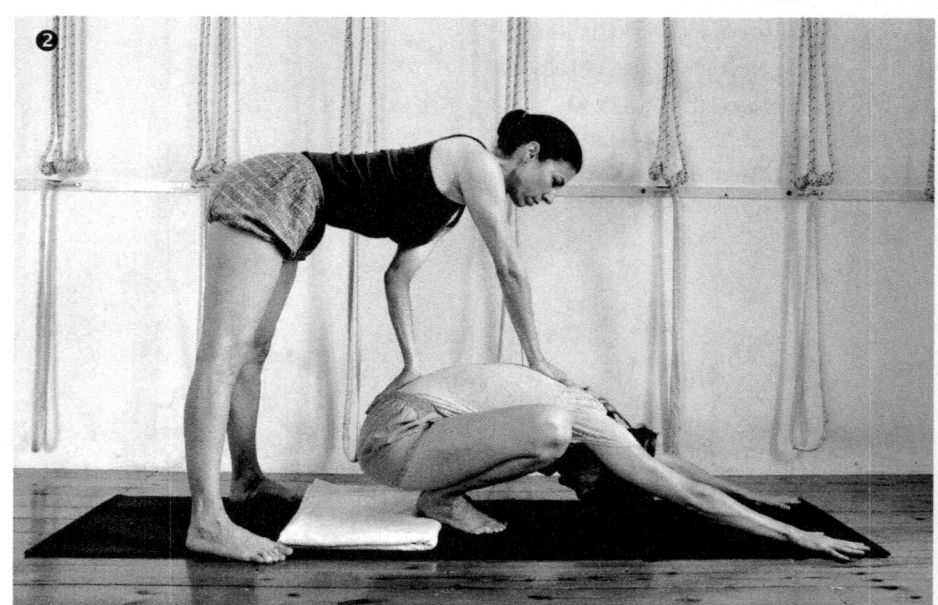

Tips

✓ In this variation your heels must be firm on the ground. If necessary use a folded blanket, a slanting plank or a rolled sticky mat under the heels.

Mālāsana

Variation 7
Mālāsana I with a belt

Effects
Grasping the hands with the help of the belt enables you to get the effects of Mālāsana I, even if you cannot clasp the fingers behind the back. This squeezing tones the abdominal organs and energizes the entire body.

Props
belt
blanket

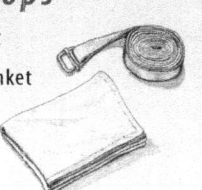

This is a more advanced variation for people who attempt Mālāsana I.

The word *Mālā* means garland; in Mālāsana I the arms embrace the body like a garland. Clasping the fingers behind the back (as in LOY Pl. 321) creates a strong squeezing effect which tones the abdominal organs. However, many people cannot grasp the hands behind the back and need a belt in order to benefit from these effects.

> Wrap a belt around your pelvis.

> Squat with feet together, knees apart and heels on the floor. If necessary, support the heels with a folded blanket.

> Wrap the arms around the bent legs and move the outer armpits to touch the shins.

> Rest the palms on the floor and lower the body down as much as possible.

> Move the hands one by one behind the back and catch the belt.

> Pull against the belt, extend the trunk forward and bring the head down.

> Move the hands as close as possible to each other. Push the shin bones with your upper arms in order to bend the trunk further down.

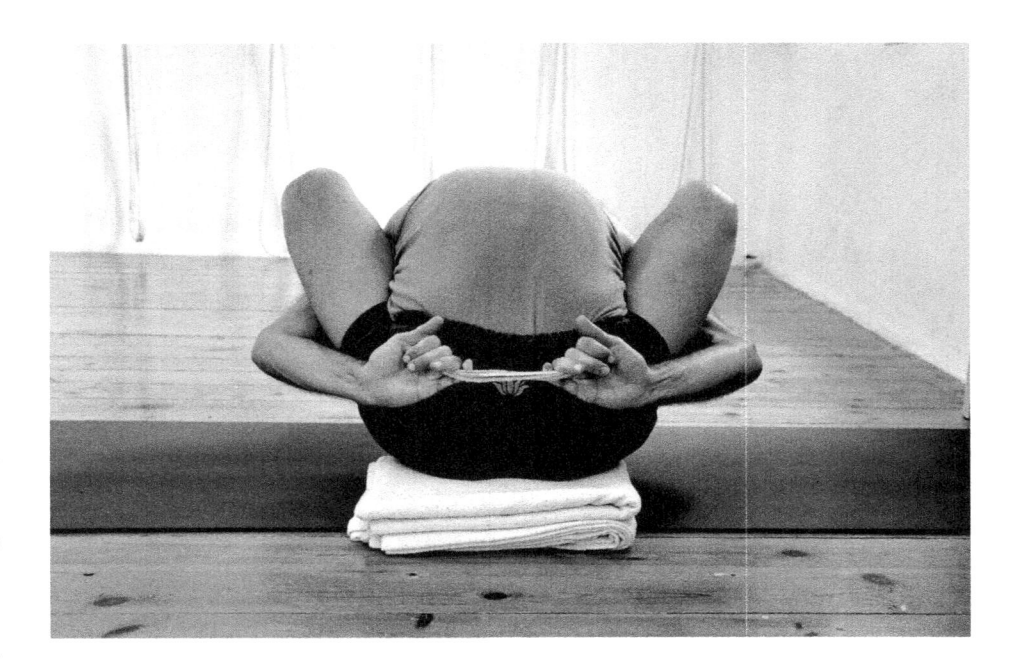

Appendix 1: A Practice Sequence

The effect of yoga practice is highly influenced by the order in which the āsanas are performed in a particular session. Correct sequencing is chosen according to the purpose and intention of the session; it takes into account one's current physical and mental condition, one's purpose in performing the sequence as well as the characteristics of the environment in which the practice takes place.

From time to time, it is interesting and enjoyable to conduct a session around one type of prop. For example, a sequence with a chair, with blocks, with a long belt, with wall ropes, or any other chosen prop. This appendix presents five sequences with differing purposes:

1. A short sequence for the busy beginner

2. A sequence of standing poses and forward extensions, using a long belt

3. A sequence of long stays in forward bends appropriate also for menstruating women

4. Sitting and forward extensions for beginners

5. Forward extensions, twists and inversions for advanced and intermediate students

For each āsana we indicate the page number where the variation can be found in this volume or in the previous one. Explanatory comments are provided for those variations that are not included in the first two volumes.

1. A Short Sequence for Beginners

Props
wall
block

Characteristics of this sequence are:

> **Duration:** 15-20 min

> **Level:** Beginners

> **Type:** A short sequence for the busy

> **Types of Asanas included:** Standing, light inversions

This short sequence can be a starting point for self-practice. Its duration is 15 to 20 minutes comprised of 7-10 minutes of active poses and 10 minutes of relaxing poses. Once you know the sequence you can change some of the standing poses and expand its content and duration to fit your needs. Because this sequence involves minimal props, it can be done anywhere.

1. Vṛkṣāsana – Next to a wall

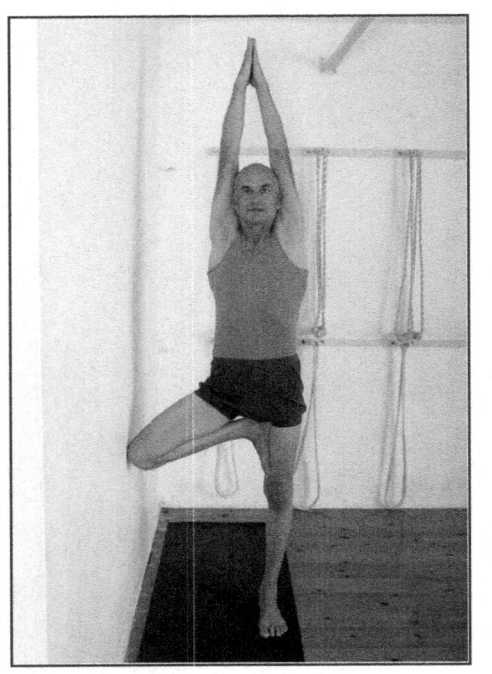

30 sec. twice on each side
See Vol. I, P. 25

2. Utthita Trikoṇāsana – Back foot against wall and palm on block

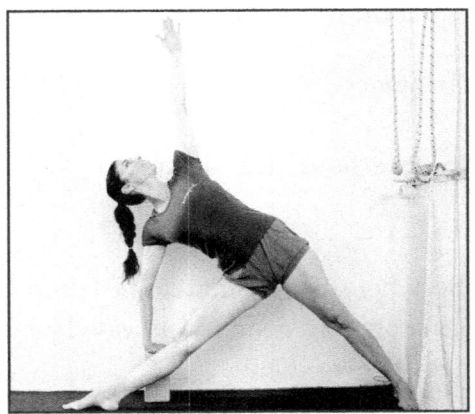

30 sec. twice on each side
See Vol. I, P. 69

3. Virabhadrāsana II – Back foot and hand against wall

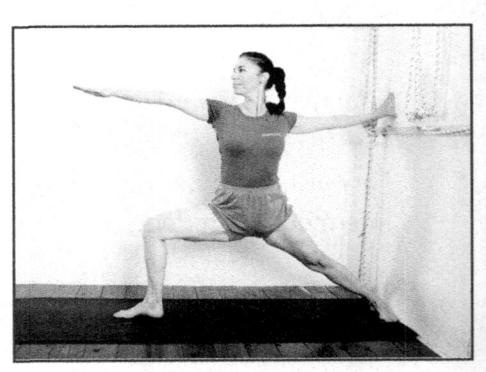

30 sec. on each side
See Vol. I, P. 99

142 Props for Yoga / Apendix 1

4. Adho Mukha Śvānāsana - Palms on blocks

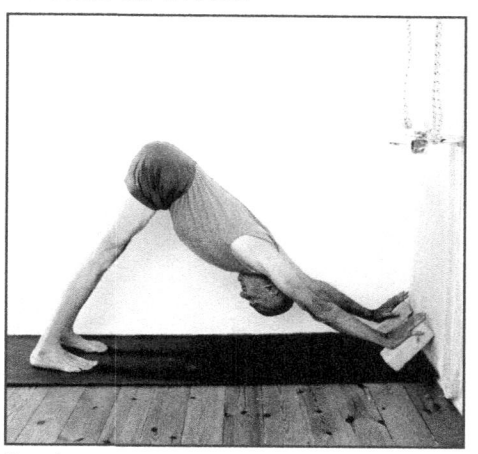

1 min.
See Vol. I, P. 32

5. Adho Mukha Śvānāsana - Head supported

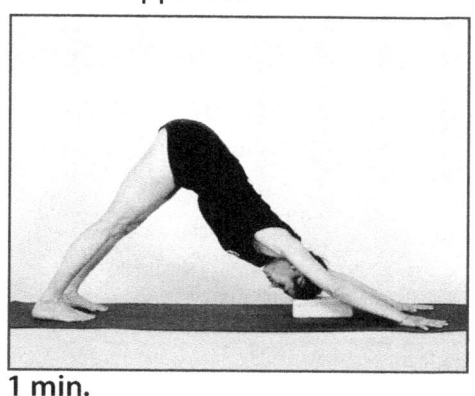

1 min.
See Vol. I, P. 52

6. Ūrdhva Prasārita Pādāsana – At the wall

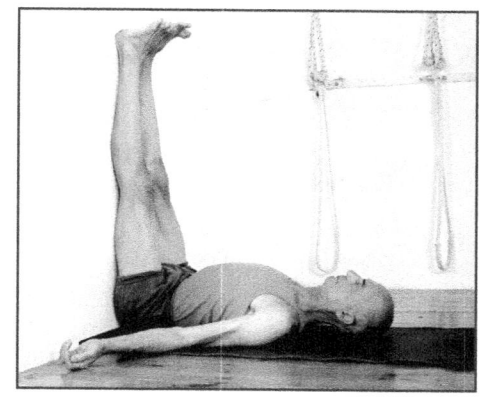

1-3 min.

Sit with your side touching the wall and roll to the side. Keep the pelvis close to the wall. To move closer to the wall, place the feet on the wall and push to lift the pelvis; then move your shoulders toward the wall. When lowering the pelvis, try to move the buttock bones as close as possible to the wall. If you cannot move the buttocks to the wall, you can place a folded blanket to support the sacral band.

7. Sālamba Chatushpādāsana – At the wall

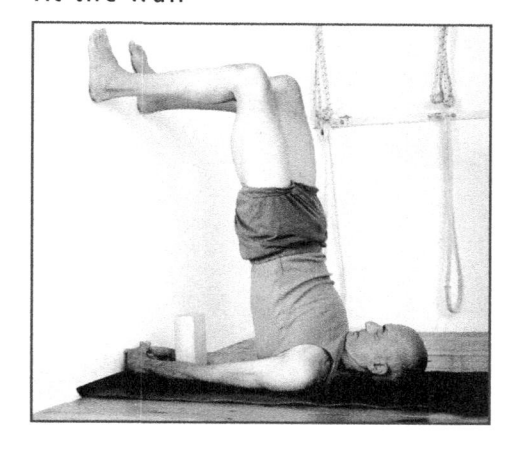

30 sec.

Bend the knees to place the feet on the wall. Push to lift the buttocks and the back. Interlock the fingers and stretch the arms and shoulders back. Push the chest forward such that the top chest is moving closer to the chin. Before releasing the pose, place the block at a distance of about 10 cm from the wall.

8. Viparita Karaṇi – With wall and block

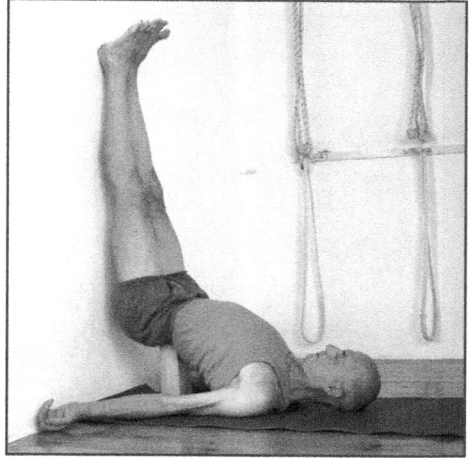

3-5 min.

The wide side of the block should be parallel to the wall. Keep lifting the top chest as you lower the pelvis until the sacrum is rested on the block. The sacrum should be parallel to the floor. Stay in the pose observing your breath.

9. Śavāsana – With optional eye cover and block on abdomen

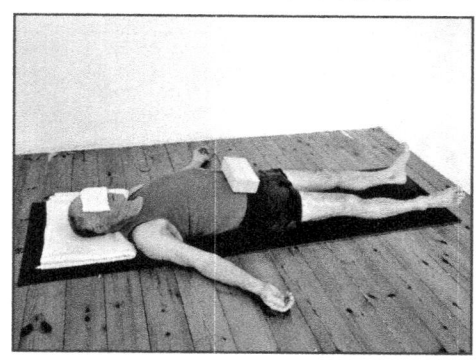

5 min.

Observe the soft, natural breath in the abdomen.

2. A Sequence with a long belt

Characteristics of this sequence are:

> **Duration:** 60 min

> **Level:** Intermediate to advanced

> **Type:** relaxing, cooling

> **Types of Asanas included:** Supine & Standing poses, forward extensions, restorative inversions

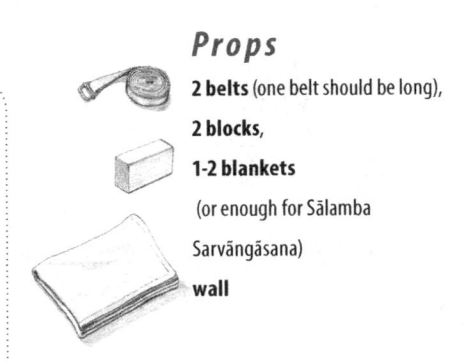

Props

2 belts (one belt should be long),
2 blocks,
1-2 blankets
(or enough for Sālamba Sarvāngāsana)
wall

1a. Supta Pādāngusthāsana I – Long belt around pelvis and heel

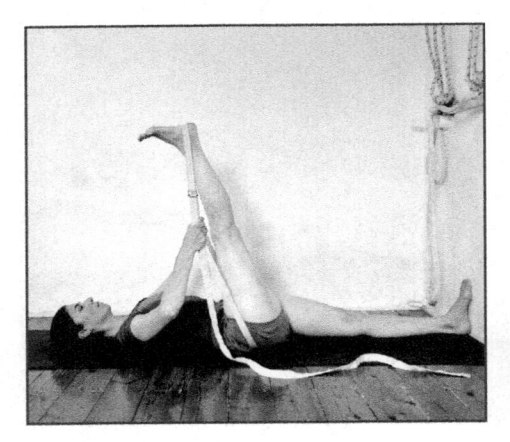

45 sec.
See Vol. II, P. 84
Start with a belt looped around the pelvis and the heel of the right leg.

1b. Supta Pādāngusthāsana I – Long belt around chest and heel

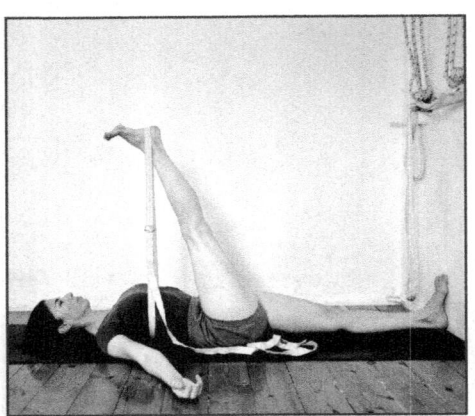

45 sec.
See Vol. II, P. 84
After 45 sec., move the belt to the middle of the back.

1c. Supta Pādāngusthāsana I – Long belt around head and heel

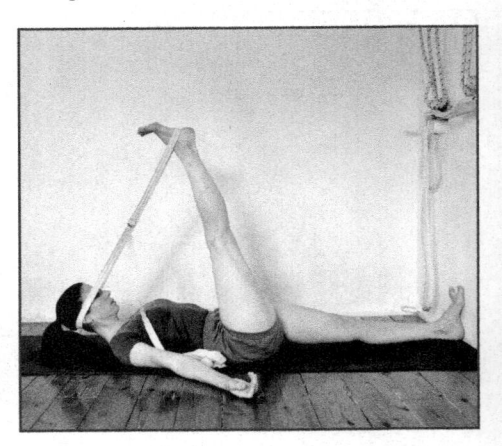

45 sec.
See Vol. II, P. 84
Then move the belt to the back of the head. Then release and do the same with the left leg.

Note: Before changing to the left leg, stay a while in Supta Tādāsana or stand in Tādāsana and compare the feelings of the legs.

2a. Supta Pādāṅguṣṭhāsana II – Long belt around pelvis and heel

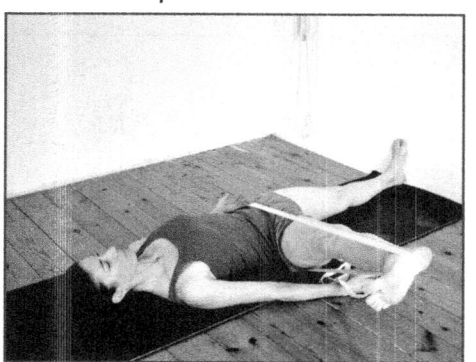

30 sec.
See Vol. II, P. 90

2b. Supta Pādāṅguṣṭhāsana II – Long belt around chest and heel

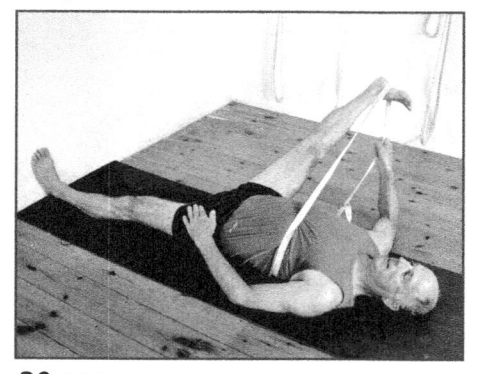

30 sec.
See Vol. II, P. 90

3. Ūrdhva Prasārita Pādāsana - Long belt around feet and pelvis

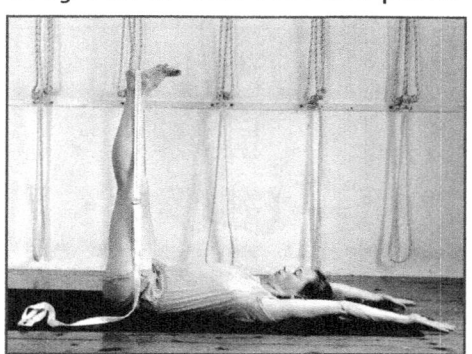

1 min.

Note: Repeat the same sequence of placing the belt on pelvis, mid-back and head. Before changing to the left leg, stay a while in Supta Tāḍāsana or stand in Tāḍāsana to compare the feelings of the legs.

4. Paripūrṇa Nāvāsana - Long belt around mid-back and feet

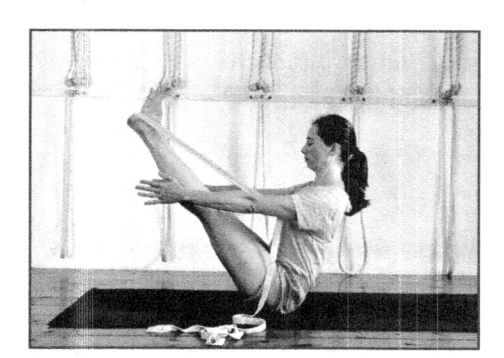

1 min.
Place the belt around the mid-back and use it to make the back concave.

5. Utthita Trikoṇāsana - Long belt from left foot to right groin

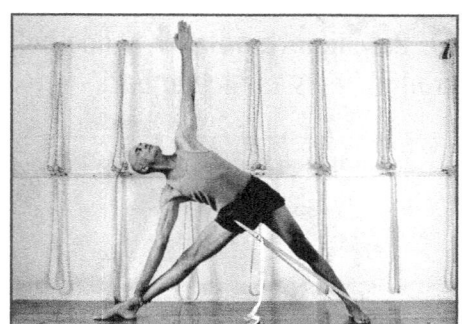

1 min.
Start with the legs spread to a medium distance; tighten the belt from the left heel to the right groin, and then slide the right leg until the belt is well stretched. Adjust the belt and the spread as needed.

6. Ardha Chandrāsana - Long belt from left foot to right groin

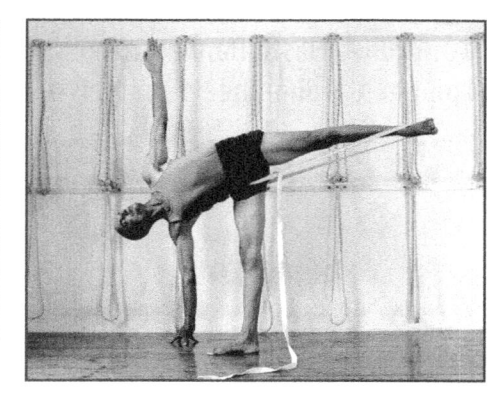

1 min.
Continue directly to Ardha Chandrāsana. If the belt is not tight, lift the leg slightly to stretch it.

Note: Do all the poses of stages 5 - 8 on the right leg and return to Tāḍāsana. Then move the belt to the left leg and repeat on the left side.

7. Virabhadrāsana III - Long belt from left foot to right groin

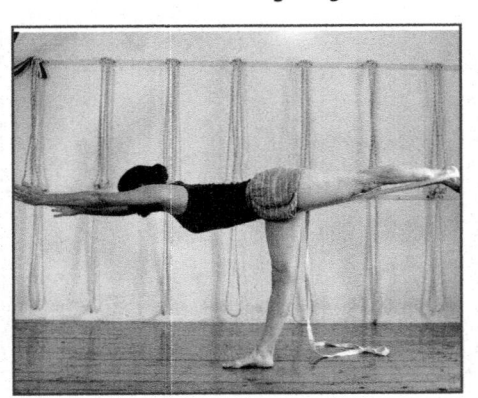

40 sec.
From there turn the body to face the floor.

8. Parivrtta Ardha Chandrāsana - Long belt from left foot to right groin

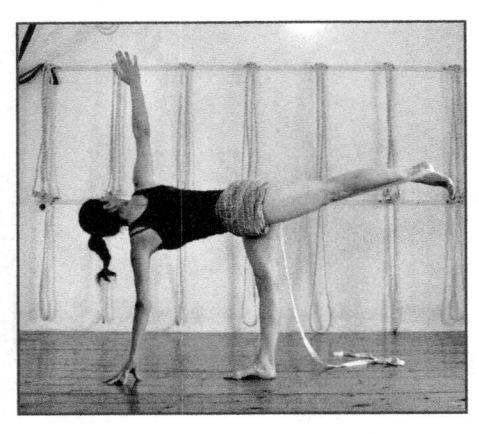

1 min.
Turn further to Parivrtta Ardha Chandrāsana

9. Daṇḍāsana – Long belt around heels and pelvis

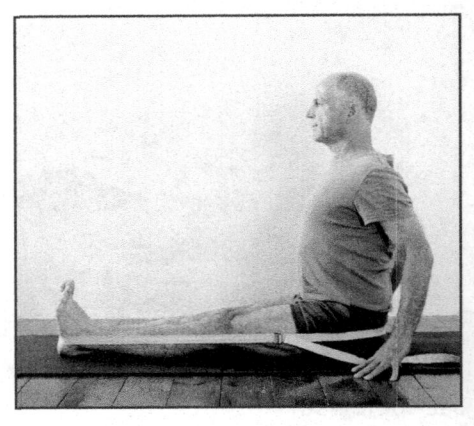

1 min.
See Vol. 2, P. 7

10. Ūrdhva Hasta Daṇḍāsana – Long belt around heels and pelvis

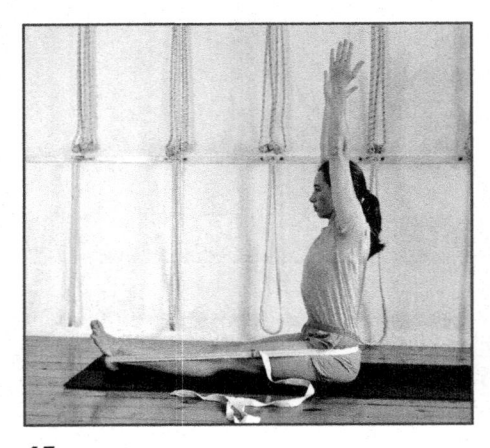

45 sec.
See Vol. 2, P. 7

11. Paschimottānāsana – Long belt around heels and lower back

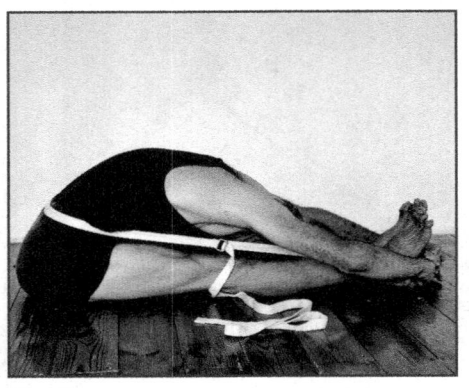

2 min.
See Vol. 2, P. 108

12. Jānu Śīrṣāsana – Long belt around heel and lower back

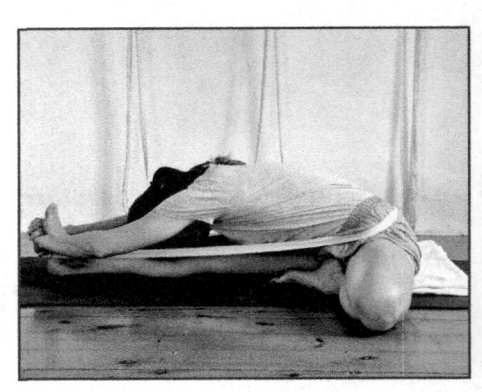

1 min. on each side

13. Paschimottānāsana – Long belt around heels and lower back

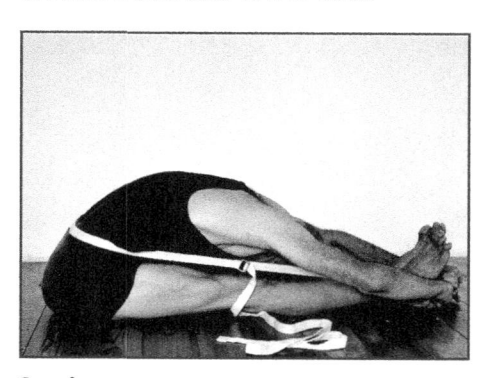

3 min.
See Vol. 2, P. 108

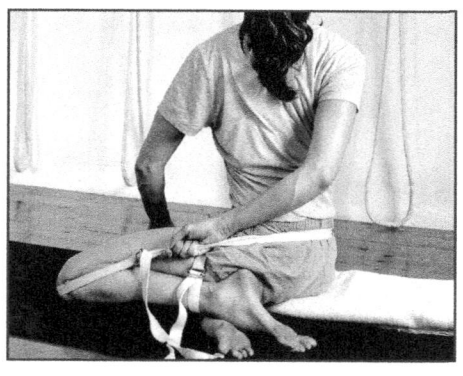

14. Bhardvājāsana I – with 2 belts

1 min. on each side
Tighten one belt around groin and ankle of the Vīrāsana leg. Then tighten another belt around the pelvis and the knee of the same leg

15. Setu Bandha Sarvāngāsana - With pelvis & chest support

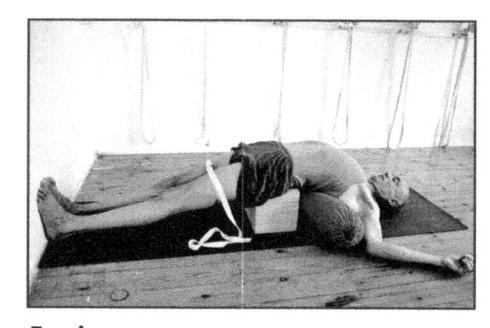

5 min.
Support the sacrum with a wooden block or several foam blocks. Tighten a belt around the upper thighs. Support the chest with a bolster. Place the feet against the wall

16. Sālamba Sarvāngāsana – On a stack of blankets

7 min.
For the Sarvāngāsana cycle set up the props as follows:
- Spread one blanket on the mat (for head cushioning) and stack five folded blankets on it to create a platform
- Place a block in the middle of the mat, where the feet should be in Halāsana; and a bolster on the other side of the platform

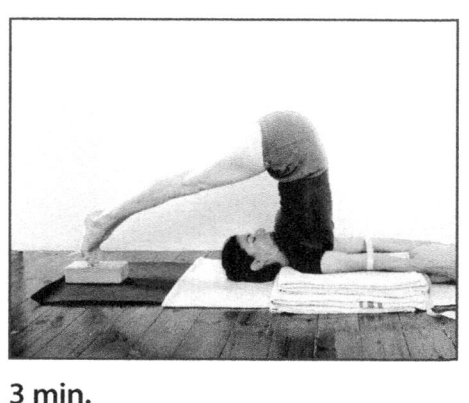

17. Halāsana – Toes on block

3 min.
Place the toes on the block and catch the bolster at the back. Make sure your arms and legs are aligned properly

18. Śavāsana

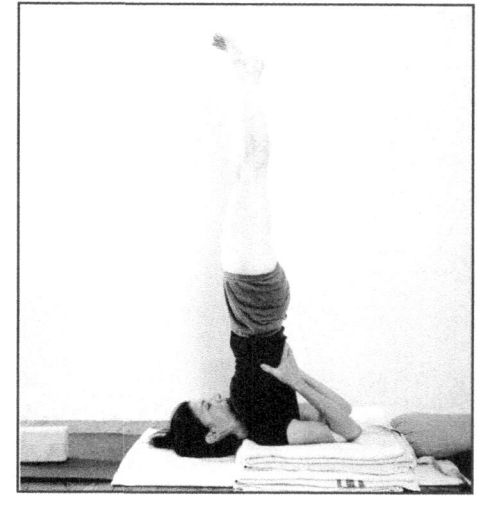

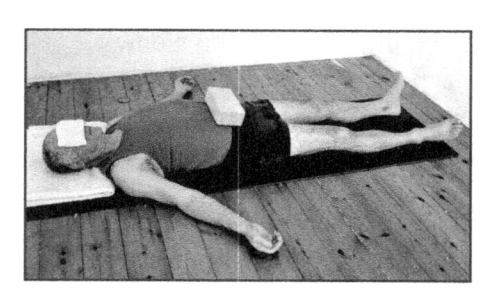

7 min.

Props for Yoga / Apendix 1 147

3. Long stays in sitting & forward extensions

Characteristics of this sequence are:

> **Duration:** 60 min

> **Level:** Intermediate to advanced

> **Type:** relaxing, cooling. Can be practiced during menstruation

> **Types of Asanas included:** forward extensions, restorative back bends

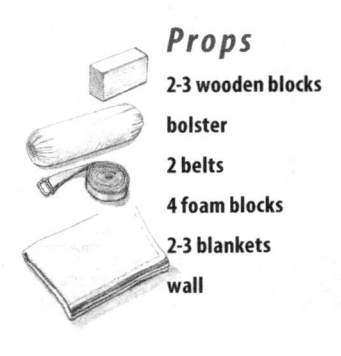

Props
2-3 wooden blocks
bolster
2 belts
4 foam blocks
2-3 blankets
wall

1. Adho Mukha Vīrāsana - With bolster to support forehead and elbows

3 min.
See Vol. II, P. 79

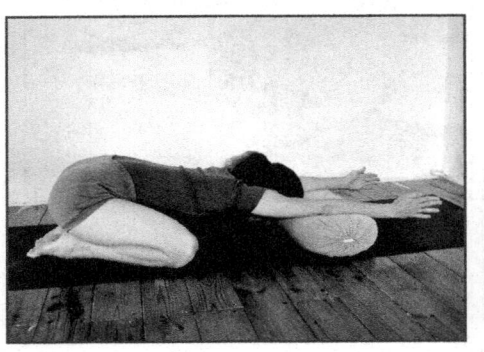

2. Supta Pādāṅguṣṭhāsana II - In a corner, both feet against wall

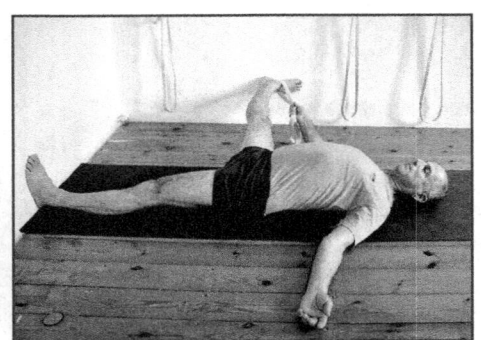

1 min. each side
See Vol. II, P. 93

3. Baddha Koṇāsana – Palms on blocks

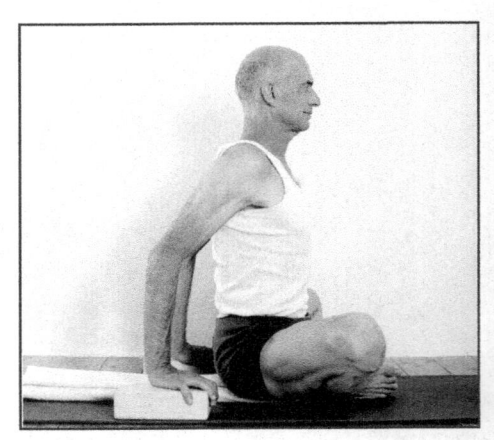

3 min.
See Vol. II, P. 15

4. Jānu Śīrṣāsana - Supported

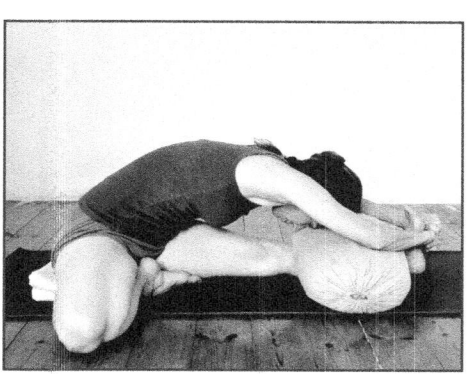

3 min. each side

5. Triaṅga Mukhaikapāda Paschimottānāsana - Supported

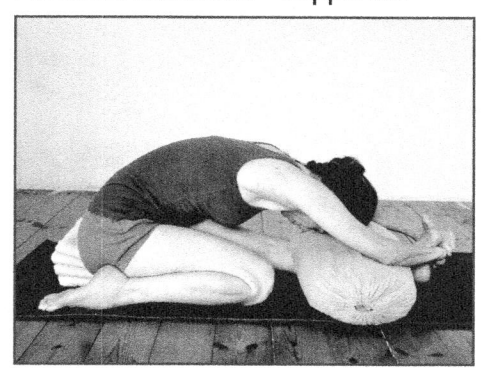

3 min. each side
Repeat the actions described for Jānu Śīrṣāsana.

6. Ardha Padma Paschimottānāsana - Supported

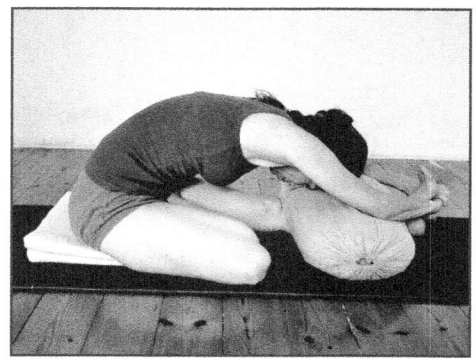

3 min. each side
If not possible, repeat Jānu Śīrṣāsana (step 4).

7. Paschimottānāsana - Supported

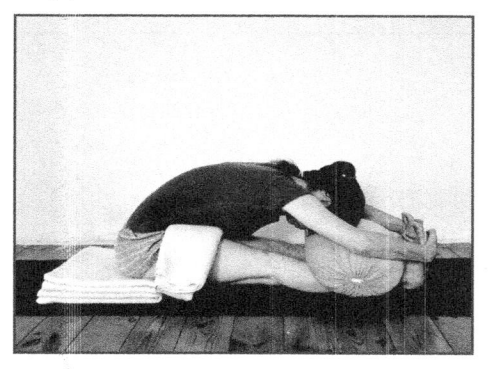

5 min.
See Vol. II, P. 114

8. Bhardvājāsana I – With two belts

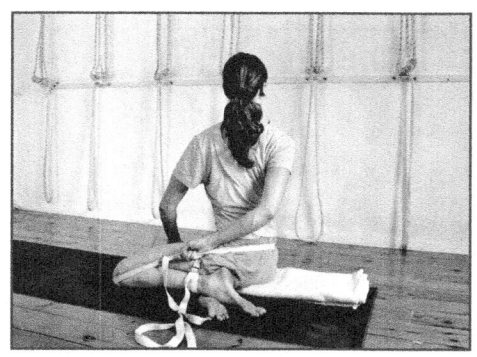

45 sec. each side. Repeat twice.
See step 14 on Sequence 2

5. Viparita Daṇḍāsana - On chair

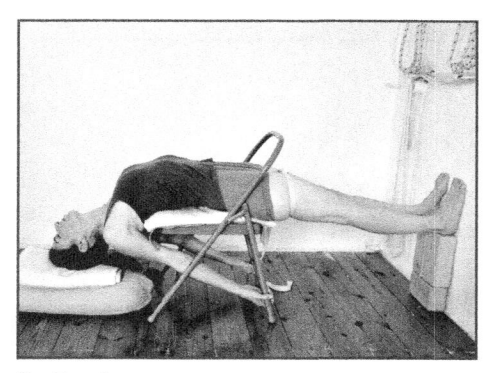

P. 5 min.
Top of head supported; heels on blocks, thighs tightened with belt

10. Setu Bandha Sarvāṅgāsana - with blocks and bolster

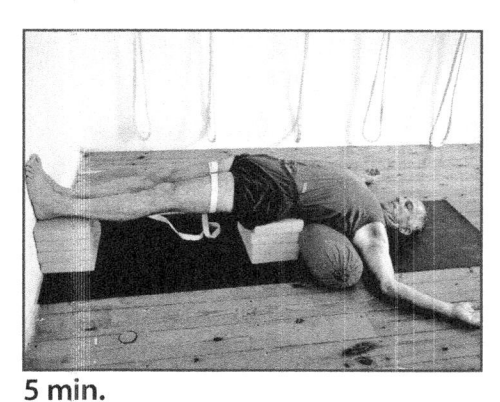

5 min.
See step 15 on Sequence 2

11. Śavāsana - With eye cover and block on abdomen

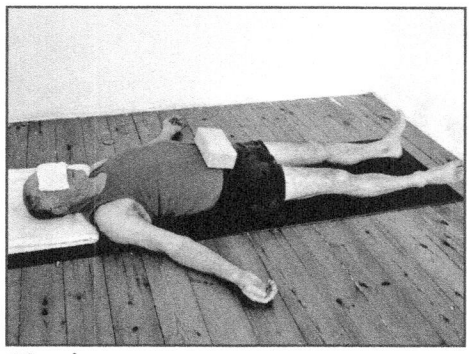

10 min.

4. Forward bends for beginners

***Characteristics** of this sequence are:*

> **Duration:** 40 min

> **Level:** Beginners to Intermediate

> **Type:** relaxing, cooling

> **Types of Asanas included:**
Standing poses, forward extensions, Sarvāngāsana cycle

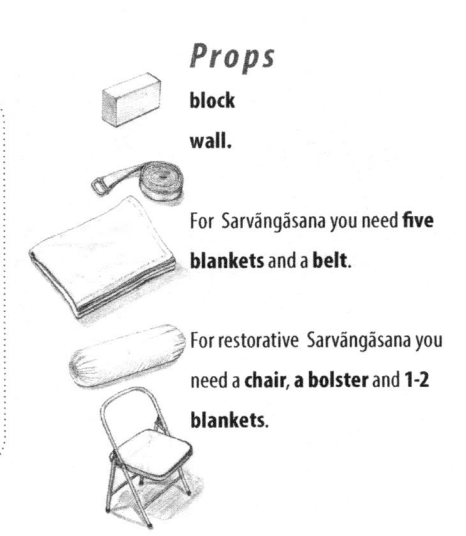

Props

block

wall.

For Sarvāngāsana you need **five blankets** and a **belt**.

For restorative Sarvāngāsana you need a **chair**, **a bolster** and **1-2 blankets**.

1. Adho Mukha Śvānāsana – Hands on inverted chair

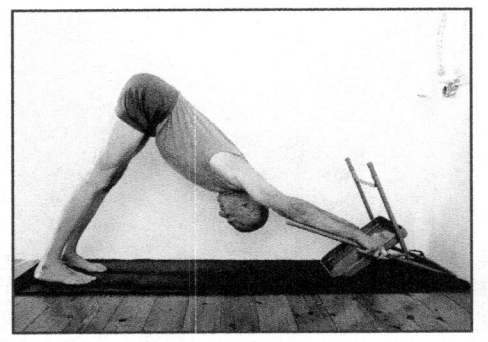

1 min.
See Vol. 1, P. 32

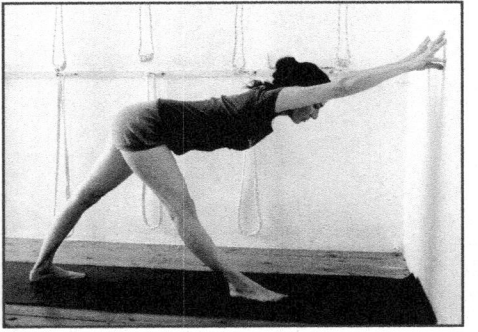

2. Pārśvōttānāsana – Hands on wall

45 sec. each side
See Vol. 1, P. 129

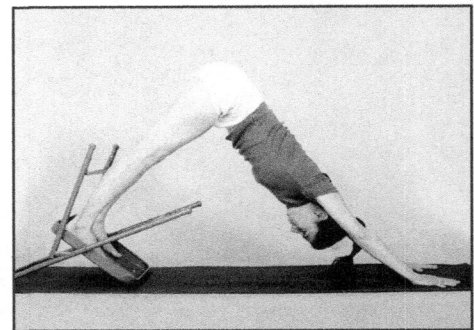

3. Adho Mukha Śvānāsana – Feet on inverted chair

1 min.
See Vol. 1, P. 39

4. Paschimottānāsana - Sitting on chair

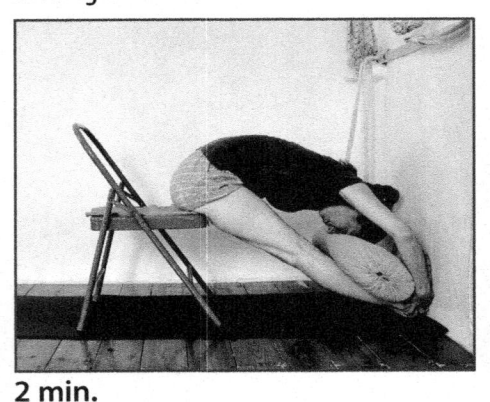

2 min.
See Vol. 2, P. 115

5. Jānu Śīrṣāsana –

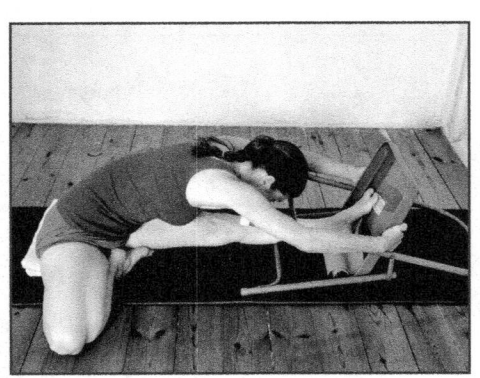

1 min. each side

6. Trianga Mukhaikapāda Paschimottānāsana –

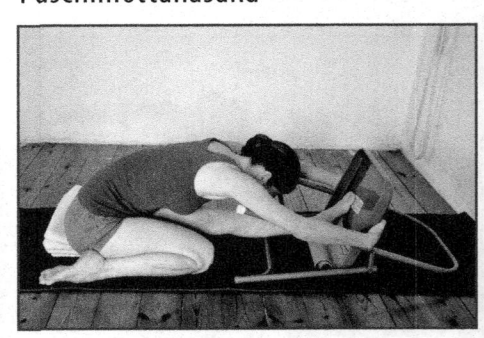

1 min. each side

150 Props for Yoga / Apendix 1

7. Paschimottānāsana – Head on chair

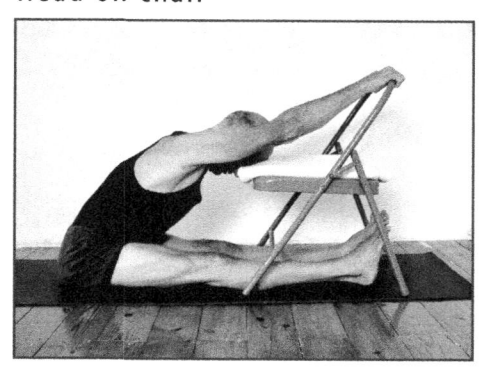

2 min.
See Vol. 2, P. 113

8. Bhardvājāsana I – Sitting on chair

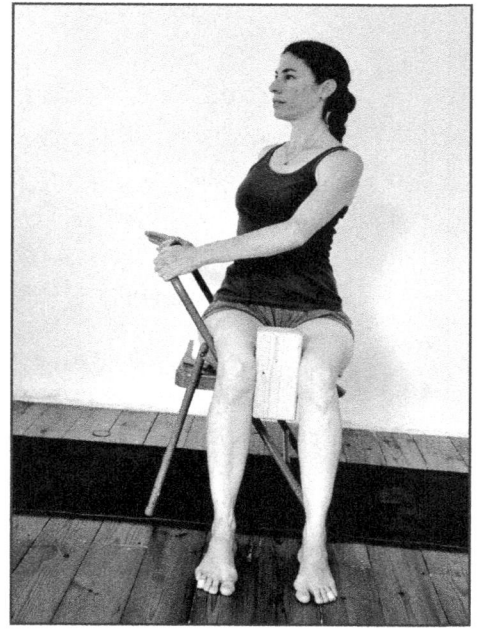

1 min. each side
Use a sticky mat on the chair. Hold a block between the knees. If the seat is lower than your knees, raise it with 1-3 folded blankets; if it is much higher, use blocks under the feet.

9. Sālamba Sarvāngāsana – On a platform

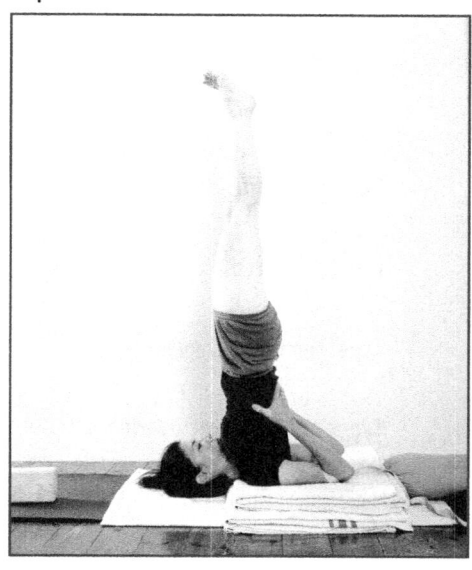

5 min.
See step 16 on Sequence 2
(If you are tired, use a chair).

10. Halāsana - Feet on chair

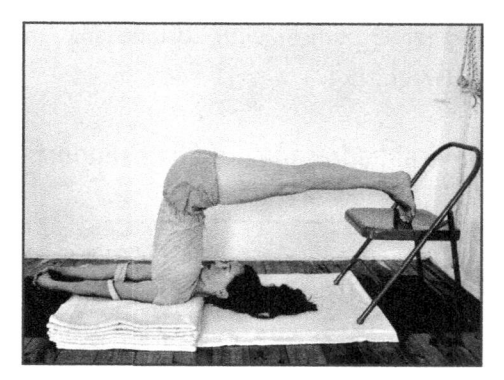

3 min.
Place the tip of the toes on the seat and push down to lift and elongate the trunk.

11. Karna Pidāsana – Feet on chair

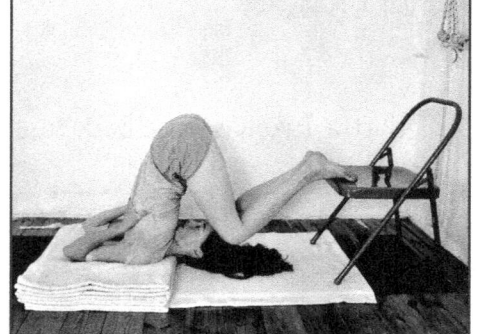

1 min.
Bent the knees and place the metatarsals on the seat.

12. Śavāsana - Lower legs on chair

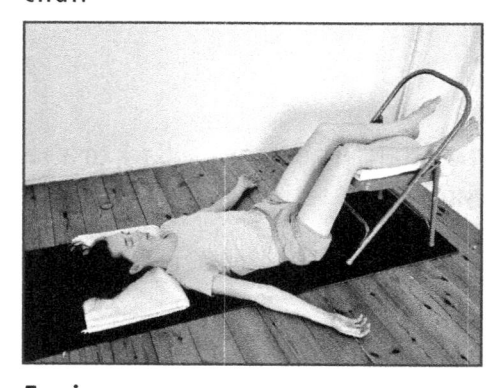

5 min.
Move the flesh of the buttocks away from the lumbar spine to lengthen and release the lower back.

Props for Yoga / Apendix 1   151

5. Forward bends & Twists – an advanced sequence

Characteristics of this sequence are:

> **Duration:** 90 min

> **Level:** Advanced

> **Type:** Energizing & opening

> **Types of Asanas included:**
> forward extensions, twists, inversions

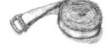

Props
chair,
2 long belts
block
wall
bandage (optional)

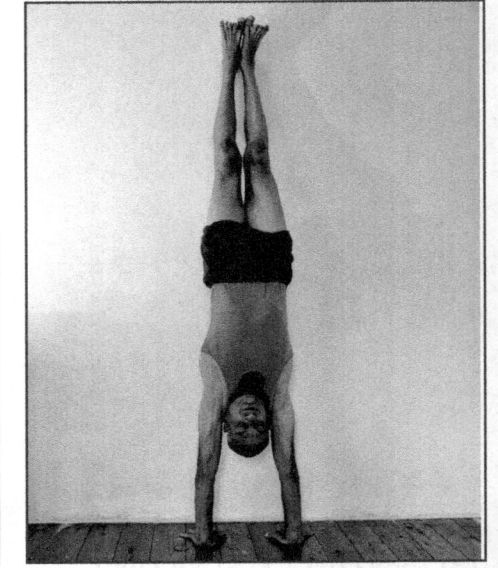

1. Adho Mukha Śvānāsana – Palms on inverted chair

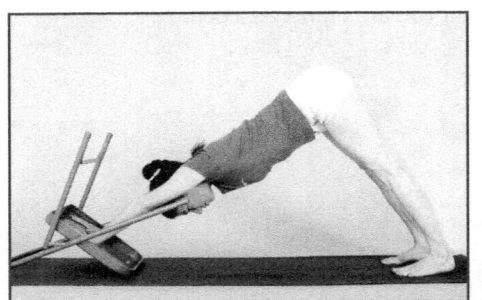

1 min.
See Vol. 1, P. 49

2. Adho Mukha Śvānāsana – Feet on inverted chair

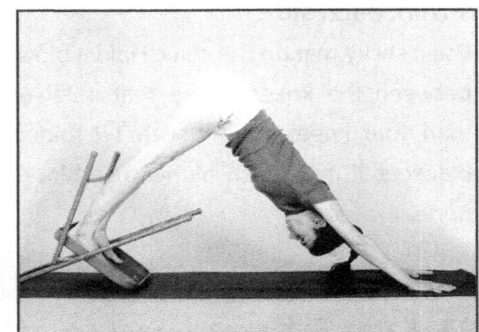

1 min.
See Vol. 1, P. 39

3. Adho Mukha Vṛkṣāsana - At the wall

40 sec.
Repeat 3 times with Uttānāsana in between.

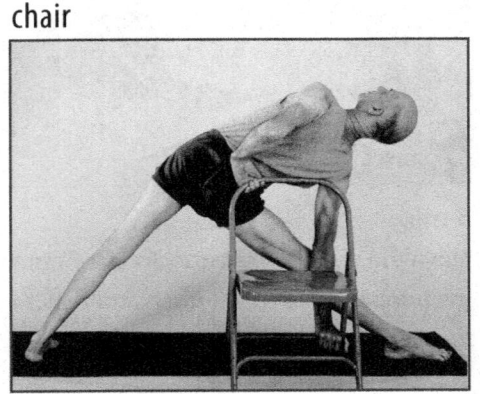

4. Utthita Trikoṇāsana – Back to a chair

1 min. each side
See Vol. 1, P. 91

5. Parivṛtta Trikoṇāsana - Back to a chair

1 min. each side
Start facing the chair, turn to the right and twist the trunk until the back faces the

6. Virabhadrāsana II – Chair support

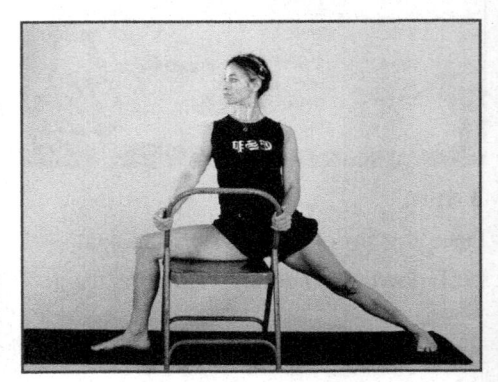

1 min. each side
See Vol. 1, P. 39

152 Props for Yoga / Apendix 1

7. Parivṛtta Pārśvakoṇāsana – Chair support

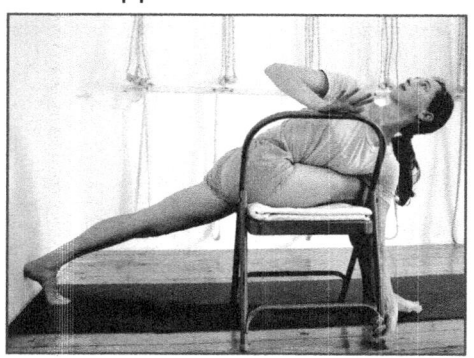

1 min. each side

8. Adho Mukha Śvānāsana – Head on block

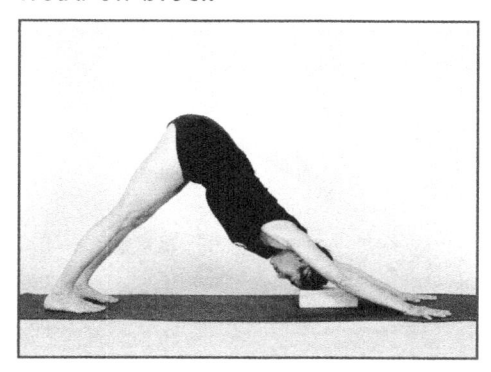

1 min.
See Vol. 1, P. 52

9. Śīrṣāsana – Blocks supporting the thoracic dorsal spine

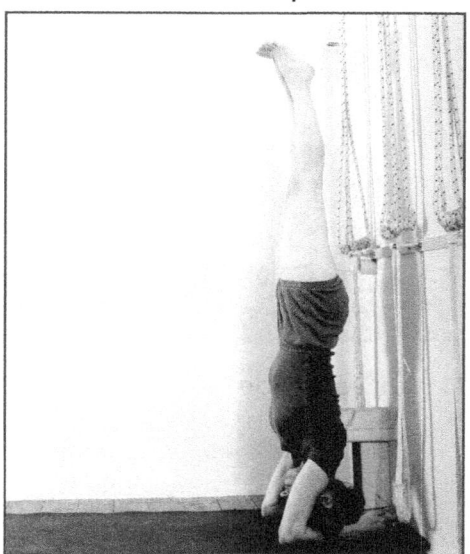

7-8 min.
Arrange 3 blocks such that they supports your thoracic dorsal spine.

10. Upaviṣṭha Koṇāsana Sitting – With two belts

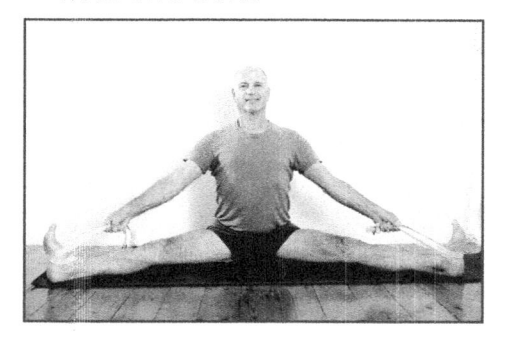

1 min.
See Vol. II, P. 22

11. Pārśva Upaviṣṭha Koṇāsana – With two belts

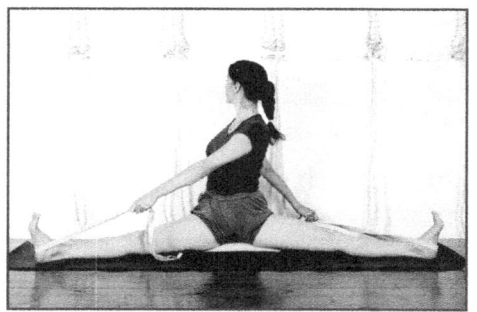

30 sec. each side
See Vol. II, P. 22

12. Pārśva Upaviṣṭha Koṇāsana – With long belts

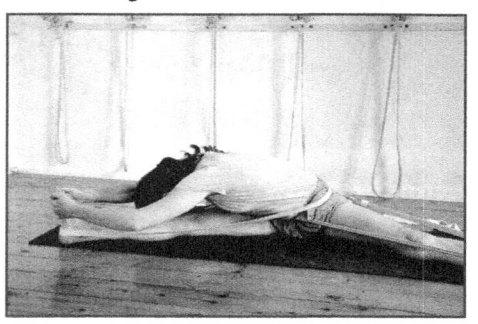

45 sec. each side

13. Parivrtta Upaviṣṭha Koṇāsana –With long belts

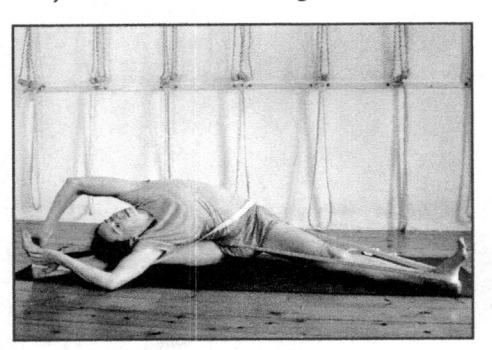

1 min. each side

14. Jānu Śīrṣāsana – With long belt

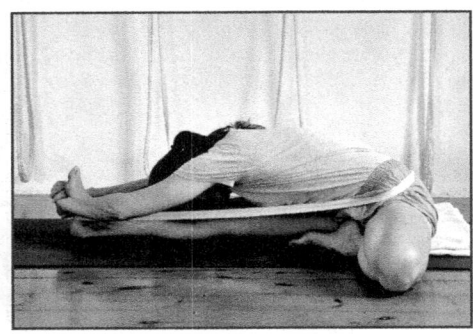

1 min. each side

15. Parivrtta Jānu Śīrṣāsana – With long belt

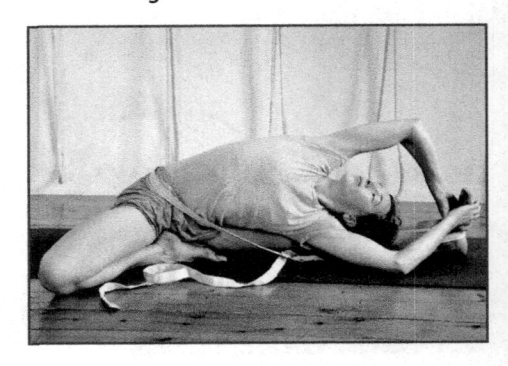

45 sec. each side

16. Paschimottānāsana –With long belt

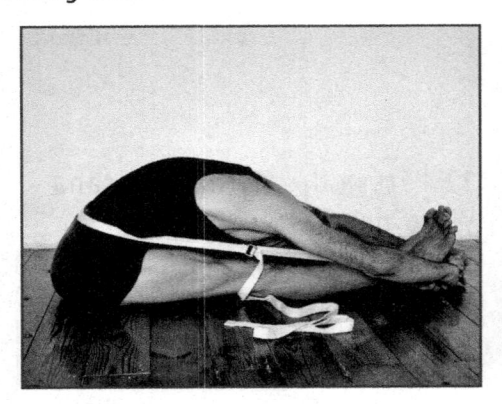

2 min.
See Vol. II, P. 108

17. Parivrtta Paschimottānāsana - With long belt

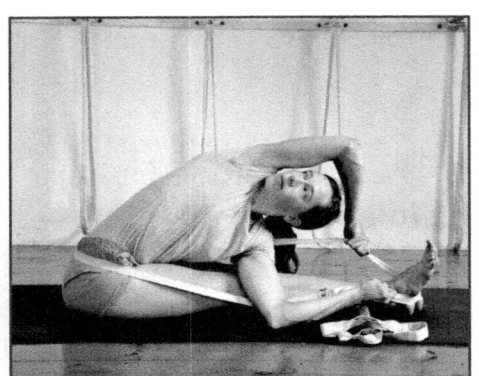

30 sec. each side

18. Pāśāsana – At the wall

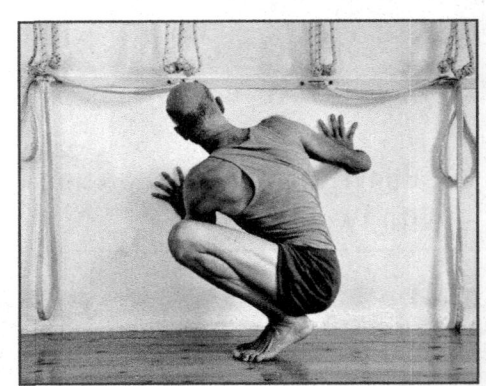

45 sec. each side

19. Adho Mukha Śvānāsana – Head on support

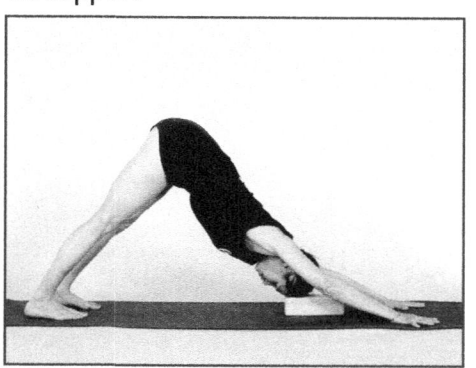

1 min.
See Vol. I, P. 52

20. Sālamba Sarvāngāsana – On a platform

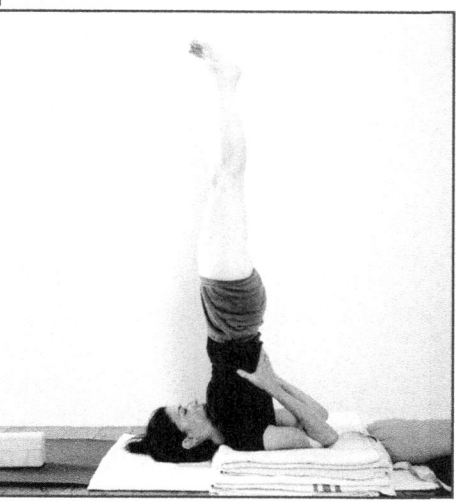

7 min.
See step 16 on Sequence 2

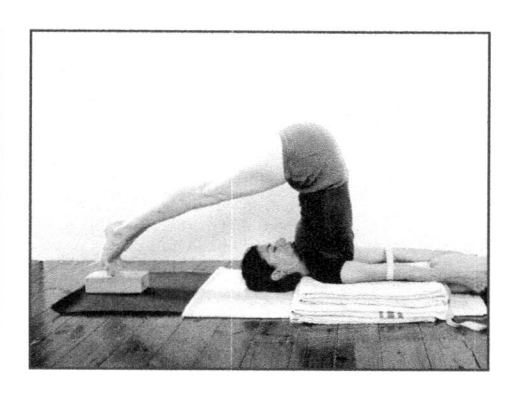

21. Halāsana – Toes on block

3 min.
See step 17 on Sequence 2

22. Setu Bandha Sarvāngāsana – With block for sacrum and belt for thighs

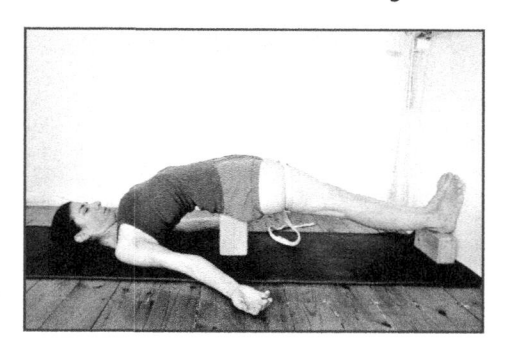

4 min.

23. Adho Mukha Swastikāsana – With block to support forehead

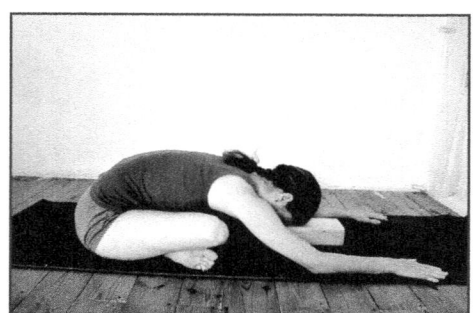

40 sec. each side

24. Śavāsana – With bandage and block on forehead

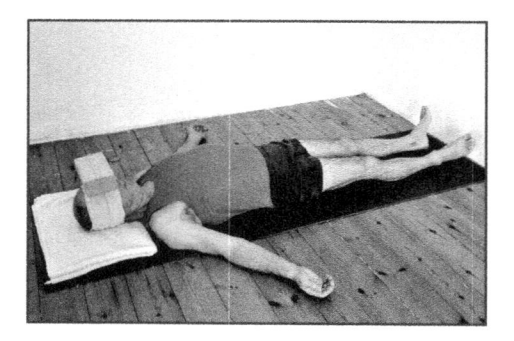

8 min.
Wrap an elastic bandage (a cotton one) around the head and after lying down, place a block (or a small weight) on the forehead.

Props for Yoga / Apendix 1   155

Index:

Below please find two sets of pointers to the book's content:

> Index 1: Pointers to specific variations of āsanas, grouped by prop type.

> Index 2: Pointers to the range of pages devoted to an āsana

Index 1: Listing by Prop Type, Asana and Variation

Belt

Asana	Variation	Page No.
> Adho Mukha Vīrāsana	2: Stretching forward: Anchoring the legs and Palms on blocks	75
Baddha Koṇāsana	1: Lifting the pelvis to descend the knees: Sitting on a height	13
	2: Moving the heels to the pelvis: Bracing the shins and the thighs	14
	4: Opening the thighs: Using belts behind the knees	16
	5: Supporting the knees: Bracing the pelvis and the knees	17
> Dandāsana	2: Making the spine Concave: Holding a belt	6
	3: Bracing the legs: Belt from heels to sacrum	7
	7: Stabilizing the legs	11
> Jānu Śīrṣāsana	1: Turning sideways: Using a belt	120
	5: Keeping the bent knee backward: Bracing the right leg	124
	7: Mālāsana I with a belt	139
> Mālāsana	4: Akunchanāsana (preparation for)	63
> Padmāsana	8: Supta Ardha Padmāsana (or Ardha Matsyāsana)	67
	9: Matsyāsana (or Supta Padmāsana)	68
> Paschimottānāsana	1: Activating the legs: Block between the thighs	97
	9: Rolling the pelvis forward: Belt around pelvis and heels	108
	10: Rolling the pelvis forward: Two belts around pelvis and heels	109
	11: Anchoring the base: Partner pulls back and down	110
	12: Bending deeper into the pose: Belt around thighs and back Using a Long Belt	111
> Practice Sequence 2	Long stays in sitting & forward extensions	144
> Practice Sequence 3	Forward bends & Twists – an advanced sequence	148

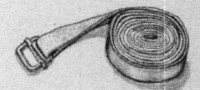

Belt (cont.)	Asana	Variation	Page No.
	▶ Practice Sequence 5	Forward bends & Twists – an advanced sequence	152
	▶ Sukhāsana	See Swastikāsana	
	▶ Supta Pādāṅguṣṭhāsana I	1: Bones vs. Muscles: Basic usage of belt	82
		2: Learning to keep the leg straight: Entering from Daṇḍāsana	83
		3: Activating the lifted leg: Bracing the body and the leg	84
		4: Creating space in the lifted leg side: Hooking a belt from heel to groin	85
		5: Creating space in the lifted leg side: Partner pulls the leg	86
		6: Supporting the leg at 90°: Using a wall corner	87
	▶ Supta Pādāṅguṣṭhāsana I (Lateral)	1: Stabilizing the pelvis: Holding a belt with two hands	89
		2: Activating the leg: Bracing the body and the leg	90
		3: Creating space in the pelvis: Hooking a belt from heel to groin	91
		4: Creating space in the stretched leg side: Partner pulls the leg	92
		5: Moving the femur head into the hip joint: Side foot against wall	93
		6: Moving the femur head into the hip joint: Partner pulls the buttock	94
		7: Restorative Supta Pādāṅguṣṭhāsana II: Supporting the outer thigh	95
	▶ Swastikāsana (Sukhāsana)	5: Arrangement for long sittings: Using a high support	32
		7: Bracing the legs	34
		8: Compacting the base: Bracing the pelvis with a belt	36
		10: Stabilizing the base: Pulling the shins	38
		14: Rolling the shoulders back: Crossed "shoulder jacket"	42
		15: Stabilizing & resting the arms: Belt on elbows	43
		17: Sensitizing the chest: A belt around the chest	45
		18: Supporting the chin in Pranayama: Using a rolled belt	46
	▶ Upaviṣṭha Koṇāsana	1: Stabilizing the back: Holding belts	22
		2: Stabilizing the legs: Bracing the pelvis and legs	23
	▶ Vajrāsana	1: Joining the ankles and knees: Using belts	48
		2: Improving feet flexibility: Stretching the toes inward	49
		3: Anchoring the roots of the legs: A belt from groins to ankles	50
	▶ Vīrāsana	2: Compacting the base: Strapping the legs	55
		3: Compacting the base: Strapping the pelvis and knees	56

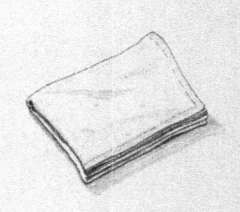

Blanket	Asana	Variation	Page No.
	Adho Mukha Vīrāsana	4: Overcoming stiffness in the ankles: Raising the shins	77
		5: Stretching the sacral band: Keeping the knees together	78
		6: Restorative Adho Mukha Vīrāsana: Supporting the body	79
	Baddha Koṇāsana	1: Lifting the pelvis to descend the knees: Sitting on a height	13
		3: Moving the pelvis to the heels: Supporting the palms with blocks	15
		4: Opening the thighs: Using belts behind the knees	16
		5: Supporting the knees: Bracing the pelvis and the knees	17
		6: Further opening of the groins: Block between soles	18
		7: Supporting the back: Using a chair	19
		8: Opening the chest: Using a wall rope	20
	Jānu Śīrṣāsana	4: Keeping the bent knee backward: Knee against wall	123
		6: A different way to enter the pose: Sliding the knee back	125
		7: Folding into the pose: Start by bending the Dandāsana leg	126
		9: Aligning the trunk: Rolled blanket on top thigh	128
	Mālāsana	2: Preparation: Supporting the heels	134
		6: Preparation: Partner pushing the knees	138
		7: Mālāsana I with a belt	139
	Padmāsana	6: Akunchanāsana with chair supporting the leg	65
		7. Standing Akunchanāsana	66
		10: From Ardha Padmāsana to full Padmāsana	69
	Paschimottānāsana	1: Activating the legs: Block between the thighs	97
		2: Activating the feet: Block against the soles	99
		7: Lifting the sides: Supporting the hips	105
		8 (old 6): Sliding back into the pose: Hands grasping hooks	107
		7: Rolling the pelvis forward: Belt around pelvis and heels	108
		14: Relaxing the head: Forehead on chair	113
		15: Relaxing the head: Forehead on bolster	114
		19: Ūrdhva Mukha Paschimottānāsana II: Helper presses down	118
	Practice Sequence 2	Using a Long Belt	144
	Practice Sequence 3	Long stays in sitting & forward extensions	148
	Practice Sequence 4	Forward bends for beginners	150
	Practice Sequence 5	Forward bends & Twists – an advanced sequence	152

Blanket (cont.)

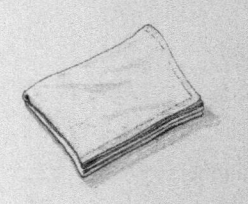

Asana	Variation	Page No.
Supta Pādāṅguṣṭhāsana II (Lateral)	7: Restorative Supta Pādāṅguṣṭhāsana II: Supporting the outer thigh	95
Swastikāsana (Sukhāsana)	2a: Supporting the palms on a folded blanket	28
	2b: Supporting the palms on blocks	29
	3: Supporting the shins with a blanket	30
	5: Arrangement for long sittings: Using a high support	32
	7: Bracing the leg	34
	9: Moving the sacrum in: Block between sacrum and wall	37
	11: Supporting the chest: A block between wall and back	39
	15: Stabilizing & resting the arms: Belt on elbows	43
	17: Sensitizing the chest: A belt around the chest	45
Upaviṣṭha Koṇāsana	1: Stabilizing the base: Supporting the lower abdomen	130
	2: Restorative bending forward: Supporting the trunk	131
Vajrāsana	1: Joining the ankles and knees: Using belts	48
	2: Improving feet flexibility: Stretching the toes inward	49
	4: Doing the pose when the ankles are stiff: Adding support for the shins	51
	5: Extending the ankles: Lifting the metatarsals	52
Vīrāsana	1: Spreading the calves from the thighs: Entering into Vīrāsana	54
	2: Compacting the base: Strapping the legs	55

Block

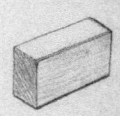

Asana	Variation	Page No.
Adho Mukha Vīrāsana	2: Stretching forward: Anchoring the legs and Palms on blocks	75
	6: Restorative Adho Mukha Vīrāsana: Supporting the body	79
Baddha Koṇāsana	1: Lifting the pelvis to descend the knees: Sitting on a height	13
	3: Moving the pelvis to the heels: Supporting the palms with blocks	15
	6: Further opening of the groins: Block between soles	18
Daṇḍāsana	1: Avoiding rounded back: Sitting on a raised plane	5
	4: Opening the backs of the legs: Heels on block	8
	6: Turning the thighs in: Block between thighs	10
Jānu Śīrṣāsana	8: Activating the straight leg: Foot against a block	127
Padmāsana	2: Baddha Koṇāsana & Adho Mukha Baddha Koṇāsana	61

Block (cont.)

Asana	Variation	Page No.
Paschimottānāsana	1: Activating the legs: Block between the thighs	97
	2: Activating the feet: Block against the soles	99
	5: Opening the backs of the legs: Heels on block	102
	13: Opening the sides of the body: Supporting the elbows with blocks	112
Practice Sequence 1	A Short Sequence for Beginners	141
Practice Sequence 2	Using a Long Belt	144
Practice Sequence 3	Long stays in sitting & forward extensions	148
Practice Sequence 5	Forward bends for beginners	152
Supta Pādāṅguṣṭhāsana II (Lateral)	7: Restorative Supta Pādāṅguṣṭhāsana II: Supporting the outer thigh	95
Swastikāsana (Sukhāsana)	2b: Supporting the palms on blocks	29
	6: Sensitizing the buttocks area: Sitting on a block	33
	9: Moving the sacrum in: Block between sacrum and wall	37
	11: Supporting the chest: A block between wall and back	39
	16: Checking the upright alignment: A block on top of the head	44

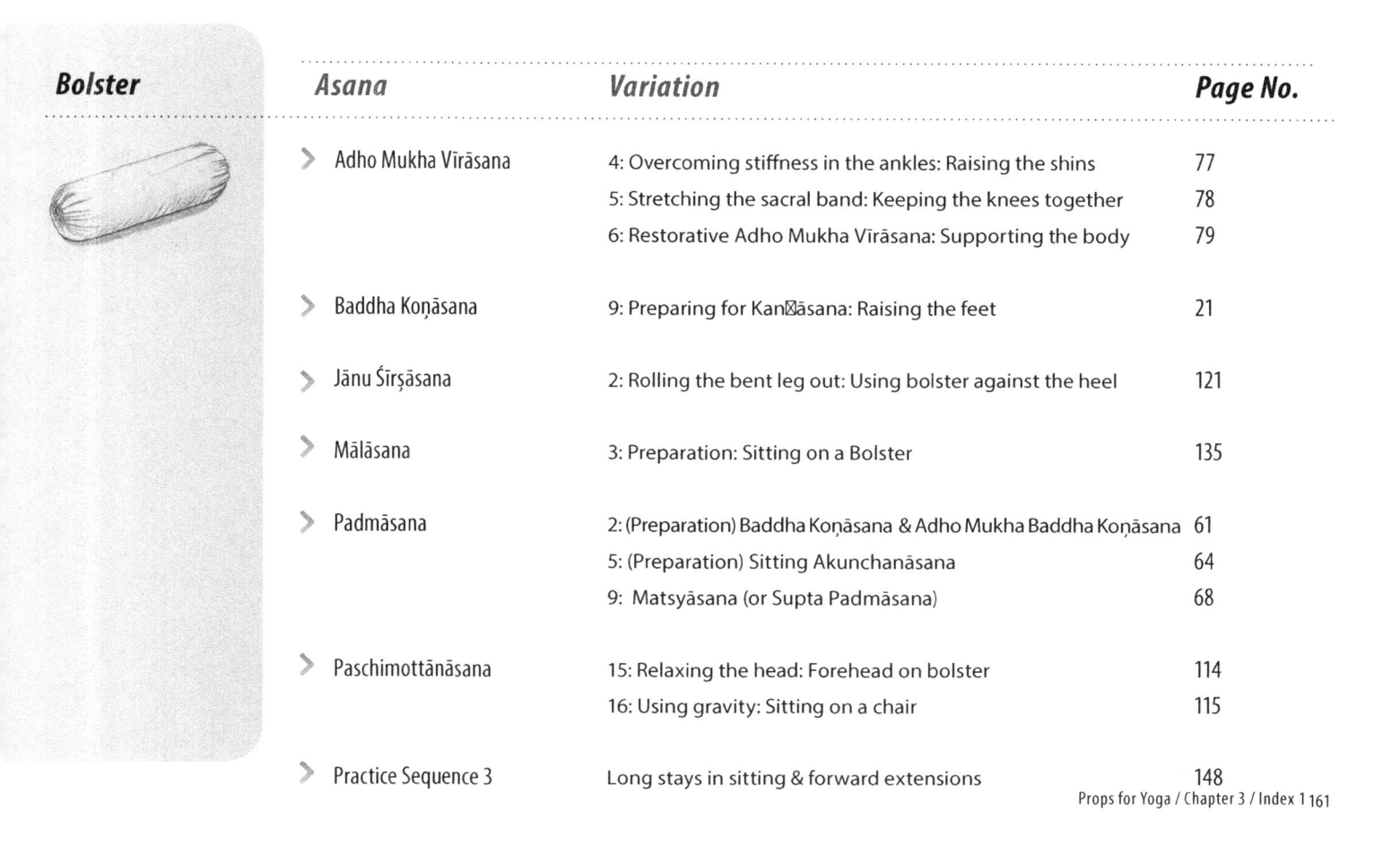

Bolster

Asana	Variation	Page No.
Adho Mukha Vīrāsana	4: Overcoming stiffness in the ankles: Raising the shins	77
	5: Stretching the sacral band: Keeping the knees together	78
	6: Restorative Adho Mukha Vīrāsana: Supporting the body	79
Baddha Koṇāsana	9: Preparing for Kanḍāsana: Raising the feet	21
Jānu Śīrṣāsana	2: Rolling the bent leg out: Using bolster against the heel	121
Mālāsana	3: Preparation: Sitting on a Bolster	135
Padmāsana	2: (Preparation) Baddha Koṇāsana & Adho Mukha Baddha Koṇāsana	61
	5: (Preparation) Sitting Akunchanāsana	64
	9: Matsyāsana (or Supta Padmāsana)	68
Paschimottānāsana	15: Relaxing the head: Forehead on bolster	114
	16: Using gravity: Sitting on a chair	115
Practice Sequence 3	Long stays in sitting & forward extensions	148

Bolster

Asana	Variation	Page No.
Swastikāsana (Sukhāsana)	5: Arrangement for long sittings: Using a high support	32
Vajrāsana	4: Doing the pose when the ankles are stiff: Adding support for the shins	51
Vīrāsana	4: Supporting the hands in Vīrāsana: Bolster on thighs	57

Chair

Asana	Variation	Page No.
Adho Mukha Vīrāsana	2: Stretching forward: Anchoring the legs and palms on blocks	75
Baddha Koṇāsana	7: Supporting the back: Using a chair	19
Dandāsana	1: Avoiding rounded back: Sitting on a raised plane	5
Mālāsana	1: Preparation: Using chair	133
Padmāsana	6: Akunchanāsana with chair supporting the leg	65
Paschimottānāsana	5: Opening the backs of the legs: Heels on block	103
	6: Anchoring the hands: Feet on inverted chair	104
	14: Relaxing the head: Forehead on chair	113
	16: Using gravity: Sitting on a chair	115
Swastikāsana (Sukhāsana)	11: Supporting the chest: A block between wall and back	39
Practice Sequence 4	Forward bends for beginners	150
Practice Sequence 5	Forward bends & Twists – an advanced sequence	152

Partner	Asana	Variation	Page No.
	Adho Mukha Vīrāsana	1: Anchoring the pelvis: Partner pulls back with a rope	74
		3: Stretching forward: Partner extends the trunk forward	76
	Baddha Koṇāsana	5: Supporting the knees: Bracing the pelvis and the knees	17
	Jānu Śīrṣāsana	3: Rolling the bent leg out: Partner pulls the thigh back	122
	Mālāsana	6: Preparation: Partner pushing the knees	138
	Paschimottānāsana	11: Anchoring the base: Partner pulls back and down	110
		17: Ūrdhva Mukha Paschimottānāsana I: Using wall ropes	116
		19: Ūrdhva Mukha Paschimottānāsana II: Helper presses down	117
	Supta Pādāṅguṣṭhāsana I	5: Creating space in the lifted leg side: Partner pulls the leg	86
	Supta Pādāṅguṣṭhāsana II (Lateral)	4: Creating space in the stretched leg side: Partner pulls the leg	92
		6: Moving the femur head into the hip joint: Partner pulls the buttock	96
	Upaviṣṭha Koṇāsana	2: Stabilizing the legs: Bracing the pelvis and legs	23
		3: Further opening of the inner legs: Feet against a wall	24

Rope	Asana	Variation	Page No.
	Adho Mukha Vīrāsana	1: Anchoring the pelvis: Partner pulls back with a rope	74
	Baddha Koṇāsana	8: Opening the chest: Using a wall rope	20
	Jānu Śīrṣāsana	3: Rolling the bent leg out: Partner pulls the thigh back	122
	Mālāsana	5: Flexing the ankles: Holding a wall anchor	137
	Paschimottānāsana	17: Ūrdhva Mukha Paschimottānāsana I: Using wall ropes	116
		18: Ūrdhva Mukha Paschimottānāsana II: Using wall ropes	117
	Supta Pādāṅguṣṭhāsana I	5: Creating space in the lifted leg side: Partner pulls the leg	86
	Supta Pādāṅguṣṭhāsana II (Lateral)	4: Creating space in the stretched leg side: Partner pulls the leg	92
		6: Moving the femur head into the hip joint: Partner pulls the buttock	94
	Swastikāsana (Sukhāsana)	13: Supporting the back: Using a hooked rope	41
	Upaviṣṭha Koṇāsana	3: Further opening of the inner legs: Feet against a wall	24

Wall	Asana	Variation	Page No.
	Baddha Koṇāsana	5: Restorative Baddha Koṇāsana	19
		9: Preparing for Kandāsana: Raising the feet	21
	Daṇḍāsana	5: Activating the feet: Feet against wall	9
	Jānu Śīrṣāsana	4: Keeping the bent knee backward: Knee against wall	123
		7: Folding into the pose: Start by bending the Dandāsana leg	126
	Mālāsana	4: Preparation: Sacrum against the wall	136
		5: Flexing the ankles: Holding a wall anchor	137
	Padmāsana	3: Ardha Baddha Padmottānāsana	62
		4: Akunchanāsana	63
	Paschimottānāsana	8: Sliding back into the pose: Hands grasping hooks	107
		16: Using gravity: Sitting on a chair	115
	Supta Pādānguṣṭhāsana I	1: Bones vs. Muscles: Basic usage of belt	81
		2: Learning to keep the leg straight: Entering from Dandāsana	83
		3: Activating the lifted leg: Bracing the body and the leg	84
		4: Creating space in the lifted leg side: Hooking a belt from heel to groin	85
		5: Creating space in the lifted leg side: Partner pulls the leg	86
		6: Supporting the leg at 900: Using a wall corner	87
	Supta Pādānguṣṭhāsana II (Lateral)	1: Stabilizing the pelvis: Holding a belt with two hands	89
		3: Creating space in the pelvis: Hooking a belt from heel to groin	91
		4: Creating space in the stretched leg side: Partner pulls the leg	92
		5: Moving the femur head into the hip joint: Side foot against wall	93
	Swastikāsana (Sukhāsana)	9: Moving the sacrum in: Block between sacrum and wall	37
		11: Supporting the chest: A block between wall and back	39
		12: Aligning the spine: Sitting against an external corner	40
	Practice Sequence 1	A Short Sequence for Beginners	142
	Practice Sequence 2	Using a Long Belt	144
	Practice Sequence 3	Long stays in sitting & forward extensions	148
	Practice Sequence 4	Forward bends for beginners	150
	Upaviṣṭha Koṇāsana	3: Further opening of the inner legs: Feet against the wall	24

164 Props for Yoga / Chapter 2 / Index 1

Weights	Asana	Variation	Page No.
	› Daṇḍāsana	7: Stabilizing the legs	12

Index 2: Listing by Asana Names

Asana Name	Asana	Page No.
	Adho Mukha Swastikāsana	60
	Adho Mukha Vīrāsana	73-79
	Akunchanāsana	63, 65, 66
	Ardha Baddha Padmottānāsana	62
	Ardha Matsyāsana	68
	Baddha Koṇāsana	12-20
	Daṇḍāsana	4-11
	Forward Extensions	72-140
	Jānu Śīrṣāsana	119-128
	Mālāsana	132-139
	Matsyāsana	68
	Padmāsana	58-69
	Paschimottānāsana	96-118
	Sitting Poses	2-70
	Sukhāsana	26
	Supta Ardha Padmāsana	67
	Supta Padmāsana	68
	Supta Pādāṅguṣṭhāsana I	80-87
	Supta Pādāṅguṣṭhāsana II (Lateral)	88-95
	Swastikāsana (Sukhāsana)	26-46
	Upaviṣṭha Koṇāsana	12, 22-25
	Vajrāsana	47-52
	Vīrāsana	53-57

Made in the USA
Coppell, TX
10 January 2022